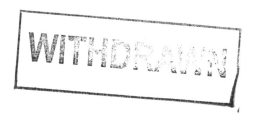

Demyelinating Disorders of the Central Nervous System in Childhood

Demyelinating Disorders of the Central Nervous System in Childhood

Edited by

Dorothée Chabas

Emmanuelle L. Waubant

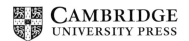

CAMBRIDGE UNIVERSITY PRESS
Cambridge, New York, Melbourne, Madrid, Cape Town,
Singapore, São Paulo, Delhi, Tokyo, Mexico City

Cambridge University Press
The Edinburgh Building, Cambridge CB2 8RU, UK

Published in the United States of America by Cambridge University
Press, New York

www.cambridge.org
Information on this title: www.cambridge.org/9780521763493

First published 2011

Printed in the United Kingdom at the University Press, Cambridge

*A catalog record for this publication is available from the British
Library*

Library of Congress Cataloging in Publication data

ISBN 978-0-521-76349-3 Hardback

Contents

Contributors

Gregory S. Aaen, MD
Division of Child Neurology,
Loma Linda University School of Medicine,
Loma Linda, CA, USA

Maria Pia Amato
Department of Neurology,
University of Florence, Florence, Italy

Laura J. Balcer, MD, MSCE
Hospital of the University of Pennsylvania,
University of Pennsylvania School of Medicine,
Philadelphia, PA, USA

Brenda Banwell, MD
Pediatric Multiple Sclerosis Clinic,
Division of Neurology,
The Hospital for Sick Children,
Toronto, Ontario, Canada

Amit Bar-Or, MD
Montreal Neurological Institute,
McGill University, Montreal,
Quebec, Canada

Khurram Bashir, MD, MPH
Department of Neurology,
University of Alabama at Birmingham,
Birmingham, Alabama, USA

Anita L. Belman, MD
Pediatric MS Center,
Department of Neurology,
Stony Brook University Medical Center,
Stony Brook, New York,
NY, USA

Susan Bennett, PT, EdD
Department of Rehabilitation Science and
Department of Neurology,
University of Buffalo, New York,
NY, USA

Dorothée Chabas, MD, PhD
Department of Neurology,
University of California,
San Francisco, CA, USA

Tanuja Chitnis, MD
Massachusetts General Hospital,
Boston, MA, USA

Russell C. Dale, MRCPCH, MSc, PhD
Neuroimmunology Group,
Institute of Neuroscience and Muscle Research,
Children's Hospital at Westmead,
University of Sydney,
Australia

Angelo Ghezzi, MD
Department of Neurology,
Centro Studi Sclerosi Multipla,
Ospedale di Gallarate,
Gallarate, Italy

Jin S. Hahn, MD
Department of Neurology and
Neurological Sciences,
Stanford University Medical Center,
Stanford, CA, USA

Folker Hanefeld, MD
Department of Pediatric Neurology,
Georg-August University,
Göttingen, Germany

Deborah Hertz, MPH
National Multiple Sclerosis Society,
New York, NY, USA

R. Q. Hintzen, MD, PhD
MS Center ErasMS,
Department of Neurology,
Erasmus MC, Rotterdam,
The Netherlands

Sunny Im-Wang, PsyD, SSP
Regional Pediatric MS Center, UCSF,
San Francisco, CA, USA

Laura J. Julian, PhD
Department of Medicine, UCSF,
San Francisco, CA, USA

Lauren B. Krupp, MD
Department of Neurology,
SUNY at Stony Brook,
Stony Brook, NY, USA

Nancy L. Kuntz, MD
Departments of Pediatrics and Neurology,
Northwestern University Feinberg
School of Medicine, Chicago, IL, USA

Grant T. Liu, MD
Division of Neuro-Ophthalmology,
Department of Neurology,
Hospital of the University of Pennsylvania, and the
Neuro-Ophthalmology Service,
Children's Hospital of Philadelphia,
University of Pennsylvania School of Medicine,
Philadelphia, PA, USA

Timothy Lotze, MD
Assistant Professor of Pediatrics and Neurology,
Baylor College of Medicine,
Texas Children's Hospital, Houston,
TX, USA

Andrew McKeon, MB, MRCPI
Department of Neurology, Mayo Clinic,
Rochester, MN, USA

Maria Milazzo, MS, CPNP
Pediatric MS Center, Department of Neurology,
Stony Brook University Medical Center,
Stony Brook, NY, USA

Ellen M. Mowry, MD, MCR
Department of Neurology, UCSF,
San Francisco, CA, USA

Jayne Ness, MD, PhD
Department of Pediatrics, Division of Pediatric
Neurology,
University of Alabama at Birmingham,
Birmingham, AL, USA

Frank S. Pidcock, MD
Department of Physical Medicine & Rehabilitation,
Johns Hopkins School of Medicine,
Baltimore,
Maryland, USA

Immacolata Plasmati, MD
Department of Neurological and Psychiatric Sciences,
University of Bari, Italy

Daniela Pohl, MD
Department of Pediatric Neurology,
Children's Hospital of Eastern Ontario,
Ottawa, Canada

Christel Renoux, MD, PhD
Department of Neurology and
Department of Epidemiology,
McGill University,
Montreal, Canada

Moses Rodriguez, MD
Departments of Neurology and Immunology,
Mayo Clinic College of Medicine,
Rochester, MN, USA

Martino Ruggieri, BA, MD, PhD
Department of Formative Processes,
University of Catania, Italy

A. D. Sadovnick, PhD
Department of Medical Genetics and Faculty of
Medicine, Division of Neurology,
University of British Columbia,
Vancouver, Canada

Guillaume Sébire, MD, PhD
Child Neurology Section,
Pediatric Department, CHU de Sherbrooke,
Université de Sherbrooke,
QC, Canada

Isabella Simone, MD
Department of Neurological and Psychiatric Sciences,
University of Bari, Italy

Bruno P. Soares, MD
Department of Radiology,
Neuroradiology Section
University of California, San Francisco,
CA, USA

Jonathan Strober, MD
Departments of Neurology and Pediatrics,
University of California,
San Francisco, CA, USA

Esther Tantsis
Neuroimmunology Group, Institute of Neuroscience
and Muscle Research,
Children's Hospital at Westmead,
University of Sydney, Australia

Marc Tardieu, MD, PhD
Service de Neurologie Pédiatrique,
Hôpital Bicêtre,
Le Kremlin Bicêtre, France

Silvia Tenembaum, MD
Pediatric MS Center,
National Pediatric Hospital,
Buenos Aires, Argentina

Maria Trojano, MD
Department of Neurological and Psychiatric Sciences,
University of Bari, Bari, Italy

Sunita Venkateswaran, MD
Department of Pediatrics,
Division of Pediatric Neurology,

Children's Hospital of Eastern Ontario,
Ottawa, Ontario, Canada

Amy T. Waldman, MD
Children's Hospital of Philadelphia,
University of Pennsylvania School of Medicine,
Philadelphia, PA, USA

Emmanuelle L. Waubant, MD, PhD
Regional Pediatric MS Center, UCSF,
San Francisco, CA, USA

Bianca Weinstock-Guttman, MD
Pediatric MS Center of Excellence at The Jacobs
Neurological Institute,
Department of Neurology,
SUNY University of Buffalo,
Buffalo, NY, USA

Max Wintermark, MD
Department of Radiology,
Neuroradiology Division, University of Virginia,
Charlottesville, VA, USA

E. Ann Yeh, MD
Pediatric MS and Demyelinating Disorders Center of
the JNI, Departments of Neurology and Pediatrics,
SUNY Buffalo, Buffalo, NY, USA

Abbreviations

9HPT, nine-hole peg test
ACE, angiotensin converting enzyme
ACT, Avonex Combination Trial
ACTH, adrenocorticotropic hormone
ADC, apparent diffusion coefficient
ADEM, acute disseminated encephalomyelitis
ADS, acquired demyelinating syndrome
AHEM, acute hemorrhagic encephalomyelitis
AHLE, acute hemorrhagic leukoencephalomyelitis
AI, antibody indices
ALD, adrenoleukodystrophy
ANHLE, acute necrotizing hemorrhagic leukoencephalitis
AQP4, aquaporin-4
ATM, acute transverse myelitis
AUNN, aunt/uncle/niece/nephew
Blimp-1, B-lymphocyte-induce maturation protein-1
BNBC, Brief Neuropsychological Battery for Children
BOT-2, Bruininks–Oseretsky Test of Motor Proficiency-2
BS, Behçet syndrome
CADASIL, cerebral autosomal dominant arteriopathy with subcortical infarcts and leukoencephalopathy
CHOP, Children's Hospital of Philadelphia
CIC, clean intermittent catheterization
CIMT, Constraint Induced Movement Therapy
CIS, clinically isolated syndrome
CMV, cytomegalovirus
CRION, chronic recurrent inflammatory optic neuritis
CSF, cerebrospinal fluid
CT, computed tomography
CVLT, California verbal learning test
DC, dendritic cells
D-KEFS, Delis–Kaplan executive function system
DMT, disease-modifying therapies
DSD, detrusor sphincter dyssynergy
DSS, disability status scale

DTI, diffusion tensor imaging
EAE, experimental autoimmune encephalomyelitis
EBV, Epstein–Barr virus
EDSS, expanded disability status scale
ENA, extractable nuclear antigen
ETC, electron transport chain
FLAIR, fluid-attenuated inversion recovery
FS, (Kurtzke's) Functional System
GA, glatiramer acetate
GBS, Guillain–Barré syndrome
GC, germinal centers
GCR, glucocorticoid receptor
GMFCS, gross motor function classification system
GWAS, genome wide association studies
HHV-6, human herpesvirus-6
HLA, human leukocyte antigen
HLH, hemophagocytic lymphohistiocytosis
HSV, herpes simplex virus
HTLV, human T-cell lymphotropic virus
HV, herpesviruses
IDE, initial demyelinating event (episode)
IEP, individualized educational plan
IFNB, interferon beta
IM, infectious mononucleosis
IMSGC, International MS Genetics Consortium
INO, internuclear ophthalmoplegia
IPMSSG, International Pediatric MS Study Group
IVIg, intravenous immunoglobulins
IVMP, intravenous methylprednisolone
KIR, killer cell immunoglobulin-like receptors
LCH, Langerhans cell histiocytosis
LCLA, low-contrast letter acuity
LETM, longitudinally extensive transverse myelitis
LFT, liver function test
LHON, Leber's hereditary optic neuropathy
MAS, macrophage activation syndrome
MBP, myelin basic protein
MDEM, multiphasic disseminated encephalomyelitis

MG, myasthenia gravis
MHC, major histocompatibility complex
MLD, metachromatic leukodystrophy
MLF, medial longitudinal fasciculus
MOG, myelin oligodendrocyte glycoprotein
MRI, magnetic resonance imaging
MRS, magnetic resonance spectroscopy
MS, multiple sclerosis
MTR, magnetization transfer ratio
MTX, methotrexate
MUGA, multigated angiocardiography
NAA, *N*-acetylaspartate
NAB, neutralizing antibody
NAWM, normal-appearing white matter
NF-κB, nuclear factor-kappa B
NF, neurofilament
NHL, non-Hodgkin's lymphoma
NK, natural killer
NMO, neuromyelitis optica
NMOSD, NMO spectrum disorders
NMSS, National Multiple Sclerosis Society
NNT, numbers needed to treat
nTreg, naturally occurring regulatory T cells
NYSMSC, New York State Multiple Sclerosis Consortium
OCB, oligoclonal bands
OCT, optical coherence tomography
ON, optic neuritis
ONTT, Optic Neuritis Treatment Trial
PARP, polyADP-ribose polymerase
PBMC, peripheral blood mononuclear cell
PE, plasma exchange
PEDI, pediatric evaluation of disability inventory
PEDSQL, pediatric quality of life
PLP, proteolipid protein
PMD, Pelizaeus–Merzbacher disease
PML, progressive multifocal leukoencephalopathy
POMS, pediatric-onset multiple sclerosis

PPMS, primary progressive multiple sclerosis
PPRF, parapontine reticular formation
PRVEP, pattern reversed visual evoked potentials
PVPOL, periventricular perpendicular ovoid lesions
RA, rheumatoid arthritis
RCT, randomized controlled trial
RNFL, retinal nerve fiber layer
RON, recurrent events of optic neuritis
RR, relapsing–remitting
SCI, spinal cord injury
SFV, Semliki Forest virus
SIADH, syndrome of inappropriate anti-diuretic hormone secretion
SLE, systemic lupus erythematosus
SP, secondary progressive
SPMS, secondary progressive multiple sclerosis
SS-A, Sjögren's syndrome antibody
SSRI, selective serotonin reuptake inhibitor
SWI, susceptibility weighted imaging
T1D, type 1 diabetes
TM, transverse myelitis
TMEV-IDD, Theiler's murine encephalomyelitis virus–induced demyelinating disease
TNF, tumor necrosis factor
VCAM, vascular cell adhesion molecule
VDR, vitamin D receptor
VDRE, vitamin D response element
VLA-4, very late antigen-4
VMI, Beery–Buktenica developmental test of visual–motor integration
VOR, vestibular ocular reflex
VZV, varicella zoster virus
WASI, Wechsler abbreviated scale of intelligence
WEBINO, wall-eyed bilateral INO
WIAT, Wechsler individual achievement test
WISC-IV, Wechsler intelligence scale for children – II
WISC-R, Wechsler intelligence scale for children revised

Preface

Pediatric multiple sclerosis (MS) was first reported by the French neurologist Pierre Marie in 1893, 15 years after his mentor Jean-Martin Charcot published the original description of the adult disease. It would take almost a century before the first cohort of data on pediatric MS was published, after more sophisticated diagnostic techniques such as magnetic resonance imaging (MRI) became broadly available. While much has been learned about pediatric MS over the past two decades, the diagnosis remains challenging and sometimes delayed, for several reasons. One issue is the broad lack of awareness that MS can affect children as well as adults. There are also a wide range of differential diagnoses specific to children, such as acute disseminated encephalomyelitis (ADEM) or metabolic diseases affecting the central nervous system, which may divert clinicians from a diagnosis of MS. In addition, the clinical, biological, and MRI presentations of pediatric versus adult MS, especially in patients under the age of 11, are distinct from the adult form of the disease, making the diagnosis even more challenging.

In 2007, an International Pediatric MS Study Group proposed for the first time operational diagnostic criteria aimed to facilitate clinical diagnosis, improve care, and foster research. Since then, our understanding of pediatric MS and related diseases has continued to grow, leading to improved care of young patients.

The purpose of this textbook is to review in detail our current knowledge of pediatric MS and related diseases, based on published data and expert practices. Forty-seven international experts, including pediatric and adult specialists, contributed to this original collaborative endeavor. Our wish is to share this knowledge with all practitioners involved in the care of pediatric patients with MS and related disorders such as ADEM, neuromyelitis optica, optic neuritis, and transverse myelitis. Our work is also intended for researchers interested in demyelinating and neurodegenerative diseases occurring in a maturing central nervous system. Pediatric MS is likely more than an adult disease in a child's body. Thus, we believe, a better understanding of pediatric MS will lead to improved understanding of the disease in general.

Dorothée Chabas
Emmanuelle L. Waubant

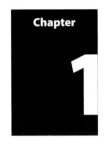

Introduction: historical perspective of pediatric multiple sclerosis and related disorders

Anita L. Belman, Deborah Hertz, and Folker Hanefeld

Why this book? Why now? We know multiple sclerosis (MS) with onset in childhood is not a newly described disease entity [1], but was in fact reported shortly after it was described in adults [2], and that was well over a century ago (Table 1.1, Figure 1.1). However, it has only been since the early 1990s that major advances in the care of adults with MS have occurred, specifically the ability to diagnosis early in the disease course (using more proficient magnetic resonance imaging (MRI) techniques), and the advent of disease-modifying therapies (DMT) [3–9]. Still, children with MS have received little attention and pediatric MS remains a challenging disease to diagnose and treat (see clinical vignettes). While MS in children is uncommon, there is an increased sense of responsibility to effectively recognize, diagnose, and treat children and adolescents with MS. This chapter briefly summarizes the history of pediatric MS and related diseases, and current clinical and research directions.

Brief history of MS origin

It has been suggested that the first reference to MS probably dates back to the age of the Vikings, with a description of a female with intermittent visual and speech disturbances [10]. Much later, in the nineteenth century, a description of MS was found in the writings of Frederick d'Este (1794–1848) [11]. At about the same time, MS pathologic findings, based on macroscopic observations of the central nervous system, were described in the respective textbooks by Cruveilhier (1793–1873) in France and Carlswell (1793–1857) in England [12,13]. The first clinical description of MS – with pathological confirmation – was proposed in 1849 by Frerichs in Goettingen [14]. Additionally, in 1868, the French neurologist Charcot characterized the disease based on its pathological

hallmark, the plaque, which led to the name "sclérose en plaque disseminée", later to be named multiple sclerosis [2] (Figure 1.1).

Pediatric MS
Initial reports

Perhaps the first documented case of pediatric MS dates back to the fourteenth century. Lidvina v. Schiedham (1380–1433), a 15-year-old Dutch girl, fell while skating shortly after recovering from an acute illness (presumably from balance and weakness problems; perhaps her first demyelinating episode). She developed recurrent headaches, left-sided visual loss, and left arm paresis. She became a nun and, history tells us, she died at age 53 having experienced recurrent and progressive disease over a 37-year period [15]. It was not until five centuries later, in 1883, that the French neurologist Pierre Marie (Charcot's student) reported the first 13 cases of pediatric MS [1] (Figure 1.1). In 1902, Schupfer, from the Institute of Neurology at Rome, summarized 58 pediatric cases published in the medical literature and added one of his own [16]. In this paper, published in German, he used the pathological criteria of focal sclerosis and disseminated sclerosis to define MS. He critically reviewed each of the 58 reported cases using these criteria, and confirmed the diagnosis in only 3. It appeared that the diagnosis of pediatric MS was inaccurate in most of these cases, since the diagnoses were based solely on clinical grounds with little or no pathological confirmation. One of these cases, Eichhorst's [17], is remarkable since both the mother and her 8-year-old son were affected. They both developed a similar pediatric-onset illness characterized by recurrent weakness and ataxia, in the context of a more complex phenotype including optic nerve involvement

Demyelinating Disorders of the Central Nervous System in Childhood, ed. Dorothée Chabas and Emmanuelle L. Waubant. Published by Cambridge University Press. © Cambridge University Press 2011.

Table 1.1 Literature milestones of the history of demyelinating diseases in childhood

Inflammatory		Year	Metabolic		
Lucas	"uncommon symptoms succeeding the measles". May be initial reported case of acute disseminated encephalomyelitis (ADEM)	1790			
Marie	"Sclérose en plaques"	1883			
Devic	Neuromyelitis Optica (NMO) (1 adult patient)	1894			
			1885	Pelizaeus	"Multiple sclerosis" (Pelizaeus–Merzbacher disease)
Müller	Monograph of 139 pediatric MS cases 1887–1902	1904			
Marburg	Acute MS (3 adult patients)	1906			
			1910	Merzbacher	"Aplasia axialis extracorticalis congenita" (Pelizaeus–Merzbacher disease)
Schilder	3 publications on "encephalitis periaxialis diffusa" (diffuse sclerosis)	1912–1924			
			1916	Krabbe	"Diffuse cerebral sclerosis" (Globoid cell leukodystrophy)
			1925	Scholz	"Diffuse cerebral sclerosis" (Metachromatic leukodystrophy)
Balo	Concentric sclerosis (adult patients)	1928			
Low/Carter	MS in children	1956			
Duquette	125 (2.7%) out of 4632 MS patients with onset before 16 years	1987			
Krupp et al.	First operational definitions of pediatic MS and related disorders proposed by the International Pediatric MS Study Group	2007			

and dementia. The child died within one year, at 9 years of age and the mother at 41 years of age. The diagnosis of pediatric MS was reportedly confirmed by pathology in both cases. The original autopsy report of the mother, issued from the Institute of Neuropathology in Zurich (pm: 401/1896) is presented in

Figure 1.2. A posteriori, the final diagnosis remains questionable. The short disease duration (at least in the boy), the clinical severity and complexity of the phenotype, its mode of inheritance, and the pathological observations, are atypical for MS according to current criteria [18].

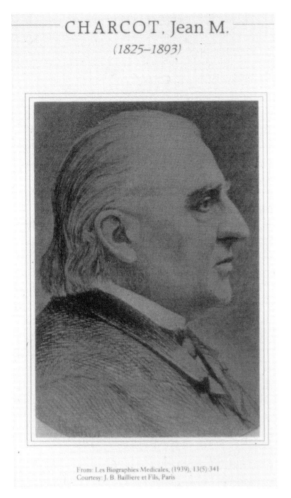
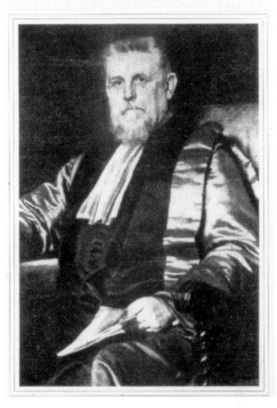

CHARCOT, Jean M.
(1825–1893)

MARIE, Pierre
(1853–1940)

From: Les Biographies Medicales, (1939), 13(5):341
Courtesy: J. B. Bailliere et Fils, Paris

Figure 1.1 Representation of Jean-Martin Charcot and Pierre Marie, two French neurologists of the nineteenth century, who initially characterized multiple sclerosis in adults and children.

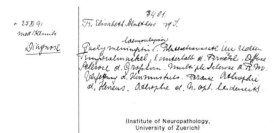

(Institute of Neuropathology,
University of Zuerich)

Figure 1.2 Autopsy report of the mother in the case of Eichhorst [17] Translation and interpretation from German by F. Hanefeld: The macroscopic evaluation showed "diffuse sclerosis" of the cerebrum, multiple sclerosis of the spinal cord, bilateral optic atrophy. However on microscopic examination no abnormalities in the cerebrum were discovered, while the spinal cord showed "multiple sclerosis".

In fact, by the end of the nineteenth century, significant confusion existed concerning the diagnosis of MS in children. Various neurological diseases such as thalamic tumors [19], Leigh's disease [20], or heterotopias [21] were misdiagnosed as MS. Marie also observed that MS in children might be related to acute infectious diseases, syphilis or trauma, suggesting that at that time, there was already some overlap with infectious or post-infectious central nervous system (CNS) diseases such as acute disseminated encephalomyelitis (ADEM).

Confusion between pediatric MS and leukodystrophies

In the early 1900s, pediatric inherited demyelinating disorders of metabolic origin (leukodystrophies) began to be described. This led to even more confusion about the nature of demyelinating diseases, given the clinical and pathological overlap with MS. It was believed that some previously reported cases of MS in children may have, in fact, been leukodystrophies. In particular, both "multiple" and "diffuse sclerosis" were pathological terms used to describe inflammatory as well as metabolic demyelination. For example, the first case of Pelizaeus–Merzbacher disease was reported as MS [22], and the initial cases of Krabbe's disease and metachromatic leukodystrophy were described as "diffuse sclerosis" [23,24].

Additional confusion resulted from the publications of three pediatric cases by Schilder (between 1912 and 1924) that he termed "diffuse sclerosis" or "encephalitis periaxialis diffusa." One case was fulminant pediatric MS, another was adrenoleukodystrophy and the third case was subacute sclerosing panencephalitis [25–27]. Despite the confusion, the term "Schilder's disease" continued to be used until the 1960s, in particular for describing adrenoleukodystrophy [28]. The reclassification of diffuse sclerosis to a metabolic rather than inflammatory etiology may even have caused some to question whether there was such a disease entity as pediatric MS, until resurgence of interest (and recognition) in the late 1950s [18].

Confusion between pediatric MS and ADEM initial events

ADEM is classically described as a monophasic illness (see Section 4), and one that predominantly occurs in childhood, as opposed to MS, a relapsing and remitting disease, which predominantly occurs in young adults. The first clinical description of ADEM probably dates back to the early eighteenth century with the recognition of the temporal relationship to the childhood exanthemata illnesses (small pox and measles) [29]. The association of ADEM with vaccines, particularly rabies vaccine, became evident towards the end of the nineteenth century. Mortality and morbidity were high, and for those who recovered, neurologic sequelae were frequent [30,31]. Clinical, pathological and epidemiological studies established the connection between ADEM and specific viruses (measles) or vaccines in the early twentieth century. Successful immunization programs for measles, mumps and rubella, the eradication of natural smallpox disease, and promotion of vaccines devoid of neural tissue, resulted in a marked decrease in the frequency of ADEM [32,33]. Currently, although a wide range of infectious illnesses and vaccines continue to be reported in association with the development of ADEM, most cases in the United States follow nonspecific (less identifiable) viral illness in the winter and spring [34].

From a historical perspective, when Marie first described pediatric MS in 1883, he noted the possible relationship to infectious illness [1]. Indeed it is probable that at least some of his 13 cases were misclassified, and were in fact due to direct infectious causes or post-infectious processes (i.e. ADEM). In contrast, Bogaert diagnosed 19 patients with ADEM, 4 of whom ultimately developed MS [35].

With no specific biologic markers, clinical or neuroimaging features, it remains very difficult to definitively distinguish ADEM from MS at disease onset. Many clinicians have acknowledged that some children with a diagnosis of ADEM may go on to have another episode, yet may have as good an outcome as children with monophasic ADEM. The period necessary to be assured of this good and perhaps theoretical outcome was, and still, is unclear. It was also recognized that a proportion of these children would continue to have attacks, and develop the lifelong illness, MS. Review of the literature highlights inconsistencies that have added to the confusion, such as:

- Different descriptions of ADEM based on pathology (perivenous), anamnestic data (post-infection, post-vaccinal) or supposed pathogenesis
- Different terminology used to describe ADEM and "its variants", often with little or no definition or consensus [36–42]
  - "biphasic ADEM", representing a protracted single episode rather than a new event
  - "multiphasic or recurrent ADEM" representing repeat episodes, if occurring within the first few months or year(s) of the initial event
  - "steroid-dependent relapse" if the event occurred as steroids were tapered.

The recent renewed interest in pediatric MS

It was only in the late 1950s that MS in the pediatric population resurfaced in the literature [43–45]. The latter half of the twentieth century led to a greater understanding of both inherited leukodystrophies and acquired CNS demyelinating disorders [46]. MRI transformed the diagnostic process, and dramatically improved early diagnosis and the ability to follow the course of the disease [47] (see Chapter 5). More recent investigations have shown that it is possible to distinguish MS from certain other CNS disorders, such as metabolic diseases or neuromyelitis optica (NMO) [48] (see Chapters 6 and 23), thus offering more specific treatment options. Despite these advancements, for the child who presents with a first CNS inflammatory demyelinating event (or at times, the second), it continues to be a challenge to predict if s/he will remain asymptomatic, or develop MS (Chapters 7 and 19).

In the past, a diagnosis of ADEM would have been considered when a physician saw a previously well child who developed new neurologic signs and symptoms (focal or multi-focal), coupled with neuroimaging evidence of demyelinating lesions (focal or multi-focal) and if cerebrospinal fluid (CSF) and other studies excluded infectious, neoplastic or metabolic etiologies (see Chapters 6, 17, and 18). Treatment with steroids and supportive care would have been recommended (even though there have been no randomized clinical trials to determine the best dose, best route of administration and best treatment duration) (see Chapter 19). Physicians often adopted a "wait and see" approach, since therapy (steroids) was the same whether the illness was labeled ADEM, clinically isolated syndrome (CIS) or MS.

However, clinical trials in adults with MS showed that use of DMT slowed the progression of the disease in some patients and early treament was recommended [7]. These treatments are now commonly used in children and adolescents, even through they have not been formally tested (see Chapters 10 and 11). Thus, the distinction between ADEM and a CIS inaugurating MS in children and adolescents is no longer a theoretical concern, since recommended early therapy for MS and CIS are markedly different from ADEM (see Chapter 19). Thus, accurate and early diagnosis has become crucial in the pediatric population.

Recent increased interest in the international scientific and medical communities

Awareness of and interest in pediatric MS have increased in the past two decades (Figure 1.3); however, information concerning diagnosis, treatment,

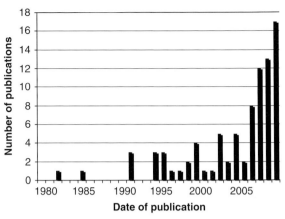

Figure 1.3 Published cases of pediatric MS. This figure represents the number of Medline publications including the term "pediatric MS" or "childhood MS" in the title or abstract over the past 30 years. By definition, this figure does not include all the publications regarding pediatric MS that have been published, but only those with the above-mentioned constraint. In 1993, Bauer and Hanefeld reported that 136 actual pediatric MS cases had been reported before 1980 (including 20 prepubertal cases), and 235 cases between 1980 and 1993 (including 43 prepubertal) [50].

epidemiology, and long-term prognosis is still limited. Since there are relatively small numbers of children in any one geographic area, especially children who develop their first symptoms before puberty (Table 1.2), it is essential to have multi-center, international collaborative efforts in order to further address these issues.

Since 2002, countries such as Australia, Canada, England, France, Germany, Italy, and the US, among others, have developed national collaborative teams of clinicians and researchers to address pediatric MS. In addition, an International Pediatric MS Study Group (IPMSSG) has evolved to include clinicians and researchers from over 18 countries, with support from MS societies throughout the world (www. ipmssg.org). The result of the initial work of the IPMSSG was the peer-reviewed supplement in the journal *Neurology* in April 2007 including a series of nine review articles. This landmark supplement included an article describing working operational definitions for acquired CNS demyelinating disorders in children including MS, CIS, ADEM, recurrent ADEM, multiphasic ADEM, and NMO [49]. These definitions were designed both to improve diagnosis in individuals under the age of 18, and to develop a platform for future research. While it was recognized that these definitions were not perfect and would need to be tested and revised with time, the uniform

Table 1.2 Early-onset cases of multiple sclerosis published by 1993 (with permission from [50])

Study	Age at onset (years)
Bauer *et al.* (1991)	3
Bejar and Ziegler (1984)	2
Boutin *et al.* (1988)	2
Brandt *et al.* (1981)	2
Bye *et al.* (1985)	3
Golden and Woody (1987)	3
Haas *et al.* (1987)	4.5
Hauser *et al.* (1982)	3
Ishahara *et al.* (1984)	5
Kesselring *et al.* (1990)	2
Maeda *et al.* (1989)	15
Mattyus and Veres	4
Miller *et al.* (1990)	2
Schneider *et al.* (1969)	4
Shaw and Alvord (1987)	2.25
Vergani *et al.* (1988)	2

classification was an important first step to accelerate international research and to advance the understanding and treatment of this disease (see Chapter 2). Today, the IPMSSG is focused on optimizing worldwide care, education and research in pediatric MS and other acquired inflammatory demyelinating disorders of the CNS, through global collaborative research.

Future research directions

Although much has been learned regarding pediatric MS, there are still more questions than answers. MS research and treatment strategies have mainly focused on adult-onset disease. It should be remembered that DMT are currently used *off-label* to treat children and adolescents with MS. Randomized clinical trials have not been conducted in children (see Chapters 10 and 11). Studies are required to better understand safety, efficacy of therapies, possible side effects, and how treatments may impact the developing nervous and immune systems. Multi-centered, prospective studies addressing natural history and long-term prognosis, treatment failures, and how best to make treatment

decisions, are essential. In addition, research is required to identify risk factors, biological and MRI disease markers, prognostic correlates, the effects of puberty, and underlying pathogenetic mechanisms.

The study of pediatric MS provides a unique opportunity to examine factors contributing to MS pathogenesis in general, since in affected children there is a close temporal proximity between the interplay of biological, genetic and environmental factors leading to clinical expression of the disease. Insights into underlying pathophysiologic mechanisms might be gained since disease expression is closer to inciting events. Pediatric MS offers an opportunity to investigate a disease at its onset and, when in the very young patient, during a time when the nervous and immune systems are still maturing (e.g. the effect on myelin damage and repair). This is also a time when exposures to infections may play an important role in the maturation and modeling of the immune system. The timing and role of immunizations as well as infection need to be explored. In addition, there are opportunities to study hormonal influences of puberty and how these may contribute to the expression of MS in this young population.

Summary

While much has been learned in the past decade, our understanding of pediatric MS remains inadequate. Increased research activity will lead to improved clinical care and better characterization of the disease in young children and adolescents. We need to advance our understanding of underlying biological and pathophysiologic mechanisms, in particular of the overlap with ADEM. The aim of this textbook is to review in detail our current knowledge of pediatric MS and related diseases, based on published data or, when unavailable, on common practices. Forty-seven authors from various geographical locations (7 countries represented) contributed to this original collaborative endeavor, including the perspectives of both pediatric and adult specialists. This textbook is written for clinicians and researchers, with an emphasis on clinical care and the most recent scientific advances in the field.

Clinical vignettes

The diagnosis of pediatric MS has been, and in large part remains, difficult at times, as demonstrated by these vignettes.

Case 1

Rosario and his parents moved to Germany from a Mediterranean country. In 1988, when he was five years old, he developed a squint, right arm weakness, and complained of dizziness and blurry vision, which resolved within a few weeks. Symptoms and signs recurred six months and then again one year later. Improvement was noted within a few weeks after each episode. The diagnosis of multiple sclerosis was established, based on clinical course, detection of IgG oligoclonal bands in CSF, and multi-focal white matter lesions visualized on brain MRI. Looking back on the historical evolution of demyelinating disorders, we would imagine that Pierre Marie in 1833 would most likely have considered MS to be the diagnosis. Schilder, in 1913, however, would have suspected diffuse sclerosis; whereas, later yet prior to introduction of CT and MRI, a neurologist might have considered a diagnosis of a metabolic–genetic demyelinating disorder such as adrenoleukodystrophy (considering the child's sex, age, and Mediterranean heritage).

Case 2

In the late 1970s, Katherine, a 14-year-old girl, had been followed in the Department of Child Psychiatry at a university hospital for two years with a diagnosis of conversion disorder (psychogenic gait disturbance). Her illness was characterized by episodes of gait instability and weakness. She used a wheelchair, since she was unable to walk independently. Because of her age, MS was not considered and the remittent and alternating nature of the paresis and ataxia led to a misdiagnosis. After two years, a pediatric neurologist found clear-cut pyramidal and cerebellar signs leading to CSF analysis showing positive IgG oligoclonal bands, and to a cranial CT scan, which led to the correct diagnosis of MS. The lack of awareness that MS can affect children and the frequent diagnosis of psychosomatic disorders in adolescent girls was, and still is, a problem. At the time of Pierre Marie, for example, hysteria might have been considered a possible diagnosis.

Case 3

In 1999, Peter, a four-year-old boy, developed an unsteady gait and clumsiness. Examination showed a mild left facial droop and left leg weakness. The CSF profile was normal, culture and PCR studies (e.g. herpesviruses) were negative. The provisional diagnosis was viral encephalitis. Signs and symptoms resolved within 10 days. He developed a left hemiparesis 16 days later. CSF examination was unremarkable. Brain MRI showed hyperintense T2 patchy lesions (some fluffy, some confluent) involving the cerebral white matter. The diagnosis of ADEM was made based on the combination of clinical course, CSF, and neuroimaging studies. He received intravenous steroids. Signs and symptoms resolved. Six months later, clumsiness and ataxia developed, lasted for two days and resolved without treatment. The diagnosis of ADEM–variant was considered. No new symptoms ensued and neurological examination remained unremarkable. Routine follow-up MRI performed one year later showed new enhancing lesions. He remained well until April 2002, when he again developed slurred speech and ataxia. The CSF profile was normal. The CSF quantity was insufficient to test for oligoclonal bands. He again received IV steroids followed by a one-month prednisone taper. Recovery was excellent. In June 2002 he had an episode of right-sided weakness. MRI showed multiple rounded ovoid and patchy T2 hyperintensities extensively involving both cerebral hemispheres, the corpus callosum, brainstem, and the cerebral and cerebellar peduncles. Repeat CSF examination showed IgG oligoclonal bands. MS was diagnosed. Neuropsychological evaluation was normal. Disease-modifying therapy was instituted. During the following years he continued to have further episodes. Changes in DMT were made. Although he had been classified as a gifted student at age 9 years he began experiencing academic difficulties necessitating special education resources. This case illustrates the challenges of distinguishing between ADEM and MS onset in children, especially when the second episode occurs within 30 days from onset and there are no IgG oligoclonal bands. It also emphasizes that cognitive problems in children with MS may have a significant impact on academic performance as well as psychosocial issues.

References

1. Marie P. De la sclérose en plaques chez les enfants. *Rev Méd* 1883;536.

2. Charcot JM. Histologie de la sclérose en plaques. *Gaz Hôp* 1868;**41**:554–566.

3. IFBN Multiple Sclerosis Study Group. Interferon beta-1b is effective in relapsing–remitting multiple sclerosis: 1. Clinical results of a multicenter,

randomized, double-blind, placebo-controlled trial. *Neurology* 1993;**43**:655–661.

4. Jacobs LD, Cookfair DL, Rudick RA, *et al.* Intramuscular interferon beta 1a for disease progression in exacerbating–remitting multiple sclerosis. *Ann Neurology* 1996;**39**:285–294.

5. Rudick RA, Goodkin DE, Jacobs LD, *et al.* Impact of interferon beta-1a on neurologic disability in relapsing multiple sclerosis. The Multiple Sclerosis Collaborative Research Group. *Neurology* 1997;**49**:358–363.

6. Johnson KP, Brooks BR, Cohen JA, *et al.* Extended use of glatiramer acetate (Copaxone) is well tolerated and maintains its clinical effect on multiple sclerosis relapse rate and degree of disability. *Neurology* 1998;**50**:701–708.

7. National Multiple Sclerosis Society. *Disease management consensus statement.* New York, NY: National Multiple Sclerosis Society 1998:1–8.

8. Oger J, Freedman M. Consensus statement of the Canadian MS Clinics Network on: the use of disease modifying agents in multiple sclerosis. *Can J Neurol Sci* 1999;**26**:274–275.

9. Freedman MS, Blumhardt LD, Brochet B, *et al.* International consensus statement on the use of disease-modifying agents in multiple sclerosis. *Multiple Sclerosis* 2002;**8**:19–23.

10. Poser CM. Viking voyages: The origin of multiple sclerosis? *Acta Neurol Scand* 1995;**161**:11–22.

11. Kesselring J. The pathogenesis of multiple sclerosis. *Schweiz Med Wochenschr* **120**:1083–1090.

12. Cruveilhier J. *Anatomie pathologique du corps humain.* Paris: J.B. Baillière 1829–1842.

13. Carswell R. *Pathological anatomy: Illustrations of the elementary forms of disease.* London: Longman, Orme, Brown, Green and Longman 1838.

14. Frerichs FT. Uber Hirnsklerose. *Arch Ges Med* 1849;**10**:334–337.

15. Maeder R. Does the history of multiple sclerosis go back as far as the 14th century? *Acta Neurol Scandinav* 1979;**60**:189–192.

16. Schupfer F. Über die infantile Herdsklerose mit Betrachtungen über sekundäre Degenerationen bei disseminierter Sklerose. *Monatsschr f Psychatr Neurol* 1902;**12**:60–122.

17. Eichhorst H. Über infantile und hereditäre multiple Sklerose. *Arch Pathol Anat Physiol* 1896;**146**:173–192.

18. Hanefeld F. Pediatric multiple sclerosis: A short history of a long story. *Neurology* 2007;**68**(Suppl 2): s3–s6.

19. Westphal A. Ein Irrthum in der Diagnose bei einem neunjährigen Knaben, der das Krankheitsbild einer multiplen Sclerose bot. *Charité-Annalen* 1889; **14**:367–371.

20. von Zenker FA. Zur Lehre von der Inselformigen Hirnsklerose. *Deutsches Archiv Klin Med* 1870;**8**:126.

21. Pollak L. Congenitale multiple Herdsklerose des Centralnervensystems; partieller Balkenmangel. *Arch Psychiatr* 1881;**12**:157.

22. Merzbacher L. Eine eigenartige familiär-hereditäre Erkrankungsform (Aplasia axialis extracorticalis congenita). *Z Ges Neurol Psychiatr* 1910;**3**:1–138.

23. Krabbe K. A new familial form of diffuse brain-sclerosis. *Brain* 1916;**39**:74–114.

24. Scholz W. Klinische, pathologisch-anatomische und erbbiologische Untersuchungen bei familiärer, diffuser Hirnskelrose im Kindesalter. (Ein Beitrag zur Lehre von den Heredodegenerationen.) *Z Ges Neurol Psychiatr* 1925;**99**:651–717.

25. Schilder P. Zur Kenntnis der sogenannten diffusen Sklerose. (Über Encephalitis periaxialis diffusa.) *Z Ges Neurol Psychiatr* 1912;**10**:1–60.

26. Schilder P. Zur Frage der Encephalitis periaxialis diffusa (sogenannte diffuse Sklerose). *Z Ges Neurol Psychiatr* 1913;**15**:359–376.

27. Schilder P. Die Encephalitis periaxialis diffusa (nebst Bemerkungen über die Apraxie des Lidschlusses). *Arch Psychiatr* 1924;**71**:327–356.

28. Crome L, Zapella M. Schilder's disease (sudanophilic leucodystrophy) in five male members of one family. *J Neurol Neurosurg Psychiatry* 1963;**26**:431–438.

29. Lucas J. An account of uncommon symptoms succeeding the measles; with some additional remarks on the infection of measles and small pox. *Lond Med J* 1790;**11**:325.

30. McAlpine D. Acute disseminated encephalomyelitis; its sequelae and its relationship to disseminated sclerosis. *Lancet* 1931:846–852.

31. Miller HG, Stanton JB, Gibbons JL. Para-infectious encephalomyelitis and related syndromes. *J MED* 1956; NS *XXV*(100);427–505.

32. Johnson, RT (ed.). *Viral infections of the nervous system.* Philadelphia, PA: Lippincott-Raven 1998:181–218.

33. Dale R. Acute disseminated encephalomyelitis. *Semin Pediatr Infect Dis* 2003;**12**:90–95.

34. Belman AL. Acute disseminated encephalomyelitis. In *Encephalitis Diagnosis and Treatment*, ed. J. Halperin. London: Informa; 2008:305–319.

35. Van Bogaert L. Post-infectious encephalomyelitis and multiple sclerosis. *J Neuropathol Exp Neurol* 1950; **9**(3):219–249.

36. Mikaeloff Y, Suissa S, Vallee L, *et al.* First episode of acute CNS inflammatory demyelination in childhood:

Prognostic factors for multiple sclerosis and disability. *J Pediatr* 2004;**144**(2):246–252.

37. Dale RC, de Sousa C, Chong WK, Cox RC, Hardings B, Neville BG. Acute disseminated encephalomyelitis, multiphasic disseminated encephalomyelitis and multiple sclerosis in children. *Brain* 2000;**123**:2407–2422.

38. Rust RS. Multiple sclerosis, acute disseminated encephalomyelitis and related conditions. *Semin Pediatr Neurol* 2000;**7**:66–90.

39. Tenembaum S, Chamoles N, Fejerman N. Acute disseminated encephalomyelitis in children: A long term follow up study of 84 pediatric patients. *Neurology* 2002;**59**:224–231.

40. Anlar b, Basaran C, Kose G, et al. Acute disseminated encephalomyelitis in children: Outcome and prognosis. *Neuropediatrics* 2003;**34**:194–199.

41. Pasternak JF, DeVivo DC, Presdky AL. Steroid-responsive encephalomyelitis in childhood. *Neurology* 1980;**30**:481–486.

42. Belman AL, Chitnas T, Renoux C, Waubant E. International Pediatric MS Study Group. Challenges in the classification of pediatric multiple sclerosis and future directions. *Neurology* 2007;**68**(Suppl 2):S70–74.

43. Low NL, Carter S. Multiple sclerosis in children. *Pediatrics* 1956;**18**:24–30.

44. Gall JC, Hayles AB, Siekert RG, et al. Multiple sclerosis in children. A clinical study of 40 cases with onset in childhood. *Pediatrics* 1958;**21**:703–709.

45. Arnouts C. La sclérose en plaques chez l'enfant: une observation anatomoclinique et une observation clinique nouvelle. *Acta Neurol Belg* 1959; **59**:796–814.

46. Duquette P, Murray TJ, PLeines J, et al. Multiple sclerosis in childhood: Clinical profile in 125 patients. *J Pediatr* 1987;**111**:359–363.

47. McDonald WI, Compston A, Edan G, et al. Recommended diagnostic criteria for multiple sclerosis: Guideline from the International Panel on the diagnosis of multiple sclerosis. *Ann Neurol* 2001;**50**:121–127.

48. Matiello M, Jacob A, Wingerchuk D, Weinshenker B. Neuromyelitis optica. *Curr Opin Neurol* 2007; **20**:255–260.

49. Krupp LB, Banwell B, Tenembaum S for the International Pediatric MS Study Group. Consensus definitions proposed for pediatric multiple sclerosis and related disorders. *Neurology* 2007;**68**(Suppl 2): s7–s12.

50. Bauer HJ, Hanefeld F. *Multiple sclerosis – Its impact from childhood to old age*. London: WB Saunders, 1993.

Controversies around the current operational definitions of pediatric MS, ADEM, and related diseases

Dorothée Chabas, Lauren B. Krupp, and Marc Tardieu

Pediatric MS has been increasingly diagnosed over the past 20 years. The increased clinical awareness has translated into growing interest in pediatric MS research in the international community, and the number of publications on pediatric MS has grown exponentially from 12 articles reported on the NIH Entrez Medline website in 1998 to 58 articles in 2008. Although diagnostic criteria for pediatric MS and related diseases have evolved in parallel, they are still debated (see Chapter 1). Until 2001, the criteria used to diagnose MS in adults were based on the clinical dissemination of symptoms in time and space [1]. In 2001, consensual MS criteria incorporating MRI findings were published [2] and then refined in 2005 [3]; they have been used in clinical practice and research settings for the past 8 years in adults.

However, these criteria may have a limited applicability in the pediatric population. In fact, MS is a challenging diagnosis in children – especially those who have not yet reached puberty – because of the atypical clinical, biological and MRI presentations, and the broader spectrum of potential differential diagnoses specific to that age range [4]. In particular, differentiating a first episode of MS from acute disseminated encephalomyelitis (ADEM) in children who present with an initial demyelinating event can be an issue for any clinician given the clinical overlap between the two entities and the absence of a reliable biomarker or MRI criteria.

In 2002, a first International Pediatric MS Study Group (subsequently referred to as Study Group) was assembled that made a first attempt to tackle the issue of operational definitions of pediatric MS and related diseases such as ADEM, clinically isolated syndrome (CIS), optic neuritis (ON), transverse myelitis (TM), and neuromyelitis optica (NMO) [5]. The goal was to improve standardization of the terminology applied to these entities to both facilitate the diagnosis and enhance communication among pediatric MS researchers across the world. This was the first attempt to speak with the same voice about pediatric MS and related diseases. The publication of these definitions in 2007 further increased the awareness of pediatric MS within the medical community and provided a framework for prospective research that could test and refine the proposed definitions [5]. At the onset, the Study Group recognized further studies would be needed to challenge and refine these definitions. As expected, both omissions and blurring of categories were identified by research studies subsequent to the publication of the operational definitions. One concept that has emerged since 2007 is that prepubertal MS patients at the time of their initial demyelinating event can have ADEM-like features even if they go on to subsequent clinical events consistent with MS. Since these MS patients have subsequent relapses, they might be misdiagnosed as multiphasic or recurrent ADEM. Two of the criteria upon which the distinctions between ADEM and MS rely, yet represent the most difficulty, are encephalopathic changes and polyregional/polysymptomatic presentation. In this chapter, we will discuss how these current operational definitions can apply to clinical practice and research settings, and we will emphasize their strengths and limitations.

The Study Group has grown in size and breadth of represented countries since the original pediatric MS and related definitions were proposed. The enlarged Study Group shares the goal to update and revise the 2007 definitions, particularly by incorporating data published since the original definitions were drafted.

Demyelinating Disorders of the Central Nervous System in Childhood, ed. Dorothée Chabas and Emmanuelle L. Waubant. Published by Cambridge University Press. © Cambridge University Press 2011.

2007 operational definitions of pediatric CIS, MS, and ADEM

The Study Group developed operational definitions for pediatric MS, CIS, ADEM, and NMO with the hope that these would facilitate collaborative work to improve our understanding of MS versus ADEM, and earlier access to appropriate care for children and adolescents [5]. These definitions have also paved the way for collaborative research projects to advance our understanding of disease specificity in young patients, including biological mechanisms.

These definitions are clinical, and include the differential of an initial demyelinating event, defined as a first acute or sub-acute clinical event with presumed inflammatory or demyelinating cause (monophasic ADEM and CIS), and diseases composed of multiple episodes of CNS demyelination (recurrent ADEM, multiphasic ADEM, MS, and NMO). They apply to patients below the age of 18 years. They are summarized below.

Diagnosis of an initial demyelinating event

According to these definitions, ADEM (monophasic) requires the presence of both encephalopathy and polysymptomatic presentation. Encephalopathy is defined as the presence of behavioral changes such as confusion, excessive irritability or alteration in consciousness, such as lethargy or coma. Polysymptomatic presentation is not specifically defined in the original definition paper, but is thought to refer to patients presenting with various neurological symptoms (e.g. visual changes and paraplegia). ADEM may last up to 3 months, with fluctuating symptoms or MRI findings.

By contrast, CIS can be either monofocal or polyfocal, but usually does not include encephalopathy (except in cases of brainstem symptoms or diffuse hemispheric involvement). Unilateral or bilateral ON, TM (typically partial) or brainstem, cerebellar, and/or hemispheric dysfunction are examples of CIS. Monofocal CIS is considered when clinical (not MRI) features are referable to a single CNS site, while multi-focal CIS refers to the involvement of more than one CNS site. The maximum length of a CIS is not specified, similarly to the adult McDonald criteria [2].

Diagnosis of diseases including multiple episodes of CNS demyelination

According to the definitions proposed in 2007, recurrent ADEM is considered when a new ADEM-like episode follows a first ADEM-like episode by at least 3 months, and occurs at least 1 month after completing steroid therapy. There should be no new anatomic CNS areas involved during the second episode by either clinical or MRI evaluation.

Multiphasic ADEM is similar to recurrent ADEM, but the second ADEM-like episode must involve new anatomic CNS areas by both clinical and MRI evaluation.

The consensus was not reached regarding the categorization of more than two ADEM-like episodes as multiphasic/recurrent ADEM or MS, although the Study Group felt that MS was highly suspicious in these cases.

Pediatric MS is defined according to the current adult MS clinical, biological, and MRI criteria [2,3]. Adult criteria specify that the second episode must occur at least one month after the previous episode, but that was not specified in the current pediatric definitions. In addition, it is specified that the demyelinating events in children must not meet criteria for ADEM, and that the criteria of dissemination in time can be met when MRI shows new lesions as early as 3 months following the initial demyelinating event. Finally, an initial demyelinating event meeting criteria for ADEM can be considered a first episode of MS in children only when the following clinical course is characterized by a second event which is later followed by new MRI lesions or by a third clinical episode three months after the second episode. In the diagnosis algorithm illustrating the definitions, it is noted that the dissemination in time may be clinically met in children below the age of 10 years, while it may be met by MRI in children of 10 years or older, but that was not noted in the text. This point arose since some clinicians considered that additional research was necessary before being willing to diagnose pediatric MS in this younger age group with one event followed only by MRI changes.

Pediatric NMO is defined according to the adult criteria: the patient must have optic neuritis and acute myelitis as major criteria, and must either have a spinal MRI lesion extending over three or more segments or be NMO antibody positive [6].

Table 2.1 Controversies around the definitions (summary)

Topic	Controversies
Prepubertal MS onset: a distinct phenotype at onset * More *common* encephalopathy * More *common* vanishing T2-bright brain MRI lesions * More *common* CSF neutrophils * Less *frequently* positive OCB *Thus* greater overlap between MS and ADEM	* Not taken into account in the current definitions
Encephalopathy criteria	* Unclear definition of behavioral changes, irritability, confusion * Encephalopathy not specific for ADEM (can be associated with MS and NMO), and more common in younger MS patients
Polysymptomatic/polyregional presentation criteria	* Unclear scientific relevance * Purely clinical, not necessarily anatomically related * Unclear whether bilateral optic neuritis is considered mono or polyregional? (may depend on chiasm involvement)
MRI criteria	* Missing for ADEM * Not specific of MS, and not validated in children, especially prepubertal * Not specific (e.g. no mention of corpus callosum involvement as a criterion for MS) * Absence of spinal cord MRI criteria
Biological (CSF) criteria	* Missing for ADEM * Not specific of MS, and not validated in children, especially prepubertal
Dissemination in time	* Absence of consensus regarding when to diagnose MS after a first ADEM-like episode * Does recurrent ADEM with ≥3 episodes exist? Or is this MS?
Other categorization issues	* Unclear whether isolated optic neuritis (normal MRI) should be considered CIS or a separate entity
Preventative treatment in MS or recurrent ADEM	* Unclear when to start (or not) DMT
Differential diagnosis	* Lack of core workup to rule out mimicking diseases * Overlap between MS, ADEM and NMO at onset

Controversies

These definitions enhance clinical care by providing consistent diagnostic tools. In particular, they may guide the clinician to recognize MS early on and therefore to promptly initiate early disease-modifying therapy. Moreover, these definitions became a reference from which multiple collaborative research studies were launched. However, there is now a recognized need for further refinement and revision (Table 2.1).

Controversies around the validity of the proposed criteria

One of the main limitations of the proposed definitions is that, although specialists from various countries came up with a consensual proposal, they based their criteria on personal and anecdotal experience and notions derived from the adult MS literature instead of analyzing a large set of patients with clinical, biological, and MRI data available to determine sensitivity and specificity. This limitation was recognized in the definition paper and the authors agreed that they would need to be validated or updated as soon as large-scale and reliable data become available.

Clinical controversies

Presence of encephalopathy

One major distinction between ADEM and CIS is that ADEM but not CIS is associated with encephalopathy [7–10]. The assumption was that encephalopathy represented a multi-focal and widespread process that was consistent with ADEM. While it was considered possible that ADEM might develop in the absence of encephalopathy, specificity rather than sensitivity was considered most important. However, the distinction is less transparent in cases of brainstem presentation, where altered consciousness might represent a clinically eloquent lesion as specified in the definitions, but also in cases of tumefactive or multi-focal involvement. Hence, in this situation encephalopathy might not distinguish CIS from ADEM. Another possible blurring of the distinction between CIS and ADEM is the patient with an ADEM-like presentation without clinically striking encephalopathy but showing only nonspecific behavioral changes and ADEM-like MRI lesions. Due to the subtle nature of the encephalopathy, CIS rather than ADEM might be mistakenly diagnosed.

Moreover, the definition of encephalopathic changes as including irritability has been controversial, especially in young children where irritability is a common and nonspecific reaction to any kind of illness. However, some clinicians consider a parent's recognition of a behavioral change which might include excessive irritability particularly in the absence of fever as a consideration in the identification of encephalopathy. Although "confusion" was included in the definition, its relation to transient cognitive change was not specified. Finally, seizures were not mentioned as examples of encephalopathy.

Subsequent to the definitions, research has challenged the importance of encephalopathy as a distinction between CIS, NMO, and ADEM. Rather, it has been suggested that the presence of encephalopathy

may actually reflect a younger age of onset rather than being specific of ADEM [7–10]. This suggests a distinct phenotype of CNS demyelination/inflammation in general in younger patients with less mature central nervous and immune systems. This idea is supported by the differences found on MRI and CSF analysis in prepubertal children versus adolescents and adults with MS (see below) [8,11].

Nonetheless, these basic considerations have clinical repercussions. If one considers that CIS is typically inaugurating MS, missing the diagnosis of CIS based on the presence of encephalopathic changes at onset may delay initiation of DMT. On the other hand, one might consider the risk of inappropriately treating an ADEM case as MS of equal concern.

An episode of ADEM, rather than representing a self-limited condition or the first clinical manifestation of MS, might also herald NMO. If NMO antibodies are absent this diagnosis can be quite difficult, since in children with NMO encephalopathic changes can occur in the initial presentation of the disorder and additional episodes of ON and/or TM may follow later [12].

Perhaps another perspective is to consider ADEM as a phenotype, which in addition to a monophasic illness could also be a first presentation of NMO or MS depending on the subsequent clinical and MRI course and the laboratory findings.

Polysymptomatic/polyregional/polyfocal presentation

Definitions for the terms "polysymptomatic", "polyregional" or "polyfocal" were not provided in the criteria for ADEM, leading to a relative confusion, while these terms refer to truly different concepts. The idea was that ADEM patients more often present with symptoms referable to more than one CNS location, given the extensiveness of typical ADEM lesions, while relapsing MS patients typically present with symptoms that can be explained by a single CNS lesion, since MS lesions are usually more limited in size and do not flare up all at the same time.

The term "polysymptomatic" refers to a purely clinical classification, and is not necessarily anatomically based. For example, a patient presenting with both tremor and dysmetria may actually have a single cerebellar lesion.

Polyfocal (also sometimes called polyregional) can be defined by the involvement of two or more anatomical areas. However, the definitions did not specify whether this term refers to purely clinical (as for adult MS) or MRI findings or both, which is an issue since there may be discrepancies between the clinical and MRI assessment of anatomic localization.

The lack of clarity among these terms explains their inconsistent use in scientific publications. To avoid the ambiguous terminology, certain authors prefer specifying the system affected by the neurological presentation, such as spinal cord/optic nerve/cerebral/brainstem/cerebellum (or sensitive/motor/cerebellum/visual) rather than using the above-mentioned categories.

Finally, in addition to considering the number of anatomical systems involved, other factors such as the localization of lesions on neuroimaging may be relevant for diagnosing MS. For example, involvement of the corpus callosum or the presence of periventricular lesions has been associated with an increased risk of a subsequent clinical event following the initial demyelinating event [13,14], and these criteria are not taken into consideration in the current definitions.

Clinical gap between CIS/MS and ADEM

According to the current definitions, it is unclear how to classify a patient with monosymptomatic presentation and encephalopathic changes, for example ON and lethargy. Indeed, this patient would not meet criteria for CIS (because of the presence of encephalopathy) or ADEM (because of the absence of polyfocal presentation). This emphasizes a gap in the definitions that should be assessed in any future revised version.

MRI controversies
Gap in the MRI definition of ADEM

The current definition of ADEM is based on encephalopathic changes and polysymptomatic presentation. It does not include MRI, as opposed to pediatric MS definition. Given the nonspecificity of encephalopathic changes and polysymptomatic features, the absence of ADEM MRI criteria in the definitions may lead to misdiagnosis. Acute cortical encephalitis of potential viral origin is a good example of an acute CNS disease that could be misdiagnosed for ADEM in the absence of guidance for more specific ADEM MRI criteria: patients may present with encephalopathic changes, polyfocal symptoms and epilepsy, as in

ADEM, while the brain MRI scan can be either normal or show only cortical lesions. Thus, it may be worth introducing a minimum of MRI requirements in ADEM criteria, such as involvement of the white matter. The reason why ADEM MRI criteria were not included in the definitions was likely because this is a highly controversial topic [13,15]. In particular, no clear distribution pattern of lesions in the white versus gray matter is agreed upon. Including spinal cord MRI criteria may be an alternate way to improve the definition of ADEM (showing extensive T2-bright lesions) versus MS/CIS [16] (see Chapters 5 and 18).

MRI overlap between ADEM, CIS/MS, and NMO

In addition, there is a potential overlap between MS, ADEM and NMO spectrum disorder based on MRI features that the current definitions do not address. Indeed, it was recently reported that pediatric, like adult, NMO can actually be associated with abnormal brain MRI scan, including potentially extensive T2-bright lesions [12]. Similarly, pediatric MS patients tend to have more tumefactive lesions, or diffuse confluent lesions at disease onset, especially before puberty, which makes the MRI differential diagnosis even more challenging [10].

Lack of validated MRI criteria in children

In conclusion, there is an urgent need to validate pediatric MRI criteria for CNS demyelinating disorders and include them in the definitions. Differences between pediatric and adult MS MRI presentations have been reported [17], and attempts to propose brain MRI criteria for MS and to differentiate MS from ADEM in children have been made, but need to be validated on a larger scale and refined given the specificities in that age range [14,15]. In particular, the MRI differences between prepubertal patients (vanishing confluent T2-bright lesions at onset) and adolescents may need to be better emphasized [10], as well as the spinal cord MRI specificities that may help in distinguishing pediatric MS from ADEM [16].

CSF controversies

Although CSF findings provide information that often helps practitioners to differentiate MS from ADEM or NMO in a clinical setting, the current definition of

ADEM does not include CSF criteria, while the definition of MS does, in an indirect way (by referring to adult MS criteria). The biological hallmarks of MS, namely the presence of CSF-restricted IgG oligoclonal bands and an elevated IgG index, are inconsistently positive in pediatric MS cases (from 10 to 90%) [18–21]. However, patients with prepubertal onset more often have a negative CSF profile compared with adolescents, especially at disease onset [22]. Similarly, prepubertal patients with MS seem to have higher white blood cell counts in the CSF, including more neutrophils [22]. Therefore, adult CSF criteria for MS may not apply to both prepubertal and postpubertal sub-groups and pediatric MS CSF criteria may be modified accordingly in future revisions. In addition, significant pleiocytosis is common in ADEM, and this may become another diagnostic criterion for ADEM, although not specific.

Controversies around the criteria of dissemination in time

Three major controversies concerning the criteria of dissemination in time relate to the fact that a consensus has not been reached about when to call pediatric MS a recurrent disease in: (1) patients with a first ADEM-like episode who further develop non-ADEM-like episodes, (2) patients with recurrent ADEM including more than two episodes, and (3) patients with recurrent non-ADEM-like events such as optic neuritis (ON) or transverse myelitis (TM) without brain MRI findings and without NMO IgG. The first two situations are fairly specific of the pediatric population, given the higher frequency of ADEM or ADEM-like presentations in children, especially before puberty. This issue is crucial not only from a clinical stand point, since practitioners may base their decision of initiating DMT when MS criteria are met, but also from a scientific perspective, since this specifically addresses the question of biological mechanisms at play in ADEM and MS. The controversy around recurrent isolated ON or recurrent TM will be discussed in the corresponding chapters (21 and 22).

MS with an initial ADEM-like episode

According to the current definitions, it is recognized that ADEM-like episodes can occur in patients who are later diagnosed with MS. Although in that case

MS diagnosis is delayed until the third clinical episode (or 3 months after the second episode if the MRI shows one or more new T2-bright or enhancing lesions) versus until the second clinical episode (or 3 months after the first episode if the MRI shows one or more new T2-bright or enhancing lesions) when the initial event is not ADEM-like. In practice, this mostly affects younger patients, since ADEM-like presentations are more frequent in that age category than in adolescents. The idea behind waiting for one more episode in order to diagnose MS in patients with an initial ADEM-like event was based on the uncertainty of the diagnosis. The solution to this dilemma would be an additional requirement that at the time of the second event certain clinical, MRI, or laboratory criteria had to be met. As the group was not in a position to specify such criteria it was considered that if the child did in fact have MS that diagnosis would become quickly apparent by the development of additional MRI lesions, and a delay of 3 months was considered reasonable.

Still, for children with a first ADEM-like episode who subsequently develop MS, waiting for an additional episode in order to confirm the diagnosis of MS may delay initiation of DMT. While DMT for MS should be initiated as early as possible, in adults, it is unclear if this is the case in pediatric patients with an initial ADEM-like episode. In particular, there is no evidence that initiating treatment right after the first ADEM-like episode decreases the chance of developing MS. In the absence of a clear consensus on this topic, the Study Group chose a conservative definition of MS following an initial ADEM-like event. Long-term management and the final decision of initiating preventative treatment in children after an ADEM-like episode remains the choice of the practitioner and the families until a better consensus is reached (see Chapter 19 regarding the treatment of ADEM).

Recurrent and multiphasic ADEM versus MS

The Pediatric MS Study Group felt that MS was highly suspected in cases of multiphasic or recurrent ADEM when more than two ADEM-like episodes occurred, although no consensus was reached. Again, this was based on the lack of understanding of underlying disease processes, although in that case the Study Group chose a less conservative approach by suggesting diagnosing such patients with MS. The implication is an encouragement to consider preventative treatment in patients with recurrent ADEM including more than 2 episodes, which is again a controversial recommendation (see Chapter 19). More fundamentally, this questions the actual existence of recurrent ADEM (see Chapters 17 and 19). This should be addressed in further revisions of the current definitions.

Differentiation of prepubertal versus postpubertal MS

As mentioned above, there is increasing evidence that younger children have a distinct MS phenotype at onset compared with adolescents, including a more even sex ratio, more frequent ADEM-like clinical presentation, more frequent brainstem/cerebellar and less frequent spinal cord symptoms, more confluent T2-bright lesions on brain MRI some of which vanish over time, and more neutrophils and less frequent oligoclonal bands in the CSF [9,10,22,23]. In contrast, older pediatric patients with MS present with clinical, MRI and biological features that are similar to adults. The age limit between the two groups has ranged between 6 and 11 years in various studies and is thought to be related to puberty, although no endocrinology evidence was provided in these reports. Because of these differences, the diagnosis of MS is obviously more challenging in younger pediatric patients, and future revisions of pediatric MS definitions may include a categorization by age sub-groups to better take into account these specificities.

Lack of a core work-up to rule out mimicking diseases

One of the major challenges to diagnosing MS in children is the broad differential diagnosis that includes a large variety of metabolic, infectious, and genetic conditions, among others. Some of these conditions may mimic the relapsing–remitting course of MS, and be associated with similar brain MRI T2 hyperintensities. It is even sometimes impossible to differentiate one from the other, questioning potential associations, such as in the case of mitochondrial mutations associated with MS. The current definitions do not include ruling out mimicking diseases as a pre-requisite to diagnosing MS or related diseases in children, and this may be addressed in further revisions. More specific recommendations may be difficult to assemble, given the clinical heterogeneity of patients, and the need to assess the differential diagnosis on a case-by-case basis.

Conclusion

The operational definitions of MS and related acquired CNS demyelinating diseases in children originally published in 2007 have been a useful tool, improving patient care and establishing the ground for uniformed collaborative research projects. However, the experience of the past years has resulted in the recognition that these current operational definitions have to be revised. It is hoped that these definitions will soon be revised by the now enlarged International Study Group on Pediatric MS, so that they better reflect recently published data suggesting in particular major differences between pediatric MS onset in prepubertal versus postpubertal patients, with broader overlap between MS and ADEM in the younger patients.

References

1. Poser CM, Paty DW, Scheinberg L, et al. New diagnostic criteria for multiple sclerosis: Guidelines for research protocols. Ann Neurol 1983;**13**:227–231.

2. McDonald WI, Compston A, Edan G, et al. Recommended diagnostic criteria for multiple sclerosis: Guidelines from the International Panel on the diagnosis of multiple sclerosis. Ann Neurol 2001;**50**:121–127.

3. Polman CH, Reingold SC, Edan G, et al. Diagnostic criteria for multiple sclerosis: 2005 revisions to the "McDonald Criteria". Ann Neurol 2005;**58**:840–846.

4. Waubant E, Chabas D. Pediatric multiple sclerosis. Curr Treat Options Neurol 2009;**11**:203–210.

5. Krupp LB, Banwell B, Tenembaum S. Consensus definitions proposed for pediatric multiple sclerosis and related disorders. Neurology 2007;**68**:S7–12.

6. Wingerchuk DM, Lennon VA, Pittock SJ, Lucchinetti CF, Weinshenker BG. Revised diagnostic criteria for neuromyelitis optica. Neurology 2006;**66**:1485–1489.

7. Tenembaum S, Chamoles N, Fejerman N. Acute disseminated encephalomyelitis: A long-term follow-up study of 84 pediatric patients. Neurology 2002;**59**:1224–1231.

8. Dale RC, de Sousa C, Chong WK, Cox TC, Harding B, Neville BG. Acute disseminated encephalomyelitis, multiphasic disseminated encephalomyelitis and multiple sclerosis in children. Brain 2000;**123**(Pt 12):2407–2422.

9. Banwell B, Krupp L, Kennedy J, et al. Clinical features and viral serologies in children with multiple sclerosis: A multinational observational study. Lancet Neurol 2007;**6**:773–781.

10. Chabas D, Castillo-Trivino T, Mowry EM, Strober J, Glenn OA, Waubant E. Vanishing MS T2-bright

lesions before puberty: A distinct MRI phenotype? *Neurology* 2008;**71**:1090–1093.

11. Ghezzi A, Pozzilli C, Liguori M, *et al.* Prospective study of multiple sclerosis with early onset. *Mult Scler* 2002;**8**:115–118.

12. Lotze TE, Northrop JL, Hutton GJ, Ross B, Schiffman JS, Hunter JV. Spectrum of pediatric neuromyelitis optica. *Pediatrics* 2008;**122**:e1039–1047.

13. Mikaeloff Y, Suissa S, Vallee L, *et al.* First episode of acute CNS inflammatory demyelination in childhood: Prognostic factors for multiple sclerosis and disability. *J Pediatr* 2004;**144**:246–252.

14. Callen DJ, Shroff MM, Branson HM, *et al.* MRI in the diagnosis of pediatric multiple sclerosis. *Neurology* 2009;**72**:961–967.

15. Callen DJ, Shroff MM, Branson HM, *et al.* Role of MRI in the differentiation of ADEM from MS in children. *Neurology* 2009;**72**:968–973.

16. Mowry EM, Gajofatto A, Blasco MR, Castillo-Trivino T, Chabas D, Waubant E. Long lesions on initial spinal cord MRI predict a final diagnosis of acute disseminated encephalomyelitis versus multiple sclerosis. *Neurology* 2008;**70**:A135.

17. Waubant E, Chabas D, Glenn OA, Okuda D, Mowry EM, Pelletier D. Pediatric patients have higher MRI lesion burden at time of MS onset compared to adults. *Arch Neurol* 2009;**66**:967–971.

18. Riikonen R. The role of infection and vaccination in the genesis of optic neuritis and multiple sclerosis in children. *Acta Neurol Scand* 1989;**80**:425–431.

19. Hanefeld F, Bauer HJ, Christen HJ, Kruse B, Bruhn H, Frahm J. Multiple sclerosis in childhood: Report of 15 cases. *Brain Dev* 1991;**13**:410–416.

20. Ruggieri M, Polizzi A, Pavone L, Grimaldi LM. Multiple sclerosis in children under 6 years of age. *Neurology* 1999;**53**:478–484.

21. Pohl D, Rostasy K, Reiber H, Hanefeld F. CSF characteristics in early-onset multiple sclerosis. *Neurology* 2004;**63**:1966–1967.

22. Chabas D, Ness J, Belman A, *et al.* Younger children with MS have a distinct CSF inflammatory profile at disease onset. *Neurology* 2010;**74**:399–405.

23. Chabas D, Deen S, McCulloch C, Erlich E, Strober J, Waubant E. Pediatric MS: A phenotype at onset influenced by ethnicity. Abstract presented at the Child Neurology Society Meeting, 2008.

Chapter 3

Epidemiology of pediatric multiple sclerosis: incidence, prevalence, and susceptibility risk factors

Martino Ruggieri, Immacolata Plasmati, and Isabella Simone

Multiple sclerosis (MS) is a relatively common neurological disorder typically affecting young adults, with a clinical onset occurring between 20 and 40 years of age [1–3] (prevalence = 1:800 or 0.12% in the general population). Over the past two decades, however, there has been an increased recognition that MS can affect children worldwide [4–9]. Although a broad spectrum of congenital and acquired diseases may occur in childhood with similar symptoms and signs and may often be confused with MS [10–12], newer clinical [13], laboratory [14] and imaging [15–17] criteria have been proposed and have facilitated the diagnosis process, including ruling out mimicking diseases and better recognizing MS at a very early age [5,8,18] such as below 6 years (reviewed in [5,19,20]). Nevertheless, there is still a need to better delineate and validate standardized clinical, laboratory, imaging, and genetic pediatric MS criteria in large pediatric cohorts.

Incidence and prevalence

The prevalence and incidence of pediatric versus adult onset MS are reported in Table 3.1a.

The prevalence of MS can exceed 200 per 100 000 in high-risk areas such as Canada [21], and ranges between 70 and 190/100 000 in the UK [22], Denmark [23], and Italy [24,25]. By contrast, the prevalence of MS in low-risk regions, such as Asia, the Middle East, and the Caribbean, is less than 5 per 100 000 [26].

Despite the consistent amount of data recently published on pediatric MS, the proportion of pediatric MS patients in the total MS population remains unclear [5–9]. Only recently, population-based and regional registry-based studies have, for the first time, succeeded in calculating and establishing reliable incidence and prevalence rate estimates in the youngest age groups [27–31].

Retrospective studies: historic difficulties and limitations

Several retrospective studies have estimated the *overall prevalence* of MS, with onset before 18 years, to range from 1.6 to 10.5% of the total MS population [15,32–39]. This wide range estimate is partially explained by the lack of consistent definitions of pediatric MS throughout time and studies, including variable age cut-off [29]. Recent progresses made in the development of consensus definitions for pediatric MS and related diseases by the International Pediatric MS Study Group, and advances in diagnostic techniques, have partially overtaken such historic difficulty [5,7,13,18,28,29,30,31].

Another critical limiting factor in estimating the proportion of pediatric MS is the lack of accurate, well-characterized clinical data derived from large cohorts of pediatric MS patients. However, progress has been made since national [9,20,31,40–43] and international [44] pediatric MS consortia and surveys gathering data from large registries and databases recently became available [28–31].

A further limitation to epidemiological studies on pediatric MS is related to the fact that a substantial amount of data were derived from neurological centers highly specialized in the diagnosis and management of MS, with a consequent recruiting bias. For example, the study by Simone *et al.* [38], which reported a particularly high frequency of pediatric-onset MS (83/793 or 10%), was issued from a single MS center located in Southern Italy [38].

Demyelinating Disorders of the Central Nervous System in Childhood, ed. Dorothée Chabas and Emmanuelle L. Waubant. Published by Cambridge University Press. © Cambridge University Press 2011.

Table 3.1a Epidemiological features in pediatric and adult MS onset: incidence and prevalence

Pediatric MS onset			Adult MS onset		
		Authors			**Authors**
Incidence	0.9/100 000/year (including ADEM, NMO)	Banwell [27], Canada	Incidence Prevalence	11.4/100 000/year 226.6/100 000	Marrie [21], Canada
Incidence	0.3/100 000/year	Pohl [31], Germany	Prevalence	73.3/100 000	Bentzen [23], Denmark
Incidence	0.12/100 000/year	Ruggieri (personal data), Italy	Incidence	6.2/100 000/year	Nicoletti [47], Italy
Prevalence	0.98/100 000 general population		Prevalence	126/100 000	
	4.6/100 000 pediatric population		Incidence Prevalence	4.18/100 000/year 144.4/100 000	Pugliatti [24], Granieri [25], Italy/Sardinia
Incidence	1.3/100 000/year	Torisu [28], Japan	Prevalence	<5 per 100 000	Lowis [26], Asia, Middle-East, Caribbean

Prospective studies, registry- and population-based surveys

Canada

The highest annual incidence rate reported so far (0.9/100 000 children) was recorded in a Canadian study that included ADEM and NMO cases. It ranged from 0.6/100 000 in Quebec (south-east Canada) and Saskatchewan (western Canada), to 1.6/100 000 in Manitoba (south-central Canada) [27]. Consistent with these data, a recent study showed that the prevalence of adult-onset MS in Manitoba was among the highest in the world [21]. Further studies are required to address whether clinical, demographic, or environmental factors might influence this south/north gradient in Canada.

A previous population (registry)-based survey, conducted in the same Canadian region of Saskatchewan (specifically, in central Saskatchewan: town of Saskatoon), from 1970 to 2004, identified 95/897 cases (10.5%) with disease onset before 20 years of age and 30/897 (3%) cases with onset before 16 years of age [30].

USA

A pediatric MS prevalence was reported by the regional Partners MS Center database, in the north-eastern US. In this study, 135 of 4399 MS patients (3.6%) seen at the Center experienced their first symptoms under 18 years of age: 3/4399 (0.06%) had an onset below the age of 10 years; 14/4399 (0.3%) between 10 and 12 years; and 118/4399 (2.6%) between 13 and 17 years [29].

Some study design characteristics may explain, at least partly, the differences in pediatric MS frequencies among the three above-mentioned studies [27,29,30]. For example, in the Canadian study run by Banwell *et al.* [27], data were obtained via the Canadian Paediatric Surveillance Program through 2400 pediatric health care providers over a 3-year period ranging from 1 April 2004 to 31 March 2007, where all Canadian pediatric MS cases were theoretically included. By contrast, the other two studies are registry-based studies, which may include a bias towards under- or over-recruitments [29,30].

Japan

A multicenter, population-based study was conducted in the Fukuoka Prefecture located in Northern Kyushu Island, the third largest island in Japan, including 4.96 million people total, with 0.73 million people under 15 years of age on 1 October 2003. At that time, the prevalence of pediatric MS (= individuals under the age of 15 years) was 1.3 per 100 000 persons [28].

Europe

Germany

The German nationwide prospective survey carried out over a 3-year period (from 1 January 1997 to 31 December 1999) estimated an annual incidence rate of pediatric MS of 0.3/100 000 children under 16 years of age, ranging from 0.1/100 000 for children under 10 years of age to 0.6/100 000 for adolescents between 10 and 15 years of age [31].

Italy

Ruggieri et al. (manuscript in preparation) conducted a prospective population-based study over an 18-year period (1 January 1992 to 31 December 2009) in the town of Catania, eastern Sicily, which includes a total population of 296 469 inhabitants, among whom 64 295 are children below 15 years of age as reported in the last Italian census [45]. The authors found, before the prevalence day, a total of 3 children with MS (1 boy, 2 girls; currently aged 10–14 years) who experienced their first symptoms before their 15th birthday compared with 380 patients with adult-onset MS recorded over a similar period of time (i.e. years 1990–2005) [46,47; Nicoletti et al., unreported data]. The prevalence of pediatric-onset MS in the general population was 0.98/100 000 (versus 126.6/100 000 for adult onset MS; Nicoletti et al., unreported data) and 4.6/100 000 in the pediatric population. From 1992 to 2009, the annual incidence rate of pediatric MS (under 15 years) was 0.12/100 000 person-years (versus 6.2/100 000 for adult-onset MS) [46,47; Nicoletti et al., unreported data]. More specifically, the pediatric MS rate was 0.78% for children aged <15 years (3/380 MS cases) and 0.26% for children aged <10 years (1/380 MS cases).

Comparison with ADEM

There is even more limited data regarding the incidence and prevalence of ADEM compared with pediatric MS.

It seems that the incidence rate of ADEM is higher in younger versus older children: 0.4/100 000/person-year in people <20 years of age, 0.64/100 000/person-year in children <15 years [28], and 0.8/100 000/person-year in children between 5 and 9 years of age [75]. The incidence rate of childhood ADEM was 1.1 per 100 000 person-years in children under the age of 10 years in a study conducted in the town of Catania, eastern Sicily, Italy over an 18-year period (mean age at presentation of ADEM, 3.6 ±2 years) [76].

The overall frequency of ADEM was 22% among Canadian children with acquired demyelinating disorders, according to a recent study [27].

Demographic characteristics

Table 3.1b shows the demographic features in pediatric-onset MS compared with adult onset MS.

Gender ratio

Adult-onset MS affects females more often than males. The female/male ratio ranges from 1.6 to 3.2 [35,38,48,49]. Recent epidemiological studies conducted on MS cohorts by date of birth have shown that the female/male ratio has remarkably increased (over 3.2) in the last 50 years [24,50,51]. The female/male ratio tends to flatten (i.e. 1.4) in adult patients with late onset MS (>50 years of age) [49,52,53].

In the pediatric population, the female/male ratio varies depending on the age at disease onset. In patients with a younger age at onset (e.g. <10 years), the ratio is reversed compared with adults, with a predominance of males (F/M = 0.42–0.7) [20,27,29, 35,38,54,55]. This is particularly evident for the rare patients with an age at onset below 24 months (F/M ratio = 0.6) [56–60; M, Ruggieri, personal observation; reviewed in 19,20]. Among pediatric MS patients whose onset of disease occurs in the peri-adolescent period (i.e. about 10–12 years of age), the female/male ratio is higher than in very young patients (2.2 to 3.0) [29,33,35,38 39,61–64]. An even higher female preponderance is recorded in patients whose onset of disease occurs at 13 (3.35) or 14 years (7.67) of age [32].

Thus, the risk of developing MS is higher for females from the age of puberty through young adulthood, while it is higher for males at a younger pediatric age or later in the adult life, after 50 years. This Gaussian gender distribution may partially support the theory that hormonal changes related to puberty, especially female sex hormones, may play an important role in MS onset ([51,65–67], reviewed in 54). There may also be a gender-specific genetic influence on immunological reactivity [68,69]. Finally, there may be an additional influence of race on gender susceptibility to pediatric MS, as suggested by the New York State Multiple Sclerosis Consortium (NYSMSC) patient registry that showed an overall increased female preponderance and a younger age at diagnosis in the African-American group [70].

Age at onset

The overall age distribution of MS patients at disease onset is bell-shaped: 10% of patients develop their first

Table 3.1b Demographic features in pediatric and adult MS onset populations

	Pediatric MS onset		Adult MS onset	
		Authors		Authors
Age at onset	0.5–18 years (includes ADEM, NMO)	Banwell [27], Canada	16–74 years	Alonso [48], UK
	5–16 years; 6.4%<11 years	Duquette [33], Canada	50–82 years (late onset)	Kis [52], Germany
	<16 years;15%<10 years	Simone [38], Italy	16.1–56 years	Simone [38], Italy
	<16 years; 5.6%<7 years 10%<10 years	Boiko [32], Canada	>50 years (late onset)	Polliack [49], Israel
	2–15 years; 10%≤4 years	Boutin [71], France	>50 years (late onset)	Review in Martinelli [53],Italy
	<16 years; 6.4%<10 years	Sindern [39], Germany		
	8–17 years; 2.2%<10 years	Chitnis [29], USA		
	≤ 16 years; 35%<10 years	Halilogu [54], Turkey		
	≤15 years; 0.5%<11 years	Ghezzi [35], Italy		
	≤ 15 years; 2.4%<10 years	Ghezzi [55], Italy		
	<18 years	Kennedy [88], Canada		
	≤16 years; 30%< 10 years	Mikaeloff [73], France		
	<16 years	Pohl [31], Germany		
	1.5–16 years; 7.6%≤10 years	Renoux [74], France, Belgium		
	<17 years; 25% <10 years	Selcen [72], Turkey		
	<6 years	Ruggieri [19], Italy		
	3 cases <18 months	Ruggieri, personal data		
Sex ratio F/M	1.07<10 years; 1.1≥10 years (includes ADEM, NMO)	Banwell [27], Canada	2.24	Alonso [48], UK
	3	Duquette [33], Canada	2	Duquette [33], Canada
	1.9; 0.6<10 years; 2.4>14 years	Simone [38], Italy	1.9	Simone [38], Italy
	2.9	Boiko [32], Canada	1.73 (late onset)	Polliack [49], Israel
	2.1	Boutin [71], France	1 (late onset)	Kis [52], Germany
	2.4	Sindern [39], Germany	2.87	Chitnis [29], USA
	3.2; 0.5<10 years; 1.8≤12 years; 3.7>13 years	Chitnis [29], USA	3.2	Orton [50], Canada
	0.75; 0.42≤10 years; 1>10 years	Halilogu [54], Turkey	1.6	Ghezzi [35], Italy
	2.2; 0.8<12 years	Ghezzi [35], Italy	2.5	Kennedy [88], Canada
	0.7<12 years; 4.7≥12 years	Ghezzi [55], Italy		
	1.32	Kennedy [88], Canada		

Table 3.1b (cont.)

Pediatric MS onset		Adult MS onset	
	Authors		Authors
1.7; 1≤10 years; 2.2>13 years	Mikaeloff [73], France		
1.2; 0.9<14 years; 2.2 >14–15 years	Pohl [31], Germany		
2.8; 2.2≤12 years; 2.9<12 years	Renoux [74], France, Belgium		
1	Selcen [72], Turkey		
2.8	Hanefeld [63], Germany		
0.6	Ruggieri [19], Italy Ruggieri, personal data		

symptoms before the age of 20 years, 70% between the ages of 20 and 40 years, and 20% after the age of 40 years.

MS patients with pediatric onset have been traditionally divided into four categories:

(1) Extremely early onset MS (i.e. before the age of 24 months) with only a few cases reported in the literature [56–60].

(2) MS in pre-school children (i.e. under 6 years of age), ranging from 0.8 to 14% of pediatric MS cases [19,33,38,71–73].

(3) Prepubertal MS (i.e. under 10–12 years of age) ranging from 0.5 to 30% of pediatric MS cases [32,33,38,62,71–74].

(4) Postpubertal or adolescent (also known as juvenile) MS (i.e. from puberty to 16 or 18 years of age), ranging from 40 to 80% of pediatric MS cases [32,33,38,63,71–74].

Extremely early onset MS

Five cases, recorded as MS with disease onset before the age of 24 months, have been reported in the literature [56–60]: three boys and two girls, who developed their first symptoms at the age of 10 months [60], 13 months (n = 2) [56,58], 15 months [57], and 18 months [59]. Two of them died after a rapid and severe disease course [56,60] and another one had a primary progressive form [59]. These extremely early onset MS cases appear to carry an unfavorable prognosis. However, in these children, ADEM could not be ruled out for certain because of the lack of long-term follow-up in unfavorable cases [56,60], the absence of brain and/or spinal cord MRI data in four cases where the diagnosis was based on pathology [56,60], or on clinical/laboratory findings [57,59], and the lack of clear-cut pathological features differentiating MS from ADEM when an autopsy was carried out [56,60]. Thus, these reported cases remain controversial.

Ruggieri et al. (manuscript in preparation) studied five additional cases: 3 males and 2 females, whose age at disease onset was 18 months, with a follow-up ranging from 17 to 21 years. Remarkably, all had seizures and motor signs (e.g. hemiparesis) at first attack and had a high relapse rate (4–9 per year). Brain and spinal cord MRI studies showed widespread white matter lesions at onset (similar to leukodystrophies), with gradual appearance of typical plaque-like lesions around the age of 6, which became confluent at age 14. The CSF and neurophysiologic analyses were typical of MS; the Extended Disability Status Scale (EDSS) scores at last follow-up were 1 (n = 1), 3 (n = 3), and 4 (n = 1).

Pre-school children

The age at onset in the group of patients who develop their first symptoms in the pre-school age fits with a

Gaussian curve. In a review analysis of 43 patients reported in literature, plus 6 additional personal cases, the mean age at presentation in this age group was 3.2 years (range = 10 months to 5.3 years), with a disease onset age younger in boys (3.0 years) than in girls (3.2 years) [19].

Prepubertal children

The mean age at presentation was 6.1 years (median 6.3 years) in a review study, which analyzed data from 87 patients (37 of whom with disease onset <6 years of age) reported in the literature [44].

Adolescents

Presentation in adolescents is similar to that of MS in the adult population.

Geographic distribution and race

Epidemiological data clearly indicate that adult MS is a geographically related disease, with disease rates rising with an increased distance from the equator in both northern and southern hemispheres. It is known that the prevalence in the adult-onset MS population can exceed 200/100 000 individuals in high-risk areas such as Scotland, Northern Ireland, and Canada, whereas the prevalence falls to under 5/100 000 in Asia, the Middle East, and the Caribbean [24,26,83]. However, data on the geographic distribution of MS in the pediatric population are lacking [82], and whether it shares the same pattern as adult MS is unknown.

Race modifies the incidence and characteristics of MS in adults [84–86]. Typically, Caucasians are more often affected while Blacks and Asians are less often affected [87]. A recent study showed that African descendants living in the USA have a smaller risk of developing MS compared to Caucasians. Nevertheless, the risk is still higher in African-Americans compared with Africans, suggesting a genetic admixture of a resistant African with a susceptible Caucasian population, or to environmental risk factors which are operative within the US [84]. Furthermore, the influence of race on MS is clinically relevant, since data suggest that non-Caucasian adult MS patients may have a more aggressive disease with a worse outcome [84].

The relative influence of race, ethnicity and ancestry on pediatric MS has been explored in only a few studies. However, these data suggest that the ethnic and racial background of patients with pediatric-onset MS may differ from adult-onset MS. A recent retrospective study conducted in a North-Eastern United States MS Center showed a lower proportion of Caucasians and more African-Americans in the pediatric compared with the adult MS population [29]. This trend was confirmed in other Canadian pediatric MS cohorts studies [27,88]. Remarkably, the disease course was more aggressive in black than in non-black pediatric MS patients [88,89], as already found in adult MS [70,84,91]. In addition, there was a higher proportion of Hispanic or Latino compared with the adult disease in the various cohorts (Boston [29]; Columbus [89]; Long Island [90] and Toronto [88]), probably reflecting current regional demographics [29]. Finally, a Canadian study conducted in Ontario compared the background of 44 pediatric-onset MS cases (<18 years at MS diagnosis) and 573 adult-onset MS patients. Ancestries originating from areas of lower MS prevalence were over-represented in children versus adult patients (e.g. Caribbean [23% vs. 3%], Asian [25% vs. 4.4%] or Middle East [12% vs. 4%]), while a European heritage was less frequent in pediatric patients [88] (Table 3.1c).

The reasons behind the greater diversity in ethnicity, race and ancestry in pediatric versus adult MS are still unclear and may include a combination of genetic and environmental factors, associated with changes in regional demographic factors occurring during childhood [27,88].

Birth place, place of residency, and role of migration

Several studies suggest that there is a critical age at migration (before 15 years of age), which impacts the overall MS susceptibility [92–96].

A Canadian study comparing pediatric-onset MS (<18 years at MS diagnosis) and adult-onset MS in Ontario reported that most patients were born in Canada (35/44 pediatric MS and 437/555 adult MS patients). Among patients born outside Canada, there were more pediatric MS patients born in Asia and less in Europe compared with adults. In part, this may be related to a strong recent immigration from Asia in Canada. For those patients who had moved to Canada, the mean age at the time of migration was 8 years (range 3–15 years) in the

Table 3.1c Race and ethnicity in pediatric and adult MS onset populations

		Pediatric MS onset		Adult MS onset	
			Authors		Authors
Race	Caucasians	100/135 (74%)	Chitnis [29], USA	1141/1356 (84%)	Chitnis [29], USA
	African-Americans	10/135 (7.4%)		58/1356 (4.3%)	
	Black	6/44 (14%)	Kennedy [88], Canada	17/573 (3%)	Kennedy [88], Canada
	European	92/219 (42%)	Banwell [27], Canada		
	African-American	16/219 (7%)			
	Caribbean	3/219 (1.4%)			
Ethnicity	Not Hispanic or Latino	76.3%	Chitnis [29], USA	86.7%	Chitnis [29], USA
	Hispanic or Latino	9.6%		2.6%	
Ancestry	Caribbean	23%	Kennedy [88], Canada	3%	Kennedy [88], Canada
	Asian	25%		4.4%	
	Middle Eastern	12%		4%	
	European	50%		91%	

pediatric-onset population versus 18 years (range <1–55 years) in the adult-onset population, and 100% of pediatric-onset versus 79% of adult-onset patients had spent at least some time in Canada as a child, suggesting that residing during childhood in Canada, a country of high MS risk, may have participated in the lifetime risk of developing MS [88]. Another study conducted in Australia showed that the prevalence of MS among migrants from high-risk UK to lower-risk Australia did not differ whether the migration occurred before or after the age of 15 years [97], suggesting a prevailing influence of the environment on MS risk rather than the age at migration [88,97].

Family history of demyelinating disorders

Overall, a family history of MS in first-degree relatives is reported in 6–8% of children and adolescents with MS [5,37,38,74,77–80]. However, retrospective studies with longer follow-up reported more frequent family history of MS (about 20%), This is likely explained by the fact that a longer follow-up allows more lifetime for patient relatives to develop the disease [33,81].

There are limited data about the relationship between age at onset of pediatric MS and a positive family history of MS. A family history of MS was present in 9.6% of children who developed their first symptoms before the age of 6 years, while there was none in those with onset of disease prior to 24 months of age after a follow-up of 17–21 years [19; and unreported data]. Similar findings (no family history) were recorded in the Japanese multi-center, population-based study on childhood MS conducted in the Prefecture of Fukuoka, which analysed observational data (years 1998–2003) on patients with MS whose mean age at onset of disease was 5.7 years (range 11 months to 15 years) [28], and in the Italian population-based study on pediatric-onset MS conducted in the town of Catania (Ruggieri *et al.*, unreported data). Thus the interaction between age of onset and a positive family history of MS is unclear in the pediatric population.

Environmental risk factors for childhood MS

Infectious agents

Environmental factors, in particular infections, have been linked with the risk of developing MS.

Herpesviridae family

Seroepidemiologic and pathologic evidences has strongly suggested that prior infection with members of the Herpesviridae family may be associated with the development of MS in adulthood [98]. One relevant characteristic of this group of viruses is its ability to remain latent. Viruses from this family with a possible MS association have included herpes simplex virus (HSV), varicella zoster virus (VZV), human herpesvirus-6 (HHV-6), Epstein–Barr virus (EBV) and cytomegalovirus (CMV) [98]. This association was first studied in the 1980s. Initially a low interferon production in MS patients was found by stimulating lymphocytes with HSV, CMV and VZV [99], and a higher frequency of HSV, HHV-6 and VZV was seen in active and inactive demyelinating plaques when compared with normal brain tissue [100]. An association between the herpesviruses (HV) and immunological alterations in MS patients was described. PCR studies revealed the presence of HSV [101], HHV-6 [102–104], VZV [105–108], and EBV [109–111] DNA in MS patients. Finally, migration studies suggested that the exposure to a non-identified environmental factor before the age of 14 increases the risk of developing MS [107].

Epstein–Barr virus

The most studied member of the Herpesviridae family in MS patients has been EBV (a member of the γ-herpesviruses). Epidemiologic evidences have suggested that prior infection (e.g. in childhood, adolescence or adulthood) with EBV may be associated with the development of MS in adulthood [118–122]. EBV infects >95% of the world's population [123]. Early age (i.e. <4 years of age) at primary EBV infection is typically asymptomatic, but primary infection during adolescence or adulthood (e.g. <40 years of age, since most individuals above 40 years of age have already been infected by EBV) manifests as infectious mononucleosis in 40–50% of cases [124], which has been associated with a two- to

threefold increased risk of MS [122,123]. Most importantly, MS risk is extremely low in individuals who are EBV-negative [122].

EBV infects resting B-lymphocytes, immortalizing them into long-lived memory B cells that survive in the peripheral circulation, largely undetected by the immune system [121,122]. In some studies, adult MS patients showed elevated (fourfold increase) serum and CSF titers of EBV antibodies (e.g. anti-EBNA, -EBNA-1 and -EBNA-2 antigens) years before developing any neurological symptom [123,125–127]. However, these findings were not reproduced in other studies [128,129]. Similar controversial findings have been recorded in post-mortem pathologic specimens of brains of adult patients with MS, which revealed intracerebral diffuse EBV-infected cells in all forms of MS in some reports [103,105–107] but not in others [128,129].

Theories about a potential pathogenic role of EBV in MS have included antigen mimicry, immortalization of B-cell clones, and cytotoxic T-cell dysfunction against viral infected B cells [121,123]. However, no data so far have unequivocally supported a direct etiologic role of the EBV virus [125–129], and there is still controversy about whether EBV could be a causative agent as opposed to an innocent bystander in the pathogenesis of MS [121,130].

There are still limited data available regarding EBV (or other neurotropic viruses) infection in pediatric patients with MS. A retrospective International study on 136 pediatric MS patients showed that over 108/136 (86%) of them were seropositive for remote EBV infection (irrespective of geographic residence) compared with only 61/95 (64%) controls matched for gender and age ($p = 0.025$), suggesting a possible role for EBV in pediatric-onset MS pathogenesis [44]. Notably, controls showed delayed infection compared with patients [44]. Pohl et al. [131,132] analyzed the frequency and intensity of CSF antibody production against EBV, VZV, and HSV (but also measles and rubella), in 43 pediatric-onset vs. 50 adult-onset MS patients and controls, by determining virus-specific CSF-to-serum antibody indices (AI). Intrathecally synthesized EBV antibodies were detectable in 26% pediatric and 10% adult onset MS patients, compared to frequencies ranging in both groups from 10 to 60% for the other viruses. Median AIs for EBV were lower than those for all other viruses, with more than twofold-higher median AI for measles, rubella and VZV [132]. Thus, the potential implication of EBV in pediatric MS remains to be investigated at a larger scale before any definite conclusion can be drawn.

Varicella zoster virus

Between 1994 and 2003, Mikealoff *et al.* [133] conducted a population-based case-control study in France to investigate whether clinically observed chickenpox increased the risk of MS in childhood. One hundred and thirty-seven pediatric-onset MS cases were matched for age, sex, and geographic origin with 1061 controls randomly selected from the general population. Information about clinically observed chickenpox in cases and controls before the index date/date of disease onset was collected with a standardized questionnaire and checked against health certificates. Clinically observed chickenpox had occurred in 76.6% of pediatric-onset MS cases compared with 84.4% of their matched controls (adjusted odds ratio of MS onset associated with chickenpox occurrence was 0.58). The authors inferred that chickenpox could be associated with a lower risk of childhood-onset MS in their French population [133]. However, these data have never been replicated in other populations, and there is no evidence of a causative relationship.

Epidemiological surveys showed that VZV and MS are more prevalent in temperate zones compared with countries closer to the equator [107]. In high-risk areas for varicella and MS, 95% of the population develops varicella before the age of 10 years [112]. In a series of six patients, the appearance of clinical varicella zoster was coincidental with the diagnosis of MS or with a relapse [113]. Another study reported the presence of VZV DNA in 95% of MS cases during relapses and only in 17% during remissions [114], suggesting that VZV activation may be either an epiphenomenon or an active participant in MS etiopathogenesis [115,116]. On the other hand, a systematic review of 40 studies from 1965 to 1999 found insufficient evidence to support an important etiological role of VZV infection in the etiopathogenesis of MS, as most of the studies lacked appropriate methodology [117]. Thus, the influence of VZV on MS is unclear.

Herpesviridae and other neurotropic viruses

In a particular study, only 1/6 of children with MS (out of 63 children with positive viral AIs tested) had positive AIs towards several of the following viruses including HSV, VZV, EBV, CMV, mumps, rubella, and measles [134].

Other microorganisms

Chlamydia pneumoniae

Chlamydia pneumoniae is an intracellular pathogen responsible for a number of different acute and chronic infections and a common cause of human respiratory disease [135]. *Chlamydia pneumoniae* infection has been shown to promote the transmigration of monocytes through human brain endothelial cells, suggesting a mechanism by which the pathogen may be able to enter the central nervous system, in particular in chronic injury [136]. During recent years, there have been seroepidemiological, cultural, molecular, immunological and therapeutic studies suggesting a possible involvement of *C. pneumoniae* in MS disease (reviewed in [135]). However, while some recent studies have suggested a role of *C. pneumoniae* only as a CNS innocent bystander epiphenomenon due to ongoing MS inflammation which favors a selective infiltration of infected mononuclear cells within the CNS, others indicate its role as a cofactor in the development and progression of the disease by enhancing a pre-existing autoimmune response in a subset of MS patients, as supported by immunological and molecular findings (reviewed in [135]).

Rostasy *et al.* [137] investigated the frequency and quantity of CSF antibody production against *C. pneumoniae* and the presence of the pathogen in the CSF in 25 children with MS: 2/25 of cases contained the *C. pneumoniae* genome, and 7/25 had positive CSF antibodies. The authors provided evidence that the positive CSF bands were only a small part of the total intrathecal immunoglobulin G (oligoclonal) profile, and inferred that the intrathecal synthesis recorded could have been part of a polyspecific, oligoclonal immune response. Krone *et al.* [138] recorded similar findings in a single MS child. Notably, a 12-year-old child reported by Pohl *et al.* [139] presented with three attacks of optic neuritis within 5 months. A positive polymerase chain reaction for *C. pneumoniae* in the CSF led to the diagnosis of a CNS infection with *C. pneumoniae*. After treatment with the antibiotic rifampicin, he experienced no further attacks during the follow-up period of 6 years.

In conclusion, the role of *Chlamydia pneumoniae* in MS pathogenesis remains controversial.

Vaccinations

Hepatitis B (HB) vaccine

The role of hepatitis B vaccine in adult MS is highly controversial [140–144]. Five studies found no increased risk but could not exclude a relative risk below 2 [145–149]. Two French case-control studies estimated a 40–70% increased risk of developing MS within 2 months following vaccination [150,151], while a study in the UK, based on the General Practitioner Research Database, reported a 60% increased risk within 1 year following immunization [152]. A nested case-control study based on that same database reported an increase in MS risk in the first 3 years after vaccination [153].

Only Mikaeloff *et al.* studied the role of hepatitis B vaccine (Engerix B; GenHevac B) in pediatric-onset MS [154–157] in a multiple population-based case-control study of children with MS [154] or with a first episode of acute CNS inflammatory demyelination [155,156] conducted in France between 1994 and 2003). The authors found no association between hepatitis B vaccination and the risk of developing a first episode of MS or a relapse over 3 years (nor over 6 months or over the entire exposure period from birth to the index date) [154,155]. The authors also found no increased risk of conversion to MS in either short- or long-term risk periods [155]. They recorded only a potential trend of increased risk, particularly for confirmed MS, in the longer term for the Engerix B vaccine [156].

In conclusion, there is no proven effect of hepatitis B vaccine on the risk of developing pediatric-onset MS.

Passive smoking

Smokers have been found to have a 40–80% higher risk of MS than non-smokers in previous epidemiological studies [157–161]. More recent surveys showed that the risk increased with cumulative doses of smoking [162], was associated with increased blood–brain barrier disruption, higher lesion volumes, and greater atrophy [163], had an adverse influence on disease progression, and accelerated conversion from a relapsing–remitting to a progressive course [164]. However, the smoking history of MS patients and the controls did not differ in a matched case-control study of 136 MS patients from 106 multiplex MS families vs. their 204 healthy siblings as control [165].

Based on these premises [157–165], Mikaeloff *et al.* [166] investigated the possible association between MS and passive smoking in the French KIDSEP pediatric MS cohort [77]. This population-based case-control study included 164 pediatric MS patients (<16 years at onset between 1 January 1994 and 31 December 2003) and 12 controls per patient, selected from the French general population, matched for age (±6 months), gender and current place of residency, who were asked to answer a standardized questionnaire regarding parents' smoking habits. Children ever exposed to parental smoking were found to have a higher risk of developing MS: exposure to parental smoking was noted in 62.0% (80/129) of pediatric-onset MS cases vs. 45.1% (468/1038) of unrelated controls. Of note, more MS patients (4.7%, 6/129) than controls (1.7%, 18/1038) had a familial history of MS ($p<0.05$), potentially biasing the results. Nonetheless, this increased risk of MS was associated with a longer duration of exposure to passive smoking in older (aged >10 years at the time of the index episode) vs. younger (<10 years) MS patients.

The postulated underlying mechanism(s) causing a potentially increased risk of developing MS in both children – exposed to passive smoking – and adults – exposed to smoke – is unclear and include direct effects of cigarette smoke components on the blood–brain barrier or a nicotine effect on microvascular blood flow in the brain [167], direct exposure to cyanide (a component of cigarette smoke) and thiocyanate (one of its metabolites), which cause demyelination in the CNS in animal models [168,169], and inhibition of interferon gamma productions by adenoid cells in children [170].

Childhood and adolescent obesity

The influence of obesity during childhood, adolescence and adulthood on the risk of developing MS was studied in two retrospective cohorts of 121 700 (Nurse's Health Study I) and 116 671 (Nurse's Health Study II) female patients followed for up to 40 years in the USA [171]. The women in the two cohorts had been asked to provide information on weight and age at age 18, from which the body mass index was derived. They were also asked to identify body silhouettes best representing themselves at ages 5, 10, and 20 years. The analysis was run on 593 confirmed MS cases identified in both cohorts. Obesity (body mass index ≥ 30 kg/m^2) at the age of 18 years was associated with a greater than twofold increased risk of developing MS (2.25; $p = 0.001$). After adjusting for body size (i.e. silhouettes) at age 20, having a large body size (i.e. a large silhouette) at ages 5 or 10 was not associated with an increased risk of developing MS, whereas a large body size at age 20 was associated with a 96% increased risk of developing MS (95% CI 1.33–2.89, $p = 0.009$). No significant association was found between adult body mass and risk of developing MS [171]. In conclusion, there were too many limitations in this study [171] to draw any definite conclusion on the potential influence of childhood obesity on the risk of developing MS.

Conclusions

Pediatric MS, once considered a rare childhood illness, has been increasingly recognized as a disabling acquired pediatric neurological disease requiring early recognition and intervention. The epidemiology of pediatric MS is distinct from adult MS in many aspects beyond its lower incidence and prevalence rates. The gender distribution seems to vary according to the age at onset, with increased risks of developing MS in males with very early age of onset (i.e. before puberty) while females are more often hit around or after puberty, suggesting hormonal or gender-specific genetic influences. Race, ethnicity, and ancestry may also influence disease susceptibility and course differently, with a higher proportion of non-Caucasian patients in the pediatric versus the adult population. However, some of these differences may also be related to changes in regional demographics (e.g. increase of migrating children from lower- to higher-risk areas). There is clear evidence that environmental factors play a role in the development of MS irrespective of age. If no single environmental factor has been consistently identified as a causal factor of MS, a few candidates have been identified as associated with pediatric MS in a few epidemiological studies (neurotropic viruses, *Chlamydia pneumonia*, passive smoking). Further, large-scale epidemiologic studies are needed to investigate the influence of environmental factors in more details on pediatric MS. Indeed, pediatric MS provides the unique opportunity to study the potential influence of recent primary infections or other pre- or perinatal environmental factors on the disease, and their interactions with the genetic background.

References

1. Compston A, Coles A. Multiple sclerosis. *Lancet* 2002;**359**:1221–1231.

2. Compston A, McDonald I, Noseworthy J, *et al. McAlpine's Multiple Sclerosis.* 4th ed. London: Churchill Livingstone, 2006.

3. Confraveaux C, Vukusic S. The clinical epidemiology of multiple sclerosis. *Neuroimag Clin N Am* 2008;**18**: 589–622.

4. Tardieu M, Mikaeloff Y. Multiple sclerosis in children. *Int MS J* 2004;**11**:36–42.

5. Banwell B, Ghezzi A, Bar-Or A, Mikaeloff Y, Tardieu M. Multiple sclerosis in children: Clinical diagnosis, therapeutic strategies, and future directions. *Lancet Neurol* 2007;**6**:887–902.

6. Hanefeld F. Pediatric multiple sclerosis: A short history of a long story. *Neurology* 2007;**68**(16 Suppl 2): S3–6.

7. Ness JM, Chabas D, Sadovnick AD, Pohl D, Banwell B, Weinstock-Gutman B for International Pediatric MS Study Group. Clinical features of children and adolescents with multiple sclerosis. *Neurology* 2007; **68**(16 Suppl 2):S37–45.

8. Chabas D, Strober J, Waubant E. Pediatric multiple sclerosis. *Curr Neurol Neurosci Rep* 2008;**8**:434–441.

9. Yeh EA, Chitnis T, Krupp L, *et al.* Pediatric multiple sclerosis. *Nat Rev Neurol* 2009;**5**:621–631.

10. Natowicz MR, Bejjani B. Genetic disorders that masquerade as multiple sclerosis. *Am J Med Genet* 1994;**49**:149–169.

11. van der Knaap MS, Valk J. *Magnetic Resonance of Myelination and Myelin Disorders.* 3rd ed. Berlin: Springer-Verlag, 2005.

12. Hahn JS, Pohl D, Rensel M, Rao S, International Pediatric MS Study Group. Differential diagnosis and evaluation in pediatric multiple sclerosis. *Neurology* 2007;**68**(16 Suppl 2):S13–22.

13. Krupp LB, Banwell B, Tenenbaum S, International Pediatric MS Study Group. Consensus definitions proposed for pediatric multiple sclerosis and related disorders. *Neurology* 2007;**68**(16 Suppl 2):S7–12.

14. Chabas D, Ness J, Belman A, *et al.* Younger children with MS have a distinct CSF inflammatory profile at disease onset. *Neurology* 2010;**74**:399–405.

15. Banwell B, Shroff M, Ness JM, *et al.* MRI features of pediatric multiple sclerosis. *Neurology* 2007;**68** (16 Suppl 2):S46–53.

16. Callen DJ, Shroff MM, Branson HM, *et al.* MRI in the diagnosis of pediatric multiple sclerosis. *Neurology* 2009;**72**:961–967.

17. Callen DJ, Shroff MM, Branson HM, *et al.* Role of MRI in the differentiation of ADEM from MS in children. *Neurology* 2009;**72**:968–973.

18. Waubant E, Chabas D. Pediatric multiple sclerosis. *Curr Treat Options Neurol* 2009; **11**:203–210.

19. Ruggieri M, Polizzi A, Pavone L, Grimaldi LM. Multiple sclerosis in children under 6 years of age. *Neurology* 1999;**53**:478–484.

20. Ruggieri M, Iannetti P, Polizzi A, Pavone L, Grimaldi LME. Italian Society of Pediatric Neurology Study Group on Childhood Multiple Sclerosis. Multiple sclerosis in children under 10 years of age. *Neurol Sci* 2004;**25**(Suppl 4):S326–335.

21. Marrie RA, Yu N, Blanchard J, Leung S, Elliott L. The rising prevalence and changing age distribution of multiple sclerosis in Manitoba. *Neurology* 2010; **74**:465–471.

22. Hill AB. The environment and disease: Association or causation? *Proc R Soc Med* 1965;**58**:295–300.

23. Bentzen J, Flachs EM, Stenager E, Brønnum-Hansen H, Koch-Henriksenb N. Prevalence of multiple sclerosis in Denmark 1950–2005. *Multiple Sclerosis* 2010;Mar 9 [Epub ahead of print].

24. Pugliatti M, Sotgiu S, Rosati G. The worldwide prevalence of multiple sclerosis. *Clin Neurol Neurosurg* 2002;**104**:182–191.

25. Granieri, Casetta I, Govoni V, *et al.* The increasing incidence and prevalence of MS in a Sardinian province. *Neurology* 2000;**55**:842–848.

26. Lowis GW. The social epidemiology of multiple sclerosis. *Sci Total Environ* **90**:163–190.

27. Banwell B, Kennedy J, Sadovnick D, *et al.* Incidence of acquired demyelination of the CNS in Canadian children. *Neurology* 2009;**72**:232–239.

28. Torisu H, Kira R, Ishizaki Y, *et al.* Clinical study of childhood acute disseminated encephalomyelitis, multiple sclerosis, and acute transverse myelitis in Fukuoka Prefecture, Japan. *Brain Dev* 2009;Nov 24 [Epub ahead of print].

29. Chitnis T, Glanz B, Jaffin S, Healy B. Demographics of pediatric onset multiple sclerosis in an MS center population from the Northeastern United States. *Mult Scler* 2009;**15**:627–631.

30. Hader WJ, Yee IM. Incidence and prevalence of multiple sclerosis in Saskatoon, Saskatchewan. *Neurology* 2007;**69**:1224–1229.

31. Pohl D, Hennemuth I, von Kries R, Hanefeld F. Pediatric multiple sclerosis and acute disseminated encephalomyelitis in Germany: Results of a nationwide survey. *Eur J Pediatr* 2007;**166**:405–412.

32. Boiko A, Vorobeychik G, Paty D, Devonshire V, Sadovnick D, University of British Columbia MS Clinic Neurologists. Early onset multiple sclerosis: a longitudinal study. *Neurology* 2002;**159**:1006–1010.

33. Duquette P, Murray TJ, Pleines J, *et al.* Multiple sclerosis in childhood: clinical profile in 125 patients. *J Pediatr* 1987; **111**:359–363.

34. Ferreira ML, Machado MI, Dantas MJ, Moreira AJ, Souza AM. Pediatric multiple sclerosis: Analysis of clinical and epidemiological aspects according to National MS Society Consensus 2007. *Arq Neuropsiquiatr* 2008;**66**:665–670.

35. Ghezzi A, Deplano V, Faroni J, *et al.* Multiple sclerosis in childhood: Clinical features of 149 cases. *Mult Scler* 1997;**3**:43–46.

36. Govender R, Wieselthaler NA, Ndondo A, Wilmshurst JM. Acquired demyelinating disorders of childhood in the Western Cape, South Africa. *J Child Neurol* 2010;**25**:48–56.

37. Ozakbas S, Idiman E, Baklan B, Yulug B. Childhood and juvenile onset multiple sclerosis: Clinical and paraclinical features. *Brain Dev* 2003;**25**:233–236.

38. Simone IL, Carrara D, Tortorella C, *et al.* Course and prognosis in early-onset MS: Comparison with adult-onset forms. *Neurology* 2002;**59**:1922–1928.

39. Sindern E, Haas J, Stark E, Wurster U. Early onset MS under the age of 16: Clinical and paraclinical features. *Acta Neurol Scand* 1992;**86**:280–284.

40. Amato MP, Goretti B, Ghezzi A, *et al.* Cognitive and psychosocial features of childhood and juvenile MS. *Neurology* 2008;**70**:1891–1987.

41. Ghassemi R, Antel SB, Narayanan S, *et al.* Lesion distribution in children with clinically isolated syndromes. *Ann Neurol* 2008;**63**:401–405.

42. Neuteboom RF, Ketelslegers IA, Boon M, Catsman-Berrevoets CE, Hintzen RQ, Dutch Study Group on Childhood Multiple Sclerosis and Acute Disseminated Encephalomyelitis. Barkhof magnetic resonance imaging criteria predict early relapse in pediatric multiple sclerosis. *Pediatr Neurol* 2010;**42**:53–55.

43. Stark W, Huppke P, Gärtner J. Pediatric multiple sclerosis: The experience of the German Centre for Multiple Sclerosis in Childhood and Adolescence. *J Neurol* 2008;**255** (Suppl 6):119–122.

44. Banwell B, Krupp L, Kennedy J, *et al.* Clinical features and viral serologies in children with multiple sclerosis: A multinational observational study. *Lancet Neurol* 2007;**6**:773–781.

45. ISTAT. *Istituto Nazionale di Statistica*. Available at http://www.istat.it.

46. Nicoletti A, Lo Bartolo ML, Lo Fermo S, *et al.* Prevalence and incidence of multiple sclerosis in Catania, Sicily. *Neurology* 2001;**56**:62–66.

47. Nicoletti A, Patti F, Lo Fermo S, *et al.* Possible increasing risk of multiple sclerosis in Catania, Sicily. *Neurology* 2005;**65**:1259–1263.

48. Alonso A, Jick SS, Olek MJ, Hernán MA. Incidence of multiple sclerosis in the United Kingdom. Findings from a population-based cohort. *J Neurol* 2004;**254**:1736–1741.

49. Polliack ML, Barak Y, Achiron A. Late-onset multiple sclerosis. *J Am Geriatr Soc* 2000;**49**:168–171.

50. Orton SM, Herrera BM, Yee IM, *et al.* Sex ratio of multiple sclerosis in Canada: A longitudinal study. *Lancet Neurol* 2006;**5**:932–936.

51. Tintorè M, Arrambide G. Early onset multiple sclerosis: The role of gender. *J Neurol Sci* 2009;**286**: 31–34.

52. Kis B, Rumberg B, Berlit P. Clinical characteristics of patients with late-onset multiple sclerosis. *J Neurol* 2008;**255**:697–702.

53. Martinelli V, Rodegher M, Moiola L, Comi G. Late onset multiple sclerosis: Clinical characteristics, prognostic factors and differential diagnosis. *Neurol Sci* 2004;**25** (Suppl 4):S350–355.

54. Haliloglu G, Anlar B, Aysun S, *et al.* Gender prevalence in childhood multiple sclerosis and myasthenia gravis. *J Child Neurol* 2002;**17**:390–392.

55. Ghezzi A, Pozzilli C, Liguori M, *et al.* Prospective study of multiple sclerosis with early onset. *Mult Scler* 2002;**8**:115–118.

56. Cole GF, Auchterlonie LA, Best PV. Very early onset multiple sclerosis. *Dev Med Child Neurol* 1995;**37**: 667–672.

57. Giroud M, Semama D, Pradeaux L, Gouyon JB, Dumas R, Nivelon JL. Hemiballismus revealing multiple sclerosis in an infant. *Childs Nerv Syst* 1990; **6**:236–238.

58. Maeda Y, Kitamoto I, Kurokawa T, Ueda K, Hasuo K, Fujioka K. Infantile multiple sclerosis with extensive white matter lesions. *Pediatr Neurol* 1989;**5**:317–319.

59. Máttyus A, Veres E. Multiple sclerosis in childhood: Long term katamnestic investigations. *Acta Paediatr Hung* 1985;**26**:193–204.

60. Shaw CM, Alvord EC Jr. Multiple sclerosis beginning in infancy. *J Child Neurol* 1987;**2**:252–256.

61. Eraksoy M, Demir GA, Yapycy Z. Multiple sclerosis in childhood: A prospective study. *Brain Dev* 1988; **20**:427 [Abstract].

62. Hanefeld F. Multiple sclerosis in childhood. *Curr Opin Neurol Neurosurg* 1992;**5**:359–363.

63. Hanefeld F, Bauer HJ, Christen HJ, Kruse B, Bruhn H, Frahm J. Multiple sclerosis in childhood: Report of 15 cases. *Brain Dev* 1991;**13**:410–416.

64. Pinhas-Hamiel O, Barak Y, Siev-Ner I, Achiron A. Juvenile multiple sclerosis: Clinical features and prognostic characteristics. *J Pediatr* 1998;**132**: 735–737.

65. Duquette P, Girard M. Hormonal factors in susceptibility to multiple sclerosis. *Curr Opin Neurol Neurosurg* 1993;**6**:195–201.

66. Shuster EA. Hormonal influences in multiple sclerosis. *Curr Top Microbiol Immunol* 2008;**318**:267–311.

67. van den Broek HH, Damoiseaux JG, De Baets MH, Hupperts RM. The influence of sex hormones on cytokines in multiple sclerosis and experimental autoimmune encephalomyelitis: A review. *Mult Scler* 2005;**11**:349–359.

68. Cocco E, Sotgiu A, Costa G, *et al.* HLA-DR, DQ and APOE genotypes and gender influence in Sardinian primary progressive MS. *Neurology* 2005;**64**:564–566.

69. Galimberti D, Scalabrini D, Fenoglio C, *et al.* Gender-specific influence of the chromosome 16 chemokine gene cluster on the susceptibility to multiple sclerosis. *J Neurol Sci* 2008;**267**:86–90.

70. Weinstock-Guttman B, Jacobs LD, Brownscheidle CM, *et al.* Multiple sclerosis characteristics in African American patients in the New York State Multiple Sclerosis Consortium. *Mult Scler* 2003,**9**:293–298.

71. Boutin B, Esquivel E, Mayer M, Chaumet S, Ponsot G, Arthuis M. Multiple sclerosis in children: Report of clinical and paraclinical features of 19 cases. *Neuropediatrics* 1987;**19**:118–123.

72. Selcen D, Banu Anlar B, Renda Y. Multiple sclerosis in childhood: Report of 16 cases. *Eur Neurol* 1996; **36**:79–84.

73. Mikaeloff Y, Caridade G, Assi S, Suissa S, Tardieu M. Prognostic factors for early severity in a childhood multiple sclerosis cohort. *Pediatrics* 2006;**118**: 1133–1139.

74. Renoux C, Vukusic S, Mikaeloff Y, *et al.* Natural history of multiple sclerosis with childhood onset. *N Engl J Med* 2007;**356**:2603–2613.

75. Leake JAD, Albani S, Kao AS, Senac MO, Billman GF, Nesepca MP. Acute disseminated encephalomyelitis in childhood: Epidemiologic, clinical and laboratory features. *Pediatr Infect Dis J* 2004;**23**:756–764.

76. Pavone P, Pettoello-Mantovano M, Le Pira A, *et al.* Acute disseminated encephalomyelitis. A long-term prospective study of 17 pediatric patients with systematic review of 750 cases and meta-analysis of 492/750 cases in the literature. *Neuropediatrics* 2010 (in press).

77. Mikaeloff Y, Suissa S, Vallée L, *et al.* First episode of acute CNS inflammatory demyelination in childhood: Prognostic factors for multiple sclerosis and disability. *J Pediatr* 2004;**144**:246–252.

78. Sadovnick AD, Armstrong H, Rice GP, *et al.* A population-based study of multiple sclerosis in twins: Update. *Ann Neurol* 1993;**33**:281–285.

79. Sadovnick AD. Multiple sclerosis and other demyelinating disorders. In *Emery and Rimoin's Principles and Practice of Medical Genetics*. 4th ed, eds. D Rimoin, JM Condor, RE Pyeritz, BR Korf. London: Churchill Livingstone; 2002:3203–3208.

80. Sadovnick AD. The genetics and genetic epidemiology of multiple sclerosis: The "hard facts". *Adv Neurol* 2006;**98**:17–25.

81. Deryck O, Ketelaer P, Dubois B. Clinical characteristics and long term prognosis in early onset multiple sclerosis. *J Neurol* 2006;**253**:720–723.

82. Pohl D. Epidemiology, immunopathogenesis and management of pediatric central nervous system inflammatory demyelinating conditions. *Curr Opin Neurol* 2008;**21**:366–372.

83. al Rajeh S, Bademosi O, Ismail H, *et al.* A community survey of neurological disorders in Saudi Arabia: The Thugbah study. *Neuroepidemiology* 1993;**12**:164–178.

84. Cree BA, Khan O, Bourdette D, *et al.* Clinical characteristics of African Americans vs Caucasian Americans with multiple sclerosis. *Neurology* 2004;**63**:2039–2045.

85. Karni A, Kahana E, Zilber N, Abramsky O, Alter M, Karussis D. The frequency of multiple sclerosis in Jewish and Arab populations in greater Jerusalem. *Neuroepidemiology* 2003;**22**:82–86.

86. Shibasaki H, McDonald WI, Kuroiwa Y. Racial modification of clinical picture of multiple sclerosis: Comparison between British and Japanese patients. *J Neurol Sci* 1981;**49**:253–271.

87. Kurtzke JF, Beebe GW, Norman JE Jr. Epidemiology of multiple sclerosis in U.S. veterans: 1. Race, sex, and geographic distribution. *Neurology* 1979;**29**:1228–1235.

88. Kennedy J, O'Connor P, Sadovnick AD, Perara M, Yee I, Banwell B. Age at onset of multiple sclerosis may be influenced by place of residence during childhood rather than ancestry. *Neuroepidemiology* 2006;**26**:162–167.

89. Boster AL, Endress CF, Hreha SA, Caon C, Perumal JS, Khan OA. Pediatric-onset multiple sclerosis in African-American black and European-origin white patients. *Pediatr Neurol* 2009;**40**:31–33.

90. Krupp L, McLinskey N, Troell R. Racial and ethnic findings in pediatric MS: an update. *Neurology* 2008;**70**(Suppl1):A135 [Abstract].

91. Kaufman MD, Johnson SK, Moyer D, Bivens J, Norton HJ. Multiple sclerosis: Severity and progression rate in African Americans compared with whites. *Am J Phys Med Rehabil* 2003;**82**:582–590.

92. Alter M, Leibowitz U, Speer J. Risk of multiple sclerosis related to age at immigration to Israel. *Arch Neurol* 1966;**15**:234–237.

93. Dean G, Kurtzke JF. On the risk of multiple sclerosis according to age at immigration to South Africa. *Br Med J* 1971;**3**:725–729.

94. Kurtzke JF, Beebe GW, Norman JE Jr. Epidemiology of multiple sclerosis in US veterans: III. Migration and the risk of MS. *Neurology* 1985;**35**:672–678.

95. Dean G, Elian M. Age at immigration to England of Asian and Caribbean immigrants and the risk of developing multiple sclerosis. *J Neurol Neurosurg Psychiatry* 1997;**63**:565–568.

96. Cabre P, Signate A, Olindo S, *et al.* Role of return migration in the emergence of multiple sclerosis in the French West Indies. *Brain* 2005;**128**:2899–2910.

97. Hammond SR, English DR, McLeod JG. The age-range of risk of developing multiple sclerosis. Evidence from a migrant population in Australia. *Brain* 2000;**123**:968–974.

98. Rodríguez-Violante M, Ordoñez G, Bermudez JR, Sotelo J, Corona T. Association of a history of varicella virus infection with multiple sclerosis. *Clin Neurol Neurosurg* 2009;**111**:54–56.

99. Haahr S, Moller-Larsen A, Pedersen E. Immunological parameters in multiple sclerosis patients with special reference to the herpes virus group. *Clin Exp Immunol* 1983;**51**:197–206.

100. Sanders V, Felisan S, Waddell A, Tourtellotte W. Detection of herpesviridae in postmortem multiple sclerosis brain tissue and controls by polimerase chain reaction. *J Neurovirol* 1996;**2**:249–258.

101. Alvarez-Lafuente R, Martin-Estefania C, De las Heras V, *et al.* Prevalence of herpes virus DNA in MS patients and healthy blood donors. *Acta Neurol Scand* 2002;**105**:95–99.

102. Al-Shammari S, Nelson R, Voevodin A. HHV-6 DNAemia in patients with multiple sclerosis in Kuwait. *Acta Neurol Scand* 2003;**107**:122–124.

103. Alvarez-La Fuente R, García-Montojo M, De la Heras V, Bartolome M, Arroyo R. Clinical parameters and HHV-6 active replication in relapsing–remitting multiple sclerosis patients. *J Clin Virol* 2006;**37** (Suppl 1):S24–26.

104. Alvarez-La Fuente R, De las Heras V, Bartolome M, García-Montojo M, Arroyo R. Human herpesvirus 6 and multiple sclerosis: A one-year follow-up study. *Brain Pathol* 2006;**16**:20–27.

105. Ross R. The varicella zoster virus and multiple sclerosis. *J Clin Epidemiol* 1998;**51**:533–535.

106. Ross R, Nicolle L, Dawood MR, Cheang M, Feschuk C. Varicella zoster antibodies after herpes zoster, varicella and multiple sclerosis. *Can J Neurol Sci* 1997;**24**:137–139.

107. Ross R, Nicolle L, Cheang M. The varicella zoster virus: A pilot trial of a potential therapeutic agent in multiple sclerosis. *J Clin Epidemiol* 1997;**50**:63–68.

108. Ross RT, Cheang M, Landry G, Klassen L, Doerksen K. Herpes zoster and multiple sclerosis. *Can J Neurol Sci* 1999;**26**:29–32.

109. Haahr S, Plesner A, Vestergaard B, Hollsberg P. A role of late Epstein Barr virus infection in multiple sclerosis. *Acta Neurol Scand* 2004;**109**:270–275.

110. Höllsberg P, Kusk M, Bech E, Hansen HJ, Jakobsen J, Haahr S. Presence of Epstein–Barr virus and Human herpesvirus 6B DNA in multiple sclerosis patients: Associations with disease activity. *Acta Neurol Scand* 2005;**112**:395–402.

111. Haahr S, Höllsberg P. Multiple sclerosis is linked to Epstein–Barr virus infection. *Rev Med Virol* 2006;**16**:297–310.

112. Ross RT, Nicolle LE, Cheang M. Varicella zoster virus and multiple sclerosis in a Hutterite population. *J Clin Epidemiol* 1995;**48**:1319–1324.

113. Perez-Cesari C, Saniger MM, Sotelo J. Frequent association of multiple sclerosis with varicella and zoster. *Acta Neurol Scand* 2005;**112**:417–419.

114. Sotelo J, Ordoñez G, Pineda B. Varicella-zoster virus at relapses of multiple sclerosis. *J Neurol* 2007;**254**: 493–500.

115. Ordoñez G, Pineda B, Garcia-Navarrete R, Sotelo J. Brief presence of varicella-zoster viral DNA in mononuclear cells during relapses of multiple sclerosis. *Arch Neurol* 2004;**61**:529–532.

116. Tarrats R, Ordoñez G, Rios C, Sotelo J. Varicella, ephemeral breastfeeding and eczema as risk factors for multiple sclerosis in Mexicans. *Acta Neurol Scand* 2002;**105**:88–94.

117. Marrie RA, Wolfson C. Multiple sclerosis and varicella zoster virus infection: A review. *Epidemiol Infect* 2001;**127**:315–325.

118. Levin LI, Munger KL, Rubertone MV, *et al.* Multiple sclerosis and Epstein–Barr virus. *JAMA* 2003;**289**:1533–1536.

119. Thacker EL, Mirzaei F, Ascherio A. Infectious mononucleosis and risk for multiple sclerosis: A meta-analysis. *Ann Neurol* 2006;**59**:499–503.

120. Alotaibi S, Kennedy J, Tellier R, Stephens D, Banwell B. Epstein–Barr virus in pediatric multiple sclerosis. *JAMA* 2004;**291**:1875–1879.

121. Pohl D. Epstein–Barr virus and multiple sclerosis. *J Neurol Sci* 2009;**286**:62–64.

122. Bagert BA. Epstein–Barr virus in multiple sclerosis. *Curr Neurol Neurosci Rep* 2009,**9**:405–410.

123. Ascherio A, Munger KL. Epstein–Barr virus infection and multiple sclerosis: A review. *J Neuroimmune Pharmacol* 2010;Apr 6 [Epub ahead of print].

124. Jenson HB. Epstein–Barr virus. In: *Nelson's Textbook of Pediatrics*. 18th ed. eds. RM Kliegman, RE Behrman, HB Jenson, BF Stanton. Philadelphia, PA: Saunders/ Elsevier; 2008: 1372–1377.

125. Lünemann JD, Huppke P, Roberts S, Brück W, Gärtner J, Münz C. Broadened and elevated humoral immune response to EBNA1 in pediatric multiple sclerosis. *Neurology* 2008;**71**:1033–1035.

126. Jaquiéry E, Jilek S, Schluep M, *et al.* Intrathecal immune responses to EBV in early MS. *Eur J Immunol* 2010;**40**:878–887.

127. Peferoen LA, Lamers F, Lodder LN, *et al.* Epstein Barr virus is not a characteristic feature in the central nervous system in established multiple sclerosis. *Brain* 2009;**132**:3318–3328.

128. Franciotta D, Bestetti A, Sala S, *et al.* Broad screening for human herpesviridae DNA in multiple sclerosis cerebrospinal fluid and serum. *Acta Neurol Belg* 2009;**109**:277–282.

129. Sargsyan SA, Shearer AJ, Ritchie AM, *et al.* Absence of Epstein–Barr virus in the brain and CSF of patients with multiple sclerosis. *Neurology* 2010;**74**:1127–1135.

130. Ramagopalan SV, Valdar W, Dyment DA, *et al.* Association of infectious mononucleosis with multiple sclerosis. A population-based study. *Neuroepidemiology* 2009;**32**:257–262.

131. Pohl D, Krone B, Rostasy K, *et al.* High seroprevalence of Epstein–Barr virus in children with multiple sclerosis. *Neurology* 2006;**67**:2063–2065.

132. Pohl D, Rostasy K, Jacobi C, *et al.* Intrathecal antibody production against Epstein–Barr and other neurotropic viruses in pediatric and adult onset multiple sclerosis. *J Neurol* 2010;**257**:212–216.

133. Mikaeloff Y, Caridade G, Suissa S, Tardieu M, KIDSEP Study Group. Clinically observed chickenpox and the risk of childhood-onset multiple sclerosis. *Am J Epidemiol* 2009;**169**:1260–1266.

134. Denne C, Kleines M, Dieckhöfer A, *et al.* Intrathecal synthesis of anti-viral antibodies in pediatric patients. *Eur J Paediatr Neurol* 2007;**11**:29–34.

135. Contini C, Seraceni S, Cultrera R, Castellazzi M, Granieri E, Fainardi E. *Chlamydophila pneumoniae* infection and its role in neurological disorders. *Interdiscip Perspect Infect Dis* 2010;**2010**:273573. Epub 2010 Feb 21.

136. MacIntyre A, Abramov R, Hammond CJ, *et al.* *Chlamydia pneumoniae* infection promotes the transmigration of monocytes through human brain endothelial cells. *J Neurosci Res* 2003;**71**: 740–750.

137. Rostasy K, Reiber H, Pohl D, *et al. Chlamydia pneumoniae* in children with MS: Frequency and quantity of intrathecal antibodies. *Neurology* 2003; **61**:125–128.

138. Krone B, Pohl D, Rostasy K, *et al.* Common infectious agents in multiple sclerosis: A case-control study in children. *Mult Scler* 2008;**14**:136–139.

139. Pohl D, Rostasy K, Gieffers J, Maass M, Hanefeld F. Recurrent optic neuritis associated with *Chlamydia pneumoniae* infection of the central nervous system. *Dev Med Child Neurol* 2006;**48**:770–772.

140. Hernán MA, Jick SS. Hepatitis B vaccination and multiple sclerosis: The jury is still out. *Pharmacoepidemiol Drug Saf* 2006;**15**:653–655.

141. Balinska MA. Hepatitis B vaccination and French Society ten years after the suspension of the vaccination campaign: How should we raise infant immunization coverage rates? *J Clin Virol* 2009;**46**:202–205.

142. Braillon A, Dubois G. Hepatitis B vaccine and the risk of CNS inflammatory demyelination in childhood. *Neurology* **2009**;72:2053.

143. Lièvre M, Members of Epidemiology Working Group of French Pharmacovigilance Commission, Costagliola D, *et al.* Hepatitis B vaccine and the risk of CNS inflammatory demyelination in childhood. *Neurology* 2009;**73**:1426–1427.

144. Ness J, Bale JF Jr. Hepatitis vaccines and pediatric multiple sclerosis: Does timing or type matter? *Neurology* 2009;**72**:870–871.

145. Zipp F, Weil JG, Einhaupl KM. No increase in demyelinating diseases after hepatitis B vaccination. *Nat Med* 1999;**5**:964–965.

146. Sadovnick AD, Scheifele DW. School-based hepatitis B vaccination programme and adolescent multiple sclerosis. *Lancet* 2000;**355**:549–550.

147. Ascherio A, Zhang SM, Hernan MA, *et al.* Hepatitis B vaccination and the risk of multiple sclerosis. *N Engl J Med* 2001;**344**:327–332.

148. DeStefano F, Verstraeten T, Jackson LA, *et al.* Vaccinations and risk of central nervous system demyelinating diseases in adults. *Arch Neurol* 2003;**60**:504–509.

149. DeStefano F, Weintraub ES, Chen RT. Recombinant hepatitis B vaccine and the risk of multiple sclerosis: A prospective study. *Neurology* 2005;**64**:1317.

150. Touzé E, Gout O, Verdier-Taillefer MH, Lyon-Caen O, Alpérovitch A. The first episode of central nervous system demyelinization and hepatitis B vaccination. *Rev Neurol (Paris)* 2000;**156**:242–246.

151. Touzé E, Fourrier A, Rue-Fenouche C, *et al.* Hepatitis B vaccination and first central nervous system demyelinating event: A case-control study. *Neuroepidemiology* 2002;**21**:180–186.

152. Sturkenboom M, Abenhaim L, Wolfson C, Roullet E, Heinzlef O, Gout O. Vaccinations, demyelination and multiple sclerosis study (VDAMS): A population-based study in the UK. *Pharmacoepidemiol Drug Saf* 1999;**8**(Suppl 2):S170–S171.

153. Hernán MA, Jick SS, Olek MJ, Jick H. Recombinant hepatitis B vaccine and the risk of multiple sclerosis: A prospective study. *Neurology* 2004;**63**:838–842.

154. Mikaeloff Y, Caridade G, Rossier M, Suissa S, Tardieu M. Hepatitis B vaccination and the risk of childhood-onset multiple sclerosis. *Arch Pediatr Adolesc Med* 2007;**161**:1176–1182.

155. Mikaeloff Y, Caridade G, Assi S, Tardieu M, Suissa S, KIDSEP study group of the French Neuropediatric Society. Hepatitis B vaccine and risk of relapse after a first childhood episode of CNS inflammatory demyelination. *Brain* 2007;**130**: 1105–1110.

156. Mikaeloff Y, Caridade G, Suissa S, Tardieu M. Hepatitis B vaccine and the risk of CNS inflammatory demyelination in childhood. *Neurology* 2009;**72**: 873–880.

157. Antonovsky A, Leibowitz U, Smith HA, *et al.* Epidemiologic study of multiple sclerosis in Israel. An overall review of methods and findings. *Arch Neurol* 1965;**13**:183–193.

158. Villard-Mackintosh L, Vessey MP. Oral contraceptives and reproductive factors in multiple sclerosis incidence. *Contraception* 1993;**47**:161–168.

159. Thorogood M, Hannaford PC. The influence of oral contraceptives on the risk of multiple sclerosis. *Br J Obstet Gynaecol* 1998;**105**:1296–1299.

160. Hernán MA, Olek MJ, Ascherio A. Cigarette smoking and incidence of multiple sclerosis. *Am J Epidemiol* 2001;**154**:69–74.

161. Riise T, Norvtvedt MW, Ascherio A. Smoking is a risk factor for multiple sclerosis. *Neurology* 2003;**61**: 1122–1124.

162. Hedstrom AK, Baarnhielm M, Olsson T, Alfredsson L. Tobacco smoking, but not Swedish snuff use, increases the risk of multiple sclerosis. *Neurology* 2009;**73**: 696–701.

163. Zivadinov R, Weinstock-Guttman B, Hashmi K, *et al.* Smoking is associated with increased lesion volumes and brain atrophy in multiple sclerosis. *Neurology* 2009;**73**:504–510.

164. Healy BC, Ali EN, Guttmann CRG, *et al.* Smoking and disease progression in multiple sclerosis. *Arch Neurol* 2009;**66**:858–864.

165. Safari N, Hoppenbrouwers IA, Hop WC, Breteler MM, Hintzen RQ. Cigarette smoking and risk of MS in multiplex families. *Mult Scl* 2009;**15**:1363–1367.

166. Mikaeloff Y, Caridade G, Tardieu M, Suissa S, KIDSEP study group. Parental smoking at home and the risk of childhood-onset multiple sclerosis in children. *Brain* 2007;**130**:2589–2595.

167. Hans FJ, Wei L, Bereczki D, *et al.* Nicotine increases microvascular blood flow and flow velocity in three groups of brain areas. *Am J Physiol* 1993;**265**:H2142–2150.

168. Smith ADM, Duckett S, Waters AH. Neuropathological changes in chronic cyanide intoxication. *Nature* 1963; **200**:179–181.

169. Bass NH. Pathogenesis of myelin lesions in experimental cyanide encephalopathy. *Neurology* 1968;**18**:167–177.

170. Avanzini MA, Ricci A, Scaramuzza C, *et al.* Deficiency of INFgamma producing cells in adenoids of children exposed to passive smoke. *Int J Immunopathol Pharmacol* 2006;**19**:609–616.

171. Munger KL, Chitnis T, Ascherio A. Body size and risk of MS in two cohorts of US women. *Neurology* 2009;**73**:1543–1550.

Clinical presentation of multiple sclerosis in children

Angelo Ghezzi and Brenda Banwell

The clinical manifestations of multiple sclerosis (MS) in children have many similarities to the relapsing–remitting symptoms described in adult-onset patients [1], but with important distinctions specific to the pediatric population. The onset of MS during childhood impacts not only established white matter and neuronal pathways, but may also negatively impact developing neural networks. The onset of MS in childhood always occurs during the period of primary acquisition of the academic substrates essential for higher-order learning, with a major concern for future academic achievement.

An essential aspect of the care of children with MS is recognition of their symptoms, coupled with appropriate investigations to ensure an accurate diagnosis and to exclude other disorders in the differential. The relative rarity of MS in children often leads to clinical uncertainty, especially amongst primary care pediatric health care providers who may never have encountered a child with demyelination, and may believe that MS is a disease exclusive to adults.

The present chapter will articulate the clinical manifestations of MS in children, review the available literature, and propose concepts for future study of the clinical manifestations of MS in children.

Methodological aspects

Defining the clinical features of MS in children is challenged by the variability of the available literature with respect to (i) consistency in the definition of clinical features and diagnostic criteria for pediatric MS; (ii) age of inclusion; (iii) duration of clinical observation, a key issue in recognizing features that may not be present at onset or may change during the course of MS in children; and (iv) definition of disease onset.

Classification of clinical features

Clinical findings of pediatric MS have been described in more than 30 single or multicenter studies from different geographic areas, including approximately 1500 children. Only 11 manuscripts [2–13] include more than 50 children with MS. Important in the review of the available data is to consider whether the study was performed in the context of a pediatric health care facility, in a dedicated pediatric MS program, or in an adult MS program. The clinical care context is influenced by referral bias, and by areas of expertise. It is likely that younger MS patients receive care in pediatric facilities, while adolescents are more likely to be referred to an established adult MS program. Few formal pediatric MS clinics exist, and serve as regional or even national resources. Table 4.1 [2–34] lists the publications reviewed for the present chapter. Only studies describing 10 or more children were included.

Further challenging the ability to accurately capture the breadth and specific features of MS in children are the inherent limitations of retrospective extraction of data from medical records. Furthermore, some studies list individual "symptoms", such as vertigo, diplopia, tremor; while others have utilized a "regional involvement" model, and would have grouped the presenting features as "brainstem or infratentorial". Thus, determination of the frequency of MS symptoms is very challenging.

Age

Controversy remains in the definition of the upper age of inclusion in pediatric MS series. The recommendations of the recently proposed International Pediatric Multiple Sclerosis Study Group (IPMSSG) is to include patients presenting with an initial central nervous system (CNS) demyelinating event prior to

Demyelinating Disorders of the Central Nervous System in Childhood, ed. Dorothée Chabas and Emmanuelle L. Waubant. Published by Cambridge University Press. © Cambridge University Press 2011.

Table 4.1 Literature review: pediatric multiple sclerosis

Author	Country, site	Setting Pediatric (P)/ Adult (A)	*n*	Mean age at onset	Retrospective (R)/ Prospective (P)	Mean Observation (yrs)	PPMS (%)	SPMS (%)
Atzori, 2009 [14]	Italy	(A) & (P)	48	14.4	R	–	–	–
Banwell, 2007 [2]	Multinational	(P)	137	11.0	R	3.1	0	4
Belopitova, 2001 [15]	Bulgaria, single center	(P)	10	11.1	P	NR	0	10
Boiko, 2002 [3]	Canada, single center	(A)	116	12.7	R	19.8	3	53
Boster, [16]	US, multicenter	(P) & (A)	43	13.6	R	About 3.3	–	–
Boutin, 1988 [17]	France, single center	(P)	19	11.0	R	variable	3	NR
Chiemchanya, 1993 [18]	Thailand	(P)	17		R	6.5	0	NR
Cole, 1995 [19]	Scotland, single center	(A)	28	11.5	R	3–47	4	10
Dale, 2000 [20]	UK, single center	(P)	13	9.4	R	5.6	0	0
Deryck, 2006 [21]	Belgium, single center	(A)	49	14.3	R	20.8	1	43
Duquette, 1987 [4]	Canada, multicenter	(A)	125	13	R	15	28	22
Ferriera, 2008 [22]	Brazil	(A)	31	11.7	R	14.2	3.2	13
Gal, 1958 [23]	USA, single center	(P)	40	11.7	R	NR	0	NR
Ghezzi, 1997 [5]	Italy, multicenter	(A)	149	12.6	R	14.2	7	29
Ghezzi, 2002 [6]	Italy, multicenter	(A)	54	12.7	P	10.9	0	28
Gorman, 2009 [24]	US, single center	(P)	21	15.0	R	3.7	0	0
Guilhoto, 1995 [25]	Brazil, single center	(P)	14	8.6	R	NR	0	0
Gusev, 2002 [7]	Russia/ Canada, 2 center comparison	(A/P)	67	11.7	R	4.9	0	11

Table 4.1 (cont.)

Author	Country, site	Setting Pediatric (P)/ Adult (A)	n	Mean age at onset	Retrospective (R)/ Prospective (P)	Mean Observation (yrs)	PPMS (%)	SPMS (%)
Hanefeld, 1991 [26]	Germany, single center	(P)	15	8.9	P	NR	4	NR
Mikaeloff, 2004 [8]	France, multicenter	(P)	116		P	4.9	0	
Mikaeloff, 2004 [9]	France, multicenter	(P)	168	12.0	P	2.9	1	5
Mikaeloff, 2006 [10]	France, multicenter	(P)	197		P	5.5	0	5
Neuteboom, 2008 [27]	Netherlands, multicenter	(P)	31[a]	8.9[b] 14.5[c]	R	need	0	0
Ozakbas, 2003 [28]	Turkey, single center	(A)	32	12.9	R	7.4	0	31
Pinhas-Hamiel, 1998 [29]	Israel, single center	(A)	13	18.5	R	NR	NR	NR
Renoux, 2007 [11]	France, multicenter	P	394	13,7	R-P	17.1	2.3	
Ruggieri, 2004 [30]	Italy (preliminary)	(P)	31		R	NR	0	NR
Selcen, 1996 [31]	Turkey, single center	(P)	16	11.4	R	NR	0	6%
Shiraishi, 2005 [32]	Japan	(P)	27	11.7	R	13.5	0	7%
Simone, 2002 [12]	Italy, single center	(A)	83	14.3	R	5.3	0	15
Sindern, 1992 [33]	Germany, single center	(A)	31	13.5	R	11.4	3	61
Trojano, 2004 [13]	Italy, multicenter	(A)	90		P	NR	0	1
Weng, 2006 [34]	Taiwan, single center	(P)	21	12.4	R	6.8	0	14

Note:
[a] In this study, patients were divided into those under age 10 years[b], and those > 11 years[c] at first attack.

age 17 years 11 months [35]. However, many studies restrict inclusion to children under the age of 16 years [2–12], and one study included patients up to the age of 21 years [29]. It is also important to clarify whether the age of inclusion refers to the age at first attack (clinical onset of MS), rather than the age at which MS was diagnosed based on clinical or MRI evidence of a second demyelinating event. While some studies have used the age at which a child was formally diagnosed with MS (rather than the age at which the second event occurred), this date reflects access to medical services rather than biological disease activity. Age at first attack also influences the clinical presentation, as discussed below.

Duration of observation

Prolonged observation and a prospective clinical care model is important for recognition of the evolution of clinical symptoms that develop over time, and provides an important view of long-term clinical outcome. Prospective observation also permits an accurate determination of the frequency of relapses over time. As has been shown in studies of adult MS, patient recall of relapses is an important factor in determination of relapse frequency [36], and for recognition of the tendency of relapse rate to decline over time. Insufficient clinical observation leads to inflation of annualized relapse rate, which has contributed to the highly variable annualized relapse rates quoted for pediatric MS.

Definition of disease onset

Descriptions of pediatric MS also differ with respect to definition of "disease onset". It can be defined by the first demyelinating event (also termed acquired or acute demyelinating syndrome (ADS) or initial demyelinating episode or event (IDE) in children; and clinically isolated syndrome (CIS) in adults), or by the second attack (first relapse). This is an important difference. If one considers the first demyelinating event to represent the clinical onset of MS, then descriptions of clinical manifestations will invariably permit inclusion of younger children. As discussed below, younger children have a greater likelihood of manifesting with polyfocal deficits and encephalopathy features that also define acute disseminated encephalomyelitis (ADEM). In contrast, if one describes the clinical features at the time of a second demyelinating event (or first relapse), the majority of children will be 10 years of age or older, and clinical manifestations are more likely to more closely resemble those of adult-onset MS.

Clinical features

Relapse-related symptoms

The findings at presentation of the most recent studies, and with large cohorts of patients, are summarized in Table 4.2. As mentioned above, brainstem and cerebellar symptoms are grouped together by some authors,

and some authors group motor and sensory disturbances together as "long tract dysfunction" [8–11].

Optic neuritis (ON) and diplopia more frequently occur in a monosymptomatic presentation. Optic neuritis associated with clinically silent white matter lesions in the brain is associated with a 68% chance of MS final diagnosis (defined by a second demyelinating event) within 2 years [37].

Motor and sensory disturbances often co-exist, and in some patients are due to a single large intracerebral lesion. Transverse myelitis occurs frequently in the context of an ADEM-like onset [2,11]. Isolated transverse myelitis is rarely the first presentation of MS [38].

Overall, 5–65% of children experience motor and sensory dysfunction as initial symptoms, 13–40% present with brainstem involvement, 3–20% have cerebellar symptoms (16–48% with brainstem–cerebellar dysfunction), and 12–37% have ON at onset. Urinary symptoms are rare (1–9% of cases). In a manuscript detailing the clinical features of 621 children, pooled from 13 studies, 42% of subjects had motor-sensory disturbances, 19% had brainstem involvement, 7% cerebellar symptoms, 19% presented ON, and 12% other symptoms, alone or in association [39].

Due to the lack of a standardized definition and classification of clinical symptoms at onset, and to the wide range of their frequency in children, it is not easy to compare these findings with those of adult MS. In studies that compared the frequency of symptoms of children with adults, brainstem dysfunction and ON occur more frequently in pediatric MS patients, while dysfunction of long tracts or motor-sensory disturbances are more common in adults [3,5,11,12]. Similar findings have been documented in a more recent study comparing pediatric and adult-onset MS patients cared for in a dedicated MS program, although differences in clinical features did not reach statistical significance [24]. MRI studies have also shown a proclivity for brainstem lesions in pediatric patients when compared to adult MS patients [40,41].

Seizures occur in about 5% of children, but are almost exclusively represented by children who are under 10 years of age [30].

Perhaps the most challenging clinical situation is represented by those children who present with an ADEM-like first attack, characterized by multiple clinical features localized to multiple areas of the CNS accompanied by encephalopathy, and often associated with headache, somnolence, lethargy, and meningism [35]. Approximately 18% of children with an

Table 4.2 The relative representation (%) of clinical features at onset in children with MS

	Banwell [2] N = 137	Boiko [3] N = 116	Deryck [21] N = 49	Gusev [7] Boys 29	Gusev [7] Girls 38	Ghezzi [5] retrospective N = 149	Ghezzi [6] (*) prospective N = 54	Mikaeloff [10] (*) N = 197	Renoux [11] N = 394	Simone [12] N = 83
Brainstem	18	12.9	28.6	41.4	13.2	25	27.7 (42.6)	24.3 (37)	16.8	40.9
Cerebellar		6.9		6.9	2.6	9	13.2 (20.4)			
Pyramidal	30	10.3	18.4	6.9	5.3	17.5	27.7 (42.6)	31.7 (65)	37.8	36.1
Sensory	30	25.9	6.1	10.3	28.9	18.3	16.8 (25.9)			18.1
Transverse myelitis								3.5 (7)		
Optic neuritis	22	21.6	14.3	27.6	36.8	16.5	12.0 (18.5)	16.6 (34)	23.4	23
Gait difficulty	NR	9.4	12.2							
Cognitive	NR							7.4 (15)		7.2
Sphincter	NR	0.9					2.4 (4)			8.4
Polyfocal	43	12.1	14.3	6.9	13.2		43	46	Other combinations 22.1	

Note:
(*)in brackets: occurrence in both mono/polysymptomatic presentations/number of subjects: it explains why the sum of percentages is >100.

ADEM-like first attack will experience relapsing disease [42], although the frequency of MS diagnosis in children with an initial ADEM-like demyelinating event is variable. In one large series of 84 children with ADEM, none were diagnosed with MS after a median period of observation of 6.6 years [43], while other studies have documented a diagnosis of MS in only one of 12 children initially diagnosed with ADEM [44]. In a prospective study, Mikaeloff *et al.* included 296 children and adolescents with an acute demyelinating event: 81 presented with focal involvement, 119 with ADEM, and 96 with symptoms highly suggestive of MS [8]. After a mean period of observation of 2.3 years, a second episode suggestive of MS occurred in 38 of 81 subjects with focal involvement (47%) and in 34 of 119 with an initial diagnosis of ADEM (29%).

Further challenging the clinician is the definition of "encephalopathy" – proposed as an absolute criterion for the diagnosis of ADEM [35] (see also Chapter 2). While the conventional definition of encephalopathy includes "impairment of consciousness or alertness unrelated to medication or recent seizure, or profound irritability", these terms are subjective. Ill children with fever are typically irritable, but may be alert or drowsy without necessarily having an impaired level of consciousness. Parents may describe their child as behaving differently from normal, but this may not be of sufficient severity as to characterize the child as encephalopathic. Even MRI studies are currently unable to reliably differentiate "true" ADEM (defined as a self-limited illness characterized by polyfocal clinical deficits, encephalopathy, typically associated with widespread lesions involving both gray and white matter) from an ADEM-like first attack of MS, although some MRI features are more typical of MS (well-defined lesions, lesions perpendicular to the long axis of the corpus callosum, and hypointense lesions on T1-weighted images – termed black holes) [45], while other features are more characteristic of monophasic ADEM (diffuse bilateral lesions, <2 periventricular lesions, and the absence of black holes) [46] (see also Chapters 5 and 18). Only careful clinical and MRI detection of new lesions reliably distinguishes children with MS from those with monophasic ADEM.

Age-related influences on clinical presentation and relapses

Clinical features at onset of the disease are influenced by age. Ataxia, encephalopathy, and fever are relatively frequent symptoms in children with disease onset prior to age 10 years, as shown in Figure 4.1. Seizures and cognitive impairment are also frequent symptoms in younger patients [30]. Polyfocal features are even more notable in children who experience the onset of MS under the age of six years (reviewed in [30,47]. Adolescents are more likely to experience monofocal features at the onset of MS. A monofocal presentation was found to be more common in European than in North/South American children, even adjusting for age at presentation [2].

The onset of MS prior to the age of 24 months is extremely rare (3 boys and 2 girls) [30] (see also Chapter 3). Symptoms in these children were predominantly motor, and were associated with encephalopathy in two children. Recovery was complete in four of the children, and the interval from the initial to second attack varied from 1 to 20 months. Three children presented seizures during the course of the disease. The importance of consideration of the differential diagnosis in the very young is highlighted by an early report of MS in a 24-month-old girl, that upon careful review is more likely to have been manifesting with pediatric Acquired Immunodeficiency Syndrome [48].

MRI studies in very young pediatric MS patients also support a predilection for widespread, large lesions with ill-defined lesion borders in children with MS onset prior to age 10 years [41,49], raising the possibility that more localized lesions and more focal clinical manifestations may be more likely with increasing CNS or immunological maturity (see also Chapter 5).

The time from acute first presentation to a second episode is quite variable, ranging from 7.5 months [2] to 71 months [3]. Mean intervals of 15 [10], 25 [6], 40 [7], and 60 [11] months have been reported. The median value was given in some papers, and varied from 8 [10] to 36 [12] months. The interval is longer in children with a first attack under age 10 years. [10,11].

Chronic symptoms

Cognitive impairment, distinct from transient encephalopathy, has been reported rarely as a feature detectable at the time of the first MS attack, with a negative prognostic effect [10]. The development of cognitive impairment during the course of childhood MS is more likely in subjects with a younger age of onset [50], although insufficient data exist to determine whether the risk for cognitive impairment increases over time as

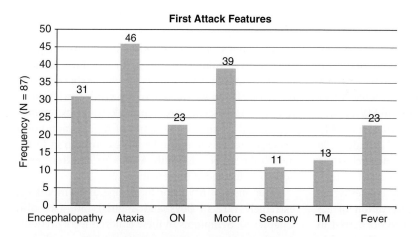

First Attack Features

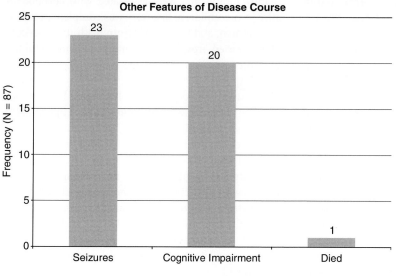

Other Features of Disease Course

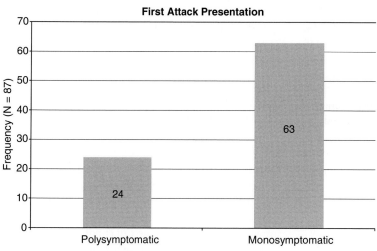

First Attack Presentation

Figure 4.1 Clinical features and outcome of MS with onset under age 10 years. These figures illustrate the frequency of disease features in 87 reported pediatric multiple sclerosis patients [46]. All children manifested with their first attack prior to age 10 years (mean 6.1; median 6.3 years). The female to male ratio was 1:23. Thirty-seven children presented under the age of 6 years. At second attack, the mean (median) age was 7.2 (7.1) years and 100% of patients followed an initial relapsing remitting multiple sclerosis disease course [47]. ON, optic neuritis; TM, transverse myelitis.

pediatric-onset MS patients mature into adulthood. Impairment of executive functions, processing speed, working memory, and low functioning in activities related to school performances have been described in children with MS, as well as deficit of attention, language [51,52], with a negative impact on academic and social activities. The impact of MS on cognition is detailed in Chapter 13.

Fatigue is a common symptom of MS, with a negative impact on disability. The occurrence of fatigue in pediatric MS has not been sufficiently investigated, and is challenged by the absence of a pediatric-specific fatigue rating scale. The fatigue measures designed for adult MS populations do not apply well to the evaluation of fatigue in children. In one study of 137 children with MS, 61 (45%) reported fatigue of sufficient severity as to interfere with daily activities [2].

Clinical outcomes

Kurtzke's Functional System (FS) and Expanded Disability Status Scale (EDSS) [53] is the most widely used scale to score neurological impairment in pediatric and adult MS patients (Table 4.3): EDSS scores below 4 indicate mild impairment, with a preserved self-sufficiency; EDSS scores of 6 indicate the need for aid with ambulation; and EDSS scores greater than 7 indicate an inability for independent ambulation. Early in the MS disease course, most children experience a complete, or near-complete, clinical recovery from the first MS attack. Studies that have evaluated EDSS in prospective pediatric MS cohorts have shown median EDSS scores of 1.3 in the first year of disease [6] and 1.5 after about 3 years of observation. In a cross-sectional study of 137 children, only 13% had an EDSS score greater than or equal to 4 after a median period of observation of 3.1 years [2].

Over 95% of children with MS experience a relapsing–remitting diseases course (reviewed in Banwell et al. [47]), with a primary progressive course being exceptionally rare (Table 4.1). Relapse rate is high in the first years of the disease, and may even be greater than that seen in adults [24].

The overall evolution and prognosis of MS is described in Chapter 7. In brief, pediatric-onset MS is associated with a longer time interval from first attack to permanent physical disability, and a longer time interval from onset to entry into the secondary progressive phase of the disease. In a longitudinal

Table 4.3 Kurtzke's Functional System (FS) and Expanded Disability Status Scale (EDSS)

The EDSS is based upon neurological testing of functional systems (CNS areas regulating body functions): *pyramidal* (ability to walk), *cerebellar* (coordination and balance), *brainstem* (speech and swallowing), *sensory* (touch and pain), *bowel and bladder; visual; mental;* and *"other"* (includes any other neurological findings due to multiple sclerosis).

Each Functional System (FS) is graded to the nearest possible grade, and V indicates an unknown abnormality; these are not additive scores and are only used for comparison of individual items, as follows:

Pyramidal function

0 – Normal

1 – Abnormal signs without disability

2 – Minimal disability

3 – Mild/moderate paraparesis of hemiparesis; severe monoparesis

4 – Marked paraparesis or hemiparesis; moderate quadraparesis or monoparesis

5 – Paraplegia, hemiplegia, or marked paraparesis

6 – Quadriplegia

V – Unknown

Cerebellar function

0 – Normal

1 – Abnormal signs without disability

2 – Mild ataxia

3 – Moderate truncal or limb ataxia

4 – Severe ataxia

5 – Unable to perform coordinated movements

V – Unknown

X – Weakness

Brainstem function

0 – Normal

1 – Signs only

2 – Moderate nystagmus or other mild disability

3 – Severe nystagmus, marked extraocular weakness or moderate disability of other cranial nerves

4 – Marked dysarthria or other marked disability

5 – Inability to speak or swallow

Table 4.3. (cont.)

V – Unknown

Sensory function

0 – Normal

1 – Vibration or figure – writing decrease only, in 1 or 2 limbs

2 – Mild decrease in touch or pain or position sense, and/or moderate decrease in Vibration in 1 or 2 limb, or vibration in 3 or 4 limbs

3 – Moderate decrease in touch or pain or proprioception, and/or essentially lost vibration in 1 or 2 limbs; or mild decrease in touch or pain and/or moderate decrease in all proprioceptive tests in 3 or 4 limbs

4 – Marked decrease in touch or pain or loss of proprioception, alone or combined in 1 or 2 limbs; or moderate decrease in touch or pain and/or severe proprioceptive decrease in more than two limbs

5 – Loss of sensation in 1 or 2 limbs; or moderate decrease in touch or pain and/or loss of proprioception for most of the body below the head

6 – Sensation essentially lost below the head

V – Unknown

Bowel and bladder function

0 – Normal

1 – Mild urinary hesitancy, urgency, or retention

2 – Moderate hesitancy, urgency, or retention of bowel or bladder, or rare urinary incontinence

3 – Frequent urinary incontinence

4 – Almost constant catheterization

5 – Loss of bladder function

6 – Loss of Bowel function

V – Unknown

Visual function

0 – Normal

1 – Scotoma with visual acuity > 20/30 (corrected)

2 – Worse eye with scotoma with maximal acuity 20/30 to 20/59

3 – Worse eye with large scotoma or decrease in fields, acuity 20/60 to 20/99

4 – Marked decrease in fields, acuity 20/100 to 20/200; grade 3 plus maximal acuity of better eye < 20/60

5 – Worse eye acuity < 20/200; grade 4 plus better eye acuity < 20/60

V – Unknown

Cerebral function

0 – Normal

1 – Mood alteration

2 – Mild decrease in mentation

3 – Moderate decrease in mentation

4 – Marked decrease in mentation

5 – Dementia

V – Unknown

Other function

0 – Normal

1 – Other neurological finding

Kurtzke Expanded Disability Status Scale (EDSS)

0.0	Normal neurological examination
1.0	No disability, minimal signs in one FS
1.5	No disability, minimal signs in more than one FS
2.0	Minimal disability in one FS
2.5	Mild disability in one FS or minimal disability in two FS
3.0	Moderate disability in one FS, or mild disability in three or four FS. Fully ambulatory
3.5	Fully ambulatory but with moderate disability in one FS and more than minimal disability in several others
4.0	Fully ambulatory without aid, self-sufficient, up and about some 12 h a day despite relatively severe disability; able to walk without aid or rest some 500 m
4.5	Fully ambulatory without aid, up and about much of the day, able to work a full day, may otherwise have some limitation of full activity or require minimal assistance; characterized by relatively severe disability; able to walk without aid or rest some 300 m
5.0	Ambulatory without aid or rest for about 200 m; disability severe enough to impair full daily activities (work a full day without special provisions)

Table 4.3. (cont.)

5.5	Ambulatory without aid or rest for about 100 m; disability severe enough to preclude full daily activities
6.0	Intermittent or unilateral constant assistance (cane, crutch, brace) required to walk about 100 m with or without resting
6.5	Constant bilateral assistance (canes, crutches, braces) required to walk about 20 m without resting
7.0	Unable to walk beyond approximately 5 m even with aid, essentially restricted to wheelchair; wheels self in standard wheelchair and transfers alone; up and about in wheelchair some 12 h a day
7.5	Unable to take more than a few steps; restricted to wheelchair; may need aid in transfer; wheels self but cannot carry on in standard wheelchair a full day; may require motorized wheelchair
8.0	Essentially restricted to bed or chair or perambulated in wheelchair, but may be out of bed itself much of the day; retains many self-care functions; generally has effective use of arms
8.5	Essentially restricted to bed much of day; has some effective use of arms retains some self care functions
9.0	Confined to bed; can still communicate and eat
9.5	Totally helpless bed patient; unable to communicate effectively or eat/swallow
10.0	Death due to MS

database study of 394 patients with MS onset prior to age 16 years, the estimated median time from onset to secondary progression was 28 years (at a median age of 41 years) and the median time to fixed disability (defined as an EDSS score greater than 4) was 20.0 years (median age 34.6 years) [11]. In adult-onset MS patients, progression to higher EDSS scores occurs earlier in the MS disease course, but at an older patient age.

The important role for acute relapse therapies on rate of clinical recovery, and the impact of disease-modifying therapies on short- and longer-term outcomes are discussed in Chapters 8 and 10.

Finally, consideration of MS impact on the psychological and emotional health, and quality of life, of the child and family is discussed in Chapters 13 and 14.

Future directions

A key consideration for future collaborative studies in pediatric MS is to establish a standardized approach to clinical assessment. Standardization of terminology and consistency of data acquisition will permit accurate assessment of the relative frequency of symptoms and clinical deficits. Such a template will also permit meaningful comparisons between patient cohorts cared for across multiple countries – an essential facet of studies aimed at determining the importance of regional and environmental contributions to pediatric MS. A recent manuscript suggesting that MS follows a more aggressive clinical course in African-American Blacks compared to European-origin Whites highlights the need to better appreciate ethnic or genetic influences on MS in children [16].

A key facet of care of children with MS involves the use of medications aimed at the reduction of relapse rate. Evaluation of efficacy would be invaluably aided by a consistent, prospective care model that records relapse-specific and chronic symptoms. As new therapies are developed, neuroprotective strategies may emerge that will require the ability to measure severity of acute and residual clinical deficits across all neurological domains. The development of such tools, specific for the pediatric MS population, will prove essential. Finally, the care of children with MS rests upon accurate recognition and prompt clinical diagnosis. Increasing awareness among pediatric health care providers remains an area of focus, and resources have been designed by national MS societies in North America and Europe, and are being developed in multiple other countries.

References

1. Noseworthy JH, Lucchinetti C, Rodriguez M, Weinshenker BG. Multiple sclerosis. *N Engl J Med* 2000;**343**:938–952.

2. Banwell B, Krupp L, Kennedy J, *et al.* Clinical features and viral serologies in children with multiple sclerosis: A multinational observational study. *Lancet Neurol* 2007;**6**:773–781.

3. Boiko A, Vorobeychik G, Paty D, Devonshire V, Sadovnick D. Early onset multiple sclerosis: A longitudinal study. *Neurology* 2002;**59**:1006–1010.

4. Duquette P, Murray TJ, Pleines J, *et al.* Multiple sclerosis in childhood: Clinical profile in 125 patients. *J Pediatr* 1987;**111**:359–363.

5. Ghezzi A, Deplano V, Faroni J, *et al*. Multiple sclerosis in childhood: Clinical features of 149 cases. *Mult Scler* 1997;**3**:43–46.

6. Ghezzi A, Pozzilli C, Liguori M, *et al*. Prospective study of multiple sclerosis with early onset. *Mult Scler* 2002;**8**:115–118.

7. Gusev E, Boiko A, Bikova O, *et al*. The natural history of early onset multiple sclerosis: Comparison of data from Moscow and Vancouver. *Clin Neurol Neurosurg* 2002;**104**:203–207.

8. Mikaeloff Y, Suissa S, Vallee L, *et al*. First episode of acute CNS inflammatory demyelination in childhood: Prognostic factors for multiple sclerosis and disability. *J Pediatr* 2004;**144**:246–252.

9. Mikaeloff Y, Adamsbaum C, Husson B, *et al*. MRI prognostic factors for relapse after acute CNS inflammatory demyelination in childhood. *Brain* 2004;**127**(Pt 9):1942–1947.

10. Mikaeloff Y, Caridade G, Assi S, Suissa S, Tardieu M. Prognostic factors for early severity in a childhood multiple sclerosis cohort. *Pediatrics* 2006;**118**:1133–1139.

11. Renoux C, Vukusic S, Mikaeloff Y, *et al*. Natural history of multiple sclerosis with childhood onset. *N Engl J Med* 2007;**365**:2603–2613.

12. Simone IL, Carrara D, Tortorella C, *et al*. Course and prognosis in early-onset MS: Comparison with adult-onset forms. *Neurology* 2002;**59**:1922–1928.

13. Trojano M, Liguori M, Bosco ZG, *et al*. Age-related disability in multiple sclerosis. *Ann Neurol* 2002; **51**:475–480.

14. Atzori M, Battistella PA, Perini P, *et al*. Clinical and diagnostic aspects of multiple sclerosis and acute monophasic encephalomielitis in pediatric patients: A single centre prospective study. *Mult Scler* 2009; **15**:363–370.

15. Belopitova L, Guergueltcheva PV, Bojinova V. Definite and suspected multiple sclerosis in children: Long-term follow-up and magnetic resonance imaging findings. *J Child Neurol* 2001; **16**(5):317–324.

16. Boster AL, Endress CF, Hreha SA, Caon C, Perumal JS, Khan OA. Pediatric-onset multiple sclerosis in African-American Black and European-origin White patients. *Pediatr Neurol* 2009;**40**:31–33.

17. Boutin B, Esquivel E, Mayer M, Chaumet S, Ponsot G, Arthuis M. Multiple sclerosis in children: Report of clinical and paraclinical features of 19 cases. *Neuropediatrics* 1988;**19**:118–123.

18. Chiemchanya S, Visudhiphan P. Multiple sclerosis in children: A report of 17 Thai pediatric patients. *J Med Assoc Thai* 1993;**76**(Suppl 2):28–33.

19. Cole GF, Stuart CA. A long perspective on childhood multiple sclerosis. *Dev Med Child Neurol* 1995; **37**:661–666.

20. Dale RC, de Sousa C, Chong WK, Cox TC, Harding B, Neville BG. Acute disseminated encephalomyelitis, multiphasic disseminated encephalomyelitis and multiple sclerosis in children. *Brain* 2000;**123**(Pt 12): 2407–2422.

21. Deryck O, Ketelaer P, Dubois B. Clinical characteristics and long term prognosis in early onset multiple sclerosis. *J Neurol* 2006;**253**:720–723.

22. Ferreira ML, Machado MI, Dantas MJ, *et al*. Pediatric multiple sclerosis: Analysis of clinical and epidemiological aspects according to National MS Society Consensus 2007. *Arq Neuropsiquiatr* 2008; **66**:665–670.

23. Gal J, Hayles A, Siekert R, Keith H. Multiple sclerosis in children: A clinical study of 40 cases with onset in childhood. *Pediatrics* 1958;**21**:703–709.

24. Gorman MP, Healy BC, Polgar-Turcsanyi M, Chitnis T. Increased relapse rate in pediatric-onset compared with adult-onset multiple sclerosis Arch. *Neurology* 2009;**66**:54–59.

25. Guilhoto LM, Osorio CA, Machado LR, *et al*. Pediatric multiple sclerosis report of 14 cases. *Brain Dev* 1995; **17**:9–12.

26. Hanefeld F, Bauer HJ, Christen HJ, Kruse B, Bruhn H, Frahm J. Multiple sclerosis in childhood: Report of 15 cases. *Brain Dev* 1991;**13**:410–416.

27. Neuteboom RF, Boon M, Catsman Berrevoets CE, Vles JS, Gooskens RH. Prognostic factors after a first attack of inflammatory CNS demyelination in children. *Neurology* 2008;**71**:967–973.

28. Ozakbas S, Idiman E, Baklan B, Yulug B. Childhood and juvenile onset multiple sclerosis: Clinical and paraclinical features. *Brain Dev* 2003;**25**:233–236.

29. Pinhas-Hamiel O, Barak Y, Siev-Ner I, Achiron A. Juvenile multiple sclerosis: clinical features and prognostic characteristics. *J Pediatr* 1998;**132**:735–737.

30. Ruggieri M, Iannetti P, Polizzi A, Pavone L, Grimaldi LM. Multiple sclerosis in children under 10 years of age. *Neurol Sci* 2004;**25**(Suppl 4):S326–S335.

31. Selcen D, Anlar B, Renda Y. Multiple sclerosis in childhood: Report of 16 cases. *Eur Neurol* 1996; **36**:79–84.

32. Shiraishi K, Higuchi Y, Ozawa K, Hao Q, Saida T. Clinical course and prognosis of 27 patients with childhood onset multiple sclerosis in Japan. *Brain Dev* 2005;**27**:224–227.

33. Sindern E, Haas J, Stark E, Wurster U. Early onset MS under the age of 16: Clinical and paraclinical features. *Acta Neurol Scand* 1992;**86**:280–284.

34. Weng WC, Yang CC, Yu TW, Shen YZ, Lee WT. Multiple sclerosis with childhood onset: Report of 21 cases in Taiwan. *Pediatr Neurol* 2006;**35**:327–334.

35. Krupp LB, Banwell B, Tenembaum S, *et al.* Consensus definitions proposed for pediatric multiple sclerosis and related disorders. *Neurology* 2007;**68**(Suppl 2):S7–S12.

36. Anderson O. Natural history of multiple sclerosis. In: *Multiple Sclerosis: A Comprehensive Text*, ed. CS Raine, HF McFarland, R Hohlfeld. Philadelphia, PA: Elsevier; 2008:100–120.

37. Wilejto M, Shroff M, Buncic JR, Kennedy J, Goia C, Banwell B. The clinical features, MRI findings, and outcome of optic neuritis in children. *Neurology* 2006;**67**:258–262.

38. Pidcock FS, Krishnan C, Crawford TO, Salorio CF, Trovato M, Kerr DA. Acute transverse myelitis in childhood: Center-based analysis of 47 cases. *Neurology* 2007;**68**:1474–1480.

39. Ghezzi A. Clinical characteristics of multiple sclerosis with early onset. *Neurol Sci* 2004;**25**:S336–S339.

40. Ghassemi R, Antel SB, Narayanan S, *et al.* Lesion distribution in children with clinically isolated syndromes. *Ann Neurol* 2008;**63**:401–405.

41. Waubant E, Chabas D, Okuda DT, *et al.* Difference in disease burden and activity in pediatric patients on brain magnetic resonance imaging at time of multiple sclerosis onset vs adults. *Arch Neurol* 2009;**66**:967–971.

42. Mikaeloff Y, Caridade G, Husson B, Suissa S, Tardieu M. Acute disseminated encephalomyelitis cohort study: Prognostic factors for relapse. *Eur J Paediatr Neurol* 2007;**11**:90–95.

43. Tenembaum S, Chamoles N, Fejerman N. Acute disseminated encephalomyelitis: A long-term follow-up study of 84 pediatric patients. *Neurology* 2002;**59**:1224–1231.

44. Dale RC, Pillai SC. Early relapse risk after a first CNS inflammatory demyelination episode: Examining international consensus definitions. *Dev Med Child Neurol* 2007;**49**:887–893.

45. Callen DJA, Shroff MM, Branson HM, *et al.* MRI in the diagnosis of pediatric multiple sclerosis. *Neurology* 2009;**72**:961–967.

46. Callen DJA, Shroff MM, Branson HM, *et al.* The role of MRI in the differentiation of ADEM from MS in children. *Neurology* 2009;**72**:968–973.

47. Banwell B, Ghezzi A, Bar-Or A, *et al.* Multiple sclerosis in children: Clinical diagnosis, therapeutic strategies, and future directions. *Lancet Neurol* 2007;**6**:887–902.

48. Shaw CM, Alvord EC Jr. Multiple sclerosis beginning in infancy. *J Child Neurol* 1987;**2**:252–256.

49. Banwell B, Shroff M, Ness JM, Jeffrey D, Schwid S, Weinstock-Guttman B, for the International Pediatric MS Study Group. MRI features of pediatric multiple sclerosis. *Neurology* 2007;**68**:S46–S53.

50. Banwell BL, Anderson PE. The cognitive burden of multiple sclerosis in children. *Neurology* 2005;**64**:891–894.

51. MacAllister WS, Belman AL, Milazzo M, *et al.* Cognitive functioning in children and adolescents with multiple sclerosis. *Neurology* 2005;**64**:1422–1425.

52. Amato M, Goretti B, Ghezzi A, *et al.* Cognitive and psychosocial features of childhood and juvanile MS. *Neurology* 2008;**70**:1891–1897.

53. Kurtzke JF. Rating neurological impairment in multiple sclerosis: An expanded disability status scale. *Neurology* 1983;**33**:1444–1452.

Chapter 5

MRI features of pediatric multiple sclerosis

Bruno P. Soares, Dorothée Chabas, and Max Wintermark

Magnetic resonance imaging (MRI) is considered an essential tool in the diagnosis and management of patients with multiple sclerosis (MS), mostly due to its high sensitivity to depict white matter lesions and characterize disease dissemination in space and time. However, the standardization of its interpretation in adult patients with MS has not yet been paralleled in the pediatric population. For instance, until recently, the diagnosis of MS in the pediatric population did not include MRI criteria as it does in adults [1–4]. This is despite the fact that MRI has been studied for more than 20 years in the diagnosis of MS in pediatric patients [5]. Similarly, the operational definitions for pediatric-onset MS [6] that aim at creating a uniform terminology to be used in future prospective studies rely on the adult MRI criteria, not specific pediatric ones (see Chapter 2).

MS in children has several characteristic features, including an almost exclusive relapsing–remitting course of disease [7,8] with more frequent relapses and seizures [9]. Involved anatomical regions differ somewhat in children and adults, with children showing more frequent involvement of the posterior fossa, and less frequent involvement of the spinal cord, although this remains to be confirmed [10]. These particularities raise questions about the ability to use the same diagnostic criteria in the children and adults with MS, especially in prepubertal patients in whom the clinical, biological, and radiological presentation seem to be distinct [11–13].

In this chapter, we describe the specific MRI features of pediatric MS. We also discuss proposed MRI criteria for pediatric MS, and compare these to the MRI diagnostic criteria already well established for adult patients who present with a first demyelinating event. Finally, we discuss the predictive value of the proposed criteria for conversion to MS, as well as the

MRI features that allow differentiating pediatric MS from acute disseminated encephalomyelitis (ADEM) and other entities.

MRI protocol for MS

MRI protocols in the pediatric population have specificities, including the need to optimize these protocols and make them as short as possible, in order to alleviate the need for sedation, or at least reduce the duration of sedation. Children above 8 years of age can usually be scanned without sedation. Pediatric imaging protocols also employ different parameters, notably slice thickness that needs to be adjusted according to age to accurately assess the brain parenchyma.

Conventional MRI sequences – including T1-weighted pre- and post-gadolinium, T2-weighted and fluid-attenuated inversion recovery (FLAIR) images in multiple planes – are helpful to establish the diagnosis of MS, monitor the disease course and treatment efficacy, and somewhat predict its evolution [14]. FLAIR images are optimal to depict supratentorial lesions, whereas the posterior fossa is optimally imaged using conventional T2-weighted sequences. Enhancement of MS lesions usually indicates recent disease activity, being caused by gadolinium accumulation in the interstitial space due to transient disruption or increase in the permeability of the blood–brain barrier. Fat-suppressed T1-weighted sequences after gadolinium administration are most sensitive to detect optic nerve involvement [15,16].

However, it must be emphasized that conventional MRI sequences lack sensitivity to detect and quantify global MS damage or tissue loss in normal-appearing white matter and gray matter [17,18]. Recently, more advanced imaging techniques such as

---

Demyelinating Disorders of the Central Nervous System in Childhood, ed. Dorothée Chabas and Emmanuelle L. Waubant. Published by Cambridge University Press. © Cambridge University Press 2011.

A B

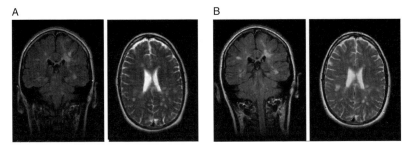

Figure 5.1 MRI findings in a postpubertal MS patient. (A) Coronal FLAIR and axial T2-weighted images of a 13-year-old boy at the time of initial presentation demonstrate bilateral T2-hyperintense lesions involving the periventricular and subcortical white matter, as well as the brainstem and cerebellum. Note the well-defined borders and ovoid shape of most lesions; this appearance is strongly suggestive of MS. (B) Coronal FLAIR and axial T2-weighted images acquired 3 months later do not show any significant decrease in the number of lesions. Adapted from [32].

magnetization transfer, diffusion tensor imaging (DTI) and MR spectroscopy have been proposed to better characterize the burden of MS lesions in adults [19]. Additionally, MRI assessment for MS may benefit from the improvement of post-processing methods. These methods include automated voxel-based measurement of lesion volume or atrophy, and subtraction imaging to display changes over time between two scans. Finally, new contrast agents are being studied with the potential to image important processes in the pathophysiology of MS, such as macrophage activity or Wallerian degeneration [19].

MRI findings in children with MS

Physiologically, there are several differences between adult and pediatric populations that contribute to the distinct clinical and MRI features of MS in these two age groups. These differences mainly relate to the stage of CNS maturation, with ongoing myelin maturation and a better capacity for repair (neuroplasticity) in children [12,20].

MRI studies in children may help us understand early pathogenic events that ultimately lead to clinical symptoms and signs of MS. Indeed, children are thought to have a shorter biological disease duration before clinical onset, and MRI plays an important role in depicting disease manifestations closer to their biological onset [21].

MRI studies in pediatric patients with the first clinical presentation of MS usually disclose multiple white matter T2-bright areas [22]. One study evaluating 41 patients with pediatric-onset MS and 35 patients with adult-onset MS found that, in contrast with prior belief [22], children had a higher disease

burden at onset than adults. Specifically, children had a higher number of total (median, 21 vs. 6) and large T2-bright lesions (median, 4 vs. 0). They also had more enhancing lesions (68.4% vs. 21.2%) and more T2-bright foci in the posterior fossa (68.3% vs. 31.4%) (Figure 5.1) [10]. These results contradict the hypothesis that the onset at a younger age is associated with limited accrual of clinically silent lesions prior to first clinical symptoms [23]. In another study of pediatric patients presenting with a clinically isolated syndrome, a greater number of brainstem lesions was found when compared to in adults, with a particular predilection for the pons in male patients [24]. The predilection for infratentorial involvement in pediatric patients may be related to the caudocranial temporal gradient in myelination, commencing in the brainstem and progressing to the cerebellum and the cerebrum [25].

The number of MS lesions that enhance in children compared with adults is controversial. At the time of their first episode of demyelination, 52% of adults fulfilling the McDonald criteria for MS had enhancing lesions [26]. In contrast, only 12 (24%) of 52 children ultimately diagnosed with MS had enhancing lesions at their first episode of demyelination. However, the number of gadolinium-enhanced MRI examinations is not reported in this study (and thus may be even lower) [27]. In another study where gadolinium was only administered to 9 children, 4 (44%) had enhancing lesions [22]. These studies are clearly limited by the low number of patients who received gadolinium. Besides, they contradict a larger comparative study where 68.4% of 41 children versus 21.2% of 35 adults with MS had enhancing lesions at disease onset ($p<0.001$) [10]. In adult MS,

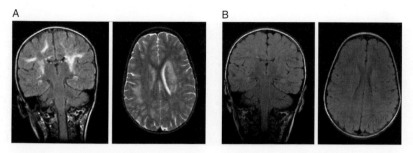

Figure 5.2 Dramatic reduction in lesion load in a prepubertal MS patient. (A) Coronal FLAIR and axial T2-weighted images of a 4-year-old girl at the time of initial presentation demonstrate bilateral ill-defined T2-hyperintense lesions involving the periventricular and subcortical white matter. Note the absence of ovoid well-defined lesions, typical of adult MS patients. (B) Coronal and axial FLAIR images acquired 3 months later demonstrate substantial improvement, with only residual T2-hyperintensity in the previously affected areas. Adapted from [32].

gadolinium-enhancing lesions have been shown to be more age-than disease duration-dependent (younger patients have more enhancing lesions). Besides, tumefactive lesions tend to more often enhance, and are more frequent in children. A few case reports indicate that, as in adults, MS in children may also present with multiple ring-enhancing lesions [28,29].

Another feature of acute demyelination in children is the propensity for large demyelinating lesions with marked perilesional edema. The appearance of tumefactive demyelinating plaques has been reported in a number of children [30,31]. In a study of 20 children with MS, review of MR images found 4 with tumefactive lesions [22].

In one study addressing differences between pre- and postpubertal MS patients, it was found that, while the overall number of T2-bright lesions was similar in the two groups, prepubertal patients had fewer well-defined ovoid lesions and more often had confluent lesions on their first brain MRI study compared to postpubertal patients. In addition, prepubertal patients tended to have fewer enhancing lesions and more deep gray matter involvement than postpubertal patients. On the follow-up MRI study, there was a reduction in the number and size of these lesions in 92% of the prepubertal patients, whereas in only 29% of the postpubertal patients this reduction was observed (Figure 5.2). These differences in MRI presentation according to age suggest that MS in prepubertal patients may have distinct underlying biologic processes and that the MRI criteria should be revised in this age group to avoid delay in diagnosis [32]. Because prepubertal children may present initially with large, bilateral and ill-defined lesions, the diagnosis of ADEM vs. MS remains difficult,

especially in younger children. An imaging pattern compatible with ADEM should be included in the spectrum of possible onsets of MS in childhood. Finally, it has been reported that children with relapsing–remitting MS, when followed for up to 8 years, may have a slower development of irreversible changes than adults, such as T1 black holes and brain atrophy [30]. However, it is still not clear whether these differences are simply due to a shorter duration of disease at the time of diagnosis than in adults.

Application of adult MRI criteria in children with MS

Earlier studies demonstrated a high sensitivity (74%) and specificity (86%) for the McDonald MRI criteria (Table 5.1) in predicting MS outcome in adults [33]. In contrast, application of adult MS criteria to MRI scans of 20 children ultimately diagnosed with MS demonstrated that, although all children had one or more T2 lesions, only 53% met the McDonald criteria for lesions dissemination in space at the time of their initial presentation [22]. Application of the McDonald MRI criteria for lesion dissemination in space in a French study of 116 children under age 16 years yielded a sensitivity of 52% with a specificity of 63% [27]. Children in these earlier studies often had less than nine lesions, perhaps reflecting a shorter subclinical period of lesion accrual, referral bias or possibly differences in MRI protocols compared to those used in adults. These results are in contrast with a more recent study, which demonstrated that children ($n = 41$) had a higher number of total T2-bright lesions at onset compared with adults ($n = 35$) [10]. The MRI scans in children failing to meet the

Table 5.1 MS MRI criteria in adults and children with their respective limitations

Operational diagnostic criteria for pediatric MS	Limitations
Barkhof criteria [1] for demonstration of dissemination in space [1–3]	– Children less often meet these criteria because of:
At least three of the following:	• Atypical locations
(1) One gadolinium-enhancing lesion or nine T2-hyperintense lesions	• Larger lesions (in younger patients)
(2) At least one infratentorial lesion	– No differentiation by age group
(3) At least one juxtacortical lesion	
(4) At least three periventricular lesions	
* A spinal cord lesion can substitute for an infratentorial lesion; an enhancing spinal cord lesion is equivalent to an enhancing brain lesion; and individual spinal cord lesions can contribute together with individual brain lesions to reach the required number of T2 lesions [4]	
MRI KIDMUS criteria [27]	– Does not consider enhancement – Does not consider spinal cord lesions
All of the following:	– Prepubertal children have ill-defined lesions
(1) Lesions with long axis perpendicular to the corpus callosum	– No differentiation by age group
(2) Sole presence of well-defined lesions	– Low number of patients studied
Callen criteria [23]	– Does not consider enhancement
At least two of the following:	– Does not consider spinal cord lesions
(1) At least five T2-hyperintense lesions	– MRI protocol not uniform
(2) At least two periventricular lesions	– No differentiation by age group
(3) At least one brainstem lesion	– Low number of patients studied
	– Does not consider enhancement
MRI criteria for the differentiation of ADEM from MS in children proposed by Callen [49]	– Does not consider spinal cord lesions
At least two of the following:	– Controversial definition of T1 black holes
(1) At least two periventricular lesions	– MRI not performed at onset of disease for pediatric MS patients
(2) Presence of T1 black holes	– No differentiation by age group
(3) Absence of bilateral lesion distribution pattern	

McDonald criteria for lesion dissemination in space typically demonstrated a low number of lesions, but also lesions in regions not considered in the McDonald criteria. When stratified by age, children younger than 10 years meeting the McDonald MRI criteria had a 27% positive predictive value for clinical recurrence, compared to 80% in children older than 10 years. This is in line with the brain MRI features found in younger pediatric MS patients, with less well-defined ovoid lesions at disease onset and more common vanishing lesions on follow-up scans.

Of note, the initial finding of high sensitivity and specificity for the McDonald MRI criteria in adults has also been questioned. A more recent study in which the criteria were applied to adults experiencing their first demyelinating event found a sensitivity of only 49% [26], similar to that observed in both the Canadian [22] and French [27] pediatric cohorts. These findings are not surprising since patients were scanned closer to disease onset, and thus, a smaller burden of disease would be expected compared to later stages of disease.

Proposed MRI criteria for children

Based on the analysis of the MRI features of 116 children enrolled in the French cohort of acute CNS demyelination with average follow-up of 4.9 ±3 years after the initial demyelinating event, the authors tested a set of 2 brain MRI criteria for pediatric MS (see Table 5.1): presence of white matter lesions located perpendicular to the long axis of the corpus callosum and sole presence of well-defined lesions [27]. Using these two features, the prediction of the occurrence of a second attack was 100% specific but only 21% sensitive. In contrast, involvement of greater than 50% of the white matter and a single large area of demyelination were more often related to monophasic disease. The presence of lesions in the basal ganglia or thalami did not help differentiate between monophasic disease and recurrent demyelination.

A recent retrospective study compared MRI scans of 38 children with MS and 45 children with nondemyelinating diseases with relapsing neurological deficits (migraine or lupus). The authors proposed the following new criteria, two of which at least should be fulfilled to diagnose pediatric MS: (a) five or more T2-bright lesions; (b) two or more periventricular lesions; (c) at least one brainstem lesion. Using these criteria, a sensitivity of 85% and specificity of 98% was achieved [23,34]. However, it is unclear whether patients with migraine and lupus represent adequate comparison cohorts. Furthermore, the MRI technique employed was not the same for all patients, with some not having contrast-enhanced sequences, and the number of patients evaluated may not be large enough to justify the proposal of new diagnostic criteria until these findings can be reproduced [35].

Predictive value of MRI for the diagnosis of MS in children

MRI is able to incidentally detect white matter pathology that represents clinically silent demyelination in adults (the radiologically isolated syndrome) [36].

In adults, the development of new clinically silent lesions is an important predictor of future MS diagnosis in patients who had an acute demyelinating episode [2]. One study in adults found that individuals with MRI findings suggestive of demyelinating disease (T2-bright foci in the corpus callosum or periventricular, ovoid, well-defined) are likely to experience subsequent radiological or clinical events related to MS [36]. This has not yet been reported in children, although the authors have seen four cases of pediatric radiologically isolated syndrome (unpublished data).

Optic neuritis (ON) is a common initial clinical presentation of MS. In both adult and pediatric patients with isolated ON, the presence of brain T2-bright foci meeting the McDonald MRI criteria is a strong predictor of future development of MS [1]. In contrast, the absence of brain or spine lesions on the initial MRI study seems to be associated with very low risk of progression to MS. In a retrospective study of 29 children with idiopathic ON followed for a mean of 50 months, none of the patients with a normal brain MRI developed MS [37]. Of the 18 patients followed for more than 24 months, 7 had white matter lesions on the initial MRI studies, 3 of whom developed MS [37]. Other studies show similar results: a prospective cohort of 35 children with isolated optic neuritis who underwent MRI studies at the time of disease onset found that 19 had one or more lesions in the brain or spine [38]. Twelve patients met the McDonald criteria, 10 of whom were diagnosed with MS during a 2.4-year follow-up. In another series of 14 children with ON, 8 demonstrated white matter lesions in the brain, 7 of whom were ultimately diagnosed with MS during a period ranging from 2 months to 14 years after the onset of symptoms [39].

Prognostic value of MRI

Studies in adult MS patients have shown that the initial lesion burden on brain imaging may be an important prognostic factor. Specifically, a higher number of brain lesions at onset or an increase in the number of lesions in the first five years of disease predict the degree of long-term disability from MS [40]. Limited data point to similar conclusions in pediatric patients [27].

In the later phases of disease, the degree of brain atrophy may be a more relevant prognostic factor than the lesion burden in adults [41]. Data from adult studies indicate that progressive global brain atrophy correlates with cognitive [42] and physical disability [43]. Even though cognitive impairment has been reported in pediatric patients beginning as early as one year from the onset of disease [44], no studies in children have correlated the degree of cognitive impairment with brain atrophy. Our own experience suggests that, as in adults, pediatric patients with a high lesion burden also tend to have brain atrophy.

"Black holes", or hypointense lesions on pre-contrast T1-weighted images, have been shown to correspond to areas of axonal loss on histopathology [45] and are considered to indicate lesion chronicity. Their presence has been correlated with clinical disability in adult patients. However, acute T1 hypointense lesions may only represent reversible tissue edema. Thus, studies of T1 hypointense foci should always include post-contrast imaging, so enhancing lesions are not accounted for as "black holes". Furthermore, the presence of T1-dark foci varies dramatically according to MRI protocols so their significance remains controversial [46]. Transient T1 hypointense lesions have also been seen on the initial MRI scan of children with monophasic disease course; therefore, it is crucial to distinguish between reversible acute T1 hypointense lesions and residual destructive lesions.

Differential diagnosis

In patients presenting with a first clinical episode involving the CNS, several differential diagnoses must be considered. The most common disease to be confused with MS is ADEM. ADEM is considered to be an isolated autoimmune attack on the CNS that leads to acute demyelination, often seen up to two weeks after a viral infection or immunization. Chapters 17 and 18 review, respectively, the clinical and radiological presentation of ADEM.

Unlike in MS, where clinically silent lesion accrual is frequently seen, in ADEM new T2-bright foci typically do not appear during asymptomatic periods [47]. Lesions are typically large with an incomplete ring of enhancement, and the degree of mass effect is less than expected for the lesion size. They may also have hemorrhage that may indicate a devastating course (acute hemorrhagic encephalomyelitis).

According to the literature, the MRI criteria for ADEM include the presence of poorly defined lesions and a high lesion load, associated with thalamus and basal ganglia involvement [48]. However, this study

was performed before the operational definition criteria were published. Unfortunately, there is some overlap between the radiological appearance of MS and ADEM, especially in prepubertal patients [12].

A recent retrospective study addressed the role of MRI to discriminate MS from ADEM in children at the time of their first demyelinating event. The evaluation of initial MRI scans from 48 children – 28 with a final diagnosis of MS, and 20 with ADEM (defined according to the International Pediatric MS Study Group operational criteria [6] and followed for at least two years) showed that periventricular involvement was more frequent in MS patients, although the total number of T2-bright foci did not differ between groups. Logistic regression analysis to define the strongest MRI predictors led to propose a set of criteria to differentiate MS from ADEM – which is fulfilled by the presence of two of the following: two or more periventricular lesions; presence of T1 black holes; and absence of a diffuse bilateral lesion pattern (Figure 5.3) [49]. Using these criteria, the authors achieved a sensitivity of 81% and specificity of 95% for distinguishing ADEM from a first attack of MS. However, the definition of black holes included all T1 hypointense lesions, when actually most of these lesions were transient and disappeared on follow-up imaging. This definition diverges from the usual definition of T1 black holes as chronic nonenhancing lesions that correspond pathologically to irreversible axonal degeneration [21].

The presence of periventricular T2-bright foci is already included in the pediatric and adult MS criteria (see Table 5.1) and is consistent with prospective data on pediatric MS published in 2008 [50]. The inclusion of black holes in the criteria, however, may not be adequate given the definitions employed in the study. The term "black holes" refers to nonenhancing hypointense lesions on pre-contrast T1-weighted images. However, the detection of black holes depends heavily on T1 pulse sequence parameters, contrast-to-noise ratios, and even magnetic field strengths. As such, how this criterion could be applied consistently in clinical practice remains unclear, because MRI protocols vary greatly from one facility to another, and even from one scanner to the other. In addition, the presence of a contrast-enhancing lesion is typically associated with breakdown of the blood–brain barrier and increase in water content (edema). The local increase in water content may by itself appear hypointense on T1-weighted images.

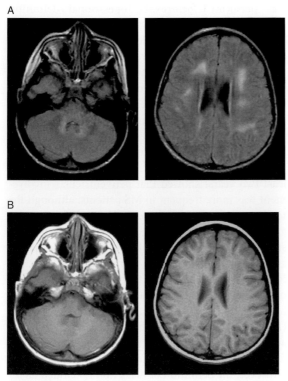

Figure 5.3 MRI Findings in a prepubertal MS patient. (A) Axial and coronal FLAIR images of a 4-year-old girl at the time of initial presentation demonstrate bilateral T2-hyperintense lesions involving the posterior pons and cerebellum, as well as bilateral confluent lesions involving mostly the periventricular regions and deep white matter. (B) Axial T1-weighted images (also at the time of initial presentation) do not demonstrate lesions. (C) The presence of a bilateral diffuse distribution on FLAIR images coupled with the absence of T1-hypointense lesion results in a failure to meet the MS criteria proposed by [49]. However, this patient has been diagnosed with definite MS with subsequent evidence of new lesions and was started on disease-modifying therapy. Adapted from [35].

Thus, if not followed with serial scans to ensure their irreversibility, T1 hypointense lesions seen on the initial MRI scans may represent acute disease activity instead of tissue destruction.

Given the preponderance of confluent lesions and the frequency of ill-defined nonovoid T2-bright foci at MS onset in prepubertal patients, a worthwhile approach might be to propose definitions that apply specifically to prepubertal patients while taking these differences into account, instead of grouping all pediatric patients together.

Another MRI feature that could help discriminate ADEM from a first episode of MS is the size of the lesions on spinal cord MRI. In clinical practice, it is generally considered that a patient with extensive T2 hyperintensity in the spinal cord is more likely to have ADEM than MS. In the UCSF pediatric cohort of patients with a first demyelinating event who underwent a spinal cord MRI within 3 months after disease onset, 24 patients with clinically isolated syndromes were less likely to have T2-bright cord foci (more than 3 vertebral bodies in height) compared with 8 ADEM patients (8.3% vs. 65%) [51]. Larger series are needed to confirm that the presence of extensive spinal cord lesions supports the diagnosis of ADEM rather than MS in children.

Other demyelinating diseases, such as neuromyelitis optica (NMO) and acute complete transverse myelitis, may have a radiological appearance similar to MS. Brain involvement may be clinically detected in NMO, along with abnormal brain MRI findings (see Chapter 23) [52–54].

Even though several other disease categories including inflammatory, infectious, metabolic, vascular, and neoplastic disorders may present in children with a combination of acute neurological problems and white matter changes on MRI, careful evaluation of clinical history, neurological examination, and laboratory studies is often helpful in narrowing the possible differential diagnoses (see Chapter 6) [55]. Analysis of MRI findings is greatly facilitated when the neuroradiologist is aware of the disease categories being considered by the clinician.

Non-conventional MRI methods

Unlike in adult MS, non-conventional MRI techniques, such as proton magnetic resonance spectroscopy (MRS), magnetization transfer imaging (MTR), diffusion tensor imaging (DTI), functional MRI (fMRI), T1 and T2 relaxometry, susceptibility weighted (SWI), and phase imaging, have not been sufficiently investigated in pediatric MS.

In a combined fMRI and DTI preliminary study comparing pediatric and adult-onset MS subjects, the authors found preserved effective connectivity in sensorimotor pathways, suggesting preservation of brain adaptation to maintain clinical functionality in pediatric-onset compared to adult-onset MS subjects [56]. However, despite effective connectivity, pediatric-onset MS patients may be at significant risk of disease progression as normal-appearing white matter DTI metrics (decreased fractional anisotropy and increased mean diffusivity) were abnormal compared to matched healthy controls [57].

Whole brain myelin water imaging using the short T2 component [58] should be ideal to study the craniocaudal temporal gradient of myelination in prepubertal MS subjects in relation with the location and distribution of white matter lesion appearance (lesion probability maps). Sustained mitochondrial dysfunction using serial NAA measurements from MRS could be assessed and potentially be used to predict permanent neuro-axonal injury. Lastly, SWI and phase imaging studies in pediatric MS subjects could shed light to the onset of excessive iron deposition found in the deep gray matter [59,60], investigate whether iron deposits accelerate tissue injury, and predict disease progression.

Conclusion

In summary, children with MS may less often meet the McDonald criteria used for MS diagnosis in adults – especially younger children – as they display less dissemination in space (smaller number of typical MS lesions in specific areas) and more atypical lesions (large or tumefactive). They also have more frequent involvement of the brainstem and cerebellum on their initial brain MRI study than adults. Moreover, even though pre- and postpubertal patients have a similar number of lesions on their initial brain MRI study, prepubertal patients tend to have less well-defined ovoid lesions that greatly reduce in number and size on the follow-up MRI study. All these particularities in the radiological presentation raise questions about the adequacy of applying adult MS MRI criteria in the pediatric population, and suggest that specific pediatric MS MRI criteria should be developed along with the revised pediatric MS diagnostic algorithm. Larger-scale collaborative prospective studies are needed, leading to criteria and definitions specific to the pediatric population, which could be ideally applied both to daily practice and research settings.

References

1. Barkhof F, Filippi M, Miller DH, *et al.* Comparison of MRI criteria at first presentation to predict conversion to clinically definite multiple sclerosis. *Brain* 1997;**120** (Pt 11):2059–2069.

2. Tintore M, Rovira A, Martinez MJ, *et al.* Isolated demyelinating syndromes: Comparison of different MR imaging criteria to predict conversion to clinically definite multiple sclerosis. *Am J Neuroradiol* 2000;**21**:702–706.

3. McDonald WI, Compston A, Edan G, *et al.* Recommended diagnostic criteria for multiple sclerosis: Guidelines from the International Panel on the diagnosis of multiple sclerosis. *Ann Neurol* 2001;**50**:121–127.

4. Polman CH, Reingold SC, Edan G, *et al.* Diagnostic criteria for multiple sclerosis: 2005 revisions to the "McDonald Criteria". *Ann Neurol* 2005;**58**:840–846.

5. Golden GS, Woody RC. The role of nuclear magnetic resonance imaging in the diagnosis of MS in childhood. *Neurology* 1987;**37**:689–693.

6. Krupp LB, Banwell B, Tenembaum S. Consensus definitions proposed for pediatric multiple sclerosis and related disorders. *Neurology* 2007;**68**:S7–12.

7. Ghezzi A, Ruggieri M, Trojano M, Filippi M. Italian studies on early-onset multiple sclerosis: The present and the future. *Neurol Sci* 2004;**25**(Suppl 4):S346–349.

8. Pinhas-Hamiel O, Barak Y, Siev-Ner I, Achiron A. Juvenile multiple sclerosis: Clinical features and prognostic characteristics. *J Pediatr* 1998;**132**:735–737.

9. Gorman MP, Healy BC, Polgar-Turcsanyi M, Chitnis T. Increased relapse rate in pediatric-onset compared with adult-onset multiple sclerosis. *Arch Neurol* 2009;**66**:54–59.

10. Waubant E, Chabas D, Okuda DT, *et al.* Difference in disease burden and activity in pediatric patients on brain magnetic resonance imaging at time of multiple sclerosis onset vs adults. *Arch Neurol* 2009;**66**:967–971.

11. Chabas D, Ness J, Belman A, *et al.* Pediatric MS before puberty: A distinct CSF inflammatory profile. *Neurology* 2010;**74**:399–405.

12. Chabas D, Strober J, Waubant E. Pediatric multiple sclerosis. *Curr Neurol Neurosci Rep* 2008;**8**:434–441.

13. Banwell B, Ghezzi A, Bar-Or A, Mikaeloff Y, Tardieu M. Multiple sclerosis in children: Clinical diagnosis, therapeutic strategies, and future directions. *Lancet Neurol* 2007;**6**:887–902.

14. Neema M, Stankiewicz J, Arora A, Guss ZD, Bakshi R. MRI in multiple sclerosis: What's inside the toolbox? *Neurotherapeutics* 2007;**4**:602–617.

15. Guy J, Mao J, Bidgood WD Jr, Mancuso A, Quisling RG. Enhancement and demyelination of the intraorbital optic nerve. Fat suppression magnetic resonance imaging. *Ophthalmology* 1992;**99**:713–719.

16. Tien RD, Hesselink JR, Szumowski J. MR fat suppression combined with Gd-DTPA enhancement in optic neuritis and perineuritis. *J Comput Assist Tomogr* 1991;**15**:223–227.

17. Miller DH, Thompson AJ, Filippi M. Magnetic resonance studies of abnormalities in the normal appearing white matter and grey matter in multiple sclerosis. *J Neurol* 2003;**250**:1407–1419.

55

18. Pirko I, Lucchinetti CF, Sriram S, Bakshi R. Gray matter involvement in multiple sclerosis. *Neurology* 2007;**68**:634–642.

19. Bakshi R, Thompson AJ, Rocca MA, *et al*. MRI in multiple sclerosis: current status and future prospects. *Lancet Neurol* 2008;**7**:615–625.

20. Banwell B, Shroff M, Ness JM, Jeffery D, Schwid S, Weinstock-Guttman B. MRI features of pediatric multiple sclerosis. *Neurology* 2007;**68**:S46–53.

21. Chitnis T, Pirko I. Sensitivity vs specificity: Progress and pitfalls in defining MRI criteria for pediatric MS. *Neurology* 2009;**72**:952–953.

22. Hahn CD, Shroff MM, Blaser SI, Banwell BL. MRI criteria for multiple sclerosis: Evaluation in a pediatric cohort. *Neurology* 2004;**62**:806–808.

23. Callen DJ, Shroff MM, Branson HM, *et al*. MRI in the diagnosis of pediatric multiple sclerosis. *Neurology* 2009;**72**:961–967.

24. Ghassemi R, Antel SB, Narayanan S, *et al*. Lesion distribution in children with clinically isolated syndromes. *Ann Neurol* 2008;**63**:401–405.

25. Barkovich AJ, Kjos BO, Jackson DE Jr, Norman D. Normal maturation of the neonatal and infant brain: MR imaging at 1.5 T. *Radiology* 1988;**166**:173–180.

26. Korteweg T, Tintore M, Uitdehaag B, *et al*. MRI criteria for dissemination in space in patients with clinically isolated syndromes: A multicentre follow-up study. *Lancet Neurol* 2006;**5**:221–227.

27. Mikaeloff Y, Adamsbaum C, Husson B, *et al*. MRI prognostic factors for relapse after acute CNS inflammatory demyelination in childhood. *Brain* 2004;**127**:1942–1947.

28. Ishihara O, Yamaguchi Y, Matsuishi T, *et al*. Multiple ring enhancement in a case of acute reversible demyelinating disease in childhood suggestive of acute multiple sclerosis. *Brain Dev* 1984;**6**:401–406.

29. Wang CH, Walsh K. Multiple ring-enhancing lesions in a child with relapsing multiple sclerosis. *J Child Neurol* 2002;**17**:69–72.

30. Balassy C, Bernert G, Wober-Bingol C, *et al*. Long-term MRI observations of childhood-onset relapsing–remitting multiple sclerosis. *Neuropediatrics* 2001;**32**:28–37.

31. McAdam LC, Blaser SI, Banwell BL. Pediatric tumefactive demyelination: Case series and review of the literature. *Pediatr Neurol* 2002;**26**:18–25.

32. Chabas D, Castillo-Trivino T, Mowry EM, Strober JB, Glenn OA, Waubant E. Vanishing MS T2-bright lesions before puberty: A distinct MRI phenotype? *Neurology* 2008;**71**:1090–1093.

33. Tintore M, Rovira A, Rio J, *et al*. New diagnostic criteria for multiple sclerosis: Application in first demyelinating episode. *Neurology* 2003;**60**:27–30.

34. Callen DJ, Shroff MM, Branson HM, *et al*. MRI in the diagnosis of pediatric multiple sclerosis. *Neurology* 2009;**72**:961–967.

35. Chabas D, Pelletier D. Sorting through the pediatric MS spectrum with brain MRI. *Nat Rev Neurol* 2009;**5**:186–188.

36. Okuda DT, Mowry EM, Beheshtian A, *et al*. Incidental MRI anomalies suggestive of multiple sclerosis: The radiologically isolated syndrome. *Neurology* 2009;**72**:800–805.

37. Bonhomme GR, Waldman AT, Balcer LJ, *et al*. Pediatric optic neuritis: Brain MRI abnormalities and risk of multiple sclerosis. *Neurology* 2009;**72**:881–885.

38. Wilejto M, Shroff M, Buncic JR, Kennedy J, Goia C, Banwell B. The clinical features, MRI findings, and outcome of optic neuritis in children. *Neurology* 2006;**67**:258–262.

39. Riikonen R, Ketonen L, Sipponen J. Magnetic resonance imaging, evoked responses and cerebrospinal fluid findings in a follow-up study of children with optic neuritis. *Acta Neurol Scand* 1988;**77**:44–49.

40. Brex PA, Ciccarelli O, O'Riordan JI, Sailer M, Thompson AJ, Miller DH. A longitudinal study of abnormalities on MRI and disability from multiple sclerosis. *N Engl J Med* 2002;**346**:158–164.

41. Kalkers NF, Bergers E, Castelijns JA, *et al*. Optimizing the association between disability and biological markers in MS. *Neurology* 2001;**57**:1253–1258.

42. Edwards SG, Liu C, Blumhardt LD. Cognitive correlates of supratentorial atrophy on MRI in multiple sclerosis. *Acta Neurol Scand* 2001;**104**:214–223.

43. Fisher E, Lee JC, Nakamura K, Rudick RA. Gray matter atrophy in multiple sclerosis: A longitudinal study. *Ann Neurol* 2008;**64**:255–265.

44. Julian L, Im-Wang S, Chabas D, *et al*. Learning and memory in pediatric multiple sclerosis. ACTRIMS/ECTRIMS meeting 2008.

45. Bruck W, Bitsch A, Kolenda H, Bruck Y, Stiefel M, Lassmann H. Inflammatory central nervous system demyelination: Correlation of magnetic resonance imaging findings with lesion pathology. *Ann Neurol* 1997;**42**:783–793.

46. Bagnato F, Jeffries N, Richert ND, *et al*. Evolution of T1 black holes in patients with multiple sclerosis imaged monthly for 4 years. *Brain* 2003;**126**:1782–1789.

47. Tenembaum S, Chamoles N, Fejerman N. Acute disseminated encephalomyelitis: A long-term follow-up study of 84 pediatric patients. *Neurology* 2002;**59**:1224–1231.

48. Gupte G, Stonehouse M, Wassmer E, Coad NA, Whitehouse WP. Acute disseminated encephalomyelitis: A review of 18 cases in childhood. *J Paediatr Child Health* 2003;**39**:336–342.

49. Callen DJ, Shroff MM, Branson HM, *et al.* Role of MRI in the differentiation of ADEM from MS in children. *Neurology* 2009;**72**:968–973.

50. Atzori M, Battistella P, Perini P, *et al.* Clinical and diagnostic aspects of multiple sclerosis and acute monophasic encephalomyelitis in pediatric patients: A single centre prospective study. *Mult Scler* 2009;**15**:363–370.

51. Mowry EM, Gajofatto A, Blasco MR, *et al.* Long lesions on initial spinal cord MRI predict a final diagnosis of acute disseminated encephalomyelitis versus multiple sclerosis in children. *Neurology* 2008;**70**:A135.

52. Pittock SJ, Lennon VA, Krecke K, Wingerchuk DM, Lucchinetti CF, Weinshenker BG. Brain abnormalities in neuromyelitis optica. *Arch Neurol* 2006;**63**:390–396.

53. Li Y, Xie P, Lu F, *et al.* Brain magnetic resonance imaging abnormalities in neuromyelitis optica. *Acta Neurol Scand* 2008;**118**:218–225.

54. Lotze TE, Northrop JL, Hutton GJ, Ross B, Schiffman JS, Hunter JV. Spectrum of pediatric neuromyelitis optica. *Pediatrics* 2008;**122**:e1039–1047.

55. Hahn JS, Pohl D, Rensel M, Rao S. Differential diagnosis and evaluation in pediatric multiple sclerosis. *Neurology* 2007;**68**:S13–22.

56. Rocca MA, Absinta M, Moiola L, *et al.* Functional and structural connectivity of the motor network in pediatric and adult-onset relapsing-remitting multiple sclerosis. *Radiology* 2010;**254**:541–550.

57. Vishwas MS, Chitnis T, Pienaar R, Healy BC, Grant PE. Tract-based analysis of callosal, projection, and association pathways in pediatric patients with multiple sclerosis: A preliminary study. *Am J Neuroradiol* 2010;**31**:121–128.

58. Deoni SCL, Peters TM, Rutt BK. High resolution T1 and T2 mapping of the brain in a clinically acceptable time with DESPOT1 and DESPOT2. *Magn Reson Med* 2005;**53**:237–241.

59. Hammond K, Metcalf M, Okuda DT, Vigneron D, Nelson SJ, Pelletier D. In vivo quantitative MRI of multiple sclerosis at 7T with sensitivity to iron. *Ann Neurol* 2008;**64**:707–713.

60. Haacke EM, Xu Y, Cheng YN, Reichenbach JR. Susceptibility weighted imaging. *Magn Reson Med* 2004;**52**:612–618.

Chapter 6

Differential diagnosis of multiple sclerosis and acquired central nervous system demyelinating disorders in children and adolescents

Nancy L. Kuntz and Jonathan Strober

Chapters in this volume describe clinical, pathologic, and diagnostic findings for a spectrum of acquired demyelinating central nervous system (CNS) disorders that occur in children. Progress toward determining triggers for these disorders in order to prevent occurrences and toward optimizing treatment in order to minimize morbidity and mortality are dependent on establishing the correct diagnosis for each child. This would not be difficult if pathologic specimens were always available for clinicopathologic correlation. However, concern regarding potential morbidity from biopsy of a central nervous system lesion makes it rare to have a pathologic specimen available for clinical diagnosis. Indirect measures, including serum and cerebrospinal fluid inflammatory markers, multimodality evoked potentials, and magnetic resonance imaging (MRI), are correlated with history and neurologic examination in order to reach a diagnosis. However, this analysis is not as universally specific as one would like. This chapter will review the spectrum of inflammatory, infectious, metabolic, and neurodegenerative disorders that can overlap or simulate the phenotype of demyelinating disorders in children, including its relapsing–remitting nature.

In 2007, a US Network of Pediatric Multiple Sclerosis Centers of Excellence funded by the National Multiple Sclerosis Society reviewed their experience regarding final diagnoses of children referred to the network for evaluation of possible pediatric multiple sclerosis (MS) [1]. Sixteen percent (67/407) of the children and adolescents presenting to this network had either alternate neurologic diagnoses or transitory symptoms that were determined to not be compatible with a demyelinating disorder. Table 6.1 lists the neurologic diagnoses or symptoms in those children who were determined to have alternative diagnoses. Diagnosis of possible MS had been offered in each of these children prior to referral for a second opinion. This experience validates the need to perform a complete personal medical history, thorough examination, extensive family history and indicated diagnostic testing to exclude other disorders that can imitate acquired CNS demyelinating disorders in children [2].

Systemic inflammatory disorders

Despite the overlap in clinical presentation, it is critical to make specific and precise diagnoses, since the treatment of the various inflammatory disorders may differ dramatically from treatment of pediatric MS.

Systemic lupus erythematosus (SLE)

SLE is a systemic autoimmune disorder characterized by inflammation of blood vessels and soft tissue [3]. The diagnostic criteria were most recently revised in 1997 [4]. CNS involvement is common and occurs over time in up to 70% of children presenting with SLE [3]. Warnatz observed that 81% of children with CNS lupus had no systemic involvement when they first presented with their CNS symptoms [5]. Neuropsychiatric SLE symptoms include cerebrovascular events (25%), psychosis (20%) and, in smaller numbers, chorea and encephalopathy [3]. There appears to be an increased frequency of vasculitic skin lesions, livedo reticularis and antiphospholipid antibodies in those children with SLE who have CNS involvement [6]. The majority of children with CNS

Demyelinating Disorders of the Central Nervous System in Childhood, ed. Dorothée Chabas and Emmanuelle L. Waubant.
Published by Cambridge University Press. © Cambridge University Press 2011.

Table 6.1 Final diagnoses of 407 children referred for evaluation of acquired CNS demyelinating disease

340 Acquired CNS demyelinating disease

67 Alternate diagnoses

    42 Other neurologic diagnoses

        13 migraine

        6 CNS vasculitis

        4 static encephalopathy

        3 cortical dysplasia

        3 mitochondrial cytopathy

        3 leukodystrophy

        3 chronic CNS infection

        3 peripheral nerve lesion

        2 CNS tumor

        1 coagulopathy

        1 cerebral folate deficiency

    25 Transient neurologic symptoms (± family history MS and ± nonspecific T2 hyperintensity brain MRI)

        12 paresthesias

        4 fatigue

        3 visual symptoms

        2 urinary incontinence

        2 involuntary movements

        1 vertigo

        1 tinnitus

lupus have cerebrospinal fluid (CSF) abnormalities including elevated total protein (30–48%), elevated IgG index (30%), oligoclonal bands (25–42%) and/or elevated white cell count (27–32%, primarily lymphocytes) [5]. A significant fraction of adolescents with SLE have MRI abnormalities consisting of white matter lesions and lesions at the white/gray matter junction. This is observed in patients with neuropsychiatric symptoms (54%) as well as in those without (39%) [7]. Serum markers of systemic SLE occur in about the same proportions as in adult SLE: 50% with positive Coombs test and 5–20% with anti-Smith, anti-RNP, anti-Ro, and anti-La antibodies [3]. Children with neuropsychiatric SLE have been observed to have higher rates of anti-dsDNA (61% vs. 25%) and anti-ribosomal P antibody (25% vs. 11%) than adults and lower rates of anti-histone antibodies (3% vs. 26%). Therefore, it is important for the clinical evaluation of children with new CNS/MRI lesions to include evaluation of the joints, skin and renal function which may be simultaneously involved in children presenting with CNS lupus. While only 19% of children proven to have CNS SLE have systemic involvement initially [5], the proportion increases to 70% over time [3]. Elevated CSF lymphocyte counts, clinical involvement of skin or joints, laboratory studies indicating renal involvement or abnormal serum markers (ANA, anti-dsDNA, anti-SM, anti-RNP) are clues that isolated neurologic symptoms in association with white matter abnormalities on MRI may be due to neuropsychiatric SLE rather than CNS demyelination.

Acute transverse myelitis occurs in 1–2% of patients with SLE [8]. Birnbaum and colleagues described two clinical sub-types of myelitis in a group of SLE patients between 15 and 70 years of age. One group consisted of patients presenting with rapid (<6 h) progression to peak of clinical deficit which included flaccid tone, decreased or absent muscle stretch reflexes, motor and sensory deficit, and urinary retention [9]. Patients with "gray matter involvement" usually presented with fever, nausea, and vomiting and were more likely to have systemic signs of SLE, elevated anti-double stranded DNA and CSF with signs of inflammation (mean of 386 white blood cells, neutrophilic predominance, mean CSF protein of 24 and mean CSF glucose of 33 mg). Spinal cord involvement of more than 4 vertebral segments and spinal cord swelling were seen in most patients with a small fraction (25%) of lesions demonstrating gadolinium enhancement [9]. The second type of clinical involvement was termed "white matter myelitis" and was more difficult to differentiate from the spectrum of neuromyelitis optica (NMO). These patients presented with spasticity and increased muscle stretch reflexes with high frequency of elevated anti-Ro/SSA autoantibodies (60%), lupus anticoagulant (55%), and anti-cardiolipin antibodies (45%). These patients' CSF was less inflammatory (mean of 10 white blood cells, lymphocytic predominance, mean CSF protein of 57 mg/dl and mean CSF glucose of 54 mg/dl). A lower incidence of systemic signs of SLE (14%) and a higher incidence of relapsing disease (71%) was noted in these patients who demonstrated a high frequency of NMO-IgG positivity (82%) [9]. In fact, the majority of their SLE patients with "white matter myelitis" met the 2006 revised diagnostic criteria for NMO, raising the possibility that their myelitis was a manifestation of two concurrent autoimmune diseases [9]. Whether these observations hold for younger children remains to be determined.

Optic neuropathy in SLE patients is often painless, progressive, sub-acute in onset and severe, responding incompletely to steroid therapy [10].

CSF oligoclonal bands can be detected in up to 50% of SLE patients, but tend to disappear when SLE activity is diminished by immune therapies [11].

In children, anti-phospholipid antibody syndrome can occur in response to viral infection, idiopathically or in association with SLE. It is the most common cause of an acquired hypercoagulable state in children [12]. It is associated with severe organ injury and renal involvement, and is a predictor of poor outcome in particular [13]. Anti-phospholipid antibodies have been reported in adult patients with NMO spectrum [14,15]. It is not known whether these are present in young children with NMO.

As isolated involvement of the optic nerves, spinal cord and brain have been noted in children eventually diagnosed with neuropsychiatric SLE, differentiation from acquired CNS demyelinating disease is important and sometimes difficult. Optic neuropathy without pain on eye movement, absence of sharply demarcated CNS MRI lesions, evidence of cord swelling without gadolinium enhancement, incomplete response to steroid therapy, and eventual development of systemic symptoms such as joint, kidney, and skin involvement should lead to suspicion of SLE. Serum anti-double stranded DNA is more specific for diagnosis of SLE and can appear up to a year prior to clinical disease onset [16]. It is important to remember that longitudinally extensive spinal cord involvement, positive serum autoantibodies (including ANA, anti-cardiolipin antibodies, lupus anticoagulant, anti-Ro/SSA), CSF inflammatory changes and CSF oligoclonal bands can be present in both SLE and acquired CNS demyelinating disorders.

Sarcoidosis

Neurosarcoidosis has an extremely variable presentation. Sarcoidosis in children (particularly pre-school-aged) has historically been termed uveoparotid fever with the combination of uveitis, swelling of the parotid gland and facial nerve palsy occurring concurrently [17]. Association of neurologic deficit with enlargement of lymph nodes, liver, and spleen as well as lung involvement or cranial neuropathy also suggests sarcoidosis. Bauman and colleagues summarized the clinical presentation for 29 children with neuro-sarcoidosis from reports in the literature. In prepubertal children, seizures were the most frequent presenting symptom (38%), while postpubertal children frequently presented with cranial nerve involvement (21%). In children of all ages, hypothalamic symptoms such as diabetes insipidus (21%), headaches (17%), motor complaints (14%), and papilledema (10%) were observed [18]. Elevated serum angiotensin converting enzyme (ACE) levels are suggestive (more specific than sensitive) of the diagnosis of sarcoidosis. It has been observed that serum ACE levels are higher in normal children than in adults [19]. CSF changes are non-specific and frequently non-diagnostic, with 19% of children with neurosarcoidosis having normal CSF findings. CSF pleocytosis (5–200 WBC, primarily lymphocytes) has been noted in 50–70%, elevated protein (up to 70 mg/dl) in 73% with increased IgG index in 37%, and oligoclonal bands noted in 19% [5]. While CSF-ACE has been found to be 94% specific, it is much less sensitive as only 33–55% of children with neurosarcoidosis have had elevated CSF ACE levels [5,18,20]. A skin test using the Kveim–Siltzbach spleen-derived antigen (the Kveim test) has historically been reported to be positive in 85% of patients but is no longer commonly available [21,22]. Tissue biopsy demonstrating a non-caseating granuloma is diagnostic [6]. Computer tomographic (CT) imaging, including spiral tomography of the chest, can help to localize involved lymph nodes to biopsy, but was diagnostic in only a fraction (28%) of cases [23]. Additional use of endobronchial ultrasound-guided transbronchial needle aspiration [24] or video-assisted cervical mediastinoscopy [25] has been reported useful for diagnosis. Fludeoxyglucose (18F) positron emission tomography (FDG-PET) scans are being used with increasing frequency in diagnosing this condition [26]. A significant fraction (24%) of children with neurosarcoidosis have been observed to have a CNS mass lesion at the time of diagnosis [18]. Multiple white matter lesions (frequently periventricular) are noted in 43% of patients with neurosarcoidosis and meningeal enhancement is frequently reported (38%) [18,22]. Differentiation of neurosarcoidosis from acquired CNS demyelinating disorders such as pediatric MS can be challenging. Involvement of other organ systems (such as eyes or reticuloendothelial tissue), positive CSF-ACE (when present) and meningeal enhancement noted on brain MRI scans should lead to consideration of sarcoidosis with search for appropriate tissue (lymph nodes, conjunctiva) to biopsy for confirmation of diagnosis.

Behçet syndrome

Behçet syndrome (BS) is a form of vasculitis that classically produces oral and genital ulcers and uveitis. There is a genetic predisposition in ethnic groups living along the historical Silk Route from the Mediteranean region to Japan. Gender frequency is equal between males and females and the disorder is infrequent in children [27]. Up to 15% of children with Behçet syndrome have neurologic involvement including an encephalomyelitis pattern [6]. Nervous system involvement in different individuals tends to either be caused by small vessel involvement with a sub-acute brainstem syndrome causing cranial nerve dysfunction, long tract motor signs, ataxia and confusion or, less frequently, involve thrombosis of large vessels with resultant intracranial hypertension and headaches. A neuropsychological profile with euphoria, disinhibition, paranoia and obsessive concerns is described in adults with BS. Virtually all of those with nervous system involvement from BS have a history of recurrent oral ulcers [27]. Standard diagnostic criteria (recurrent oral ulcers with at least two of the following findings: recurrent genital ulcers, uveitis, skin lesions and/or positive pathergy test) are delineated by Siva and Saip [27]. The skin pathergy test is specific for BS and involves puncturing the dermis with an 18 G needle and observing for the formation of sterile pustules indicative of neutrophil hyperreactivity at 48 h [28]. CSF can be normal in 25–30% of patients with neuro BS. Other individuals have a lymphocytic pleocytosis (mean WBC count of 80 but elevations to 1100 have been reported), elevated protein (73% with increased IgG index) and up to 20% with CSF oligoclonal bands [5]. The pattern of MRI lesions can be nonspecific, but T2 hyperintensities in the basal ganglia and brainstem are most common [17]. Lesions in the periventricular white matter and subcortical white matter are uncommon in BS. In summary, in patients presenting with new CNS lesions, the history of or a clinical examination demonstrating uveitis or mucosal ulcers in the mouth or genital region can suggest Behçet disease. While uveitis can occur in individuals with MS,

sometimes even prior to clinical onset of MS, it is uncommon and tends to be a chronic granulomatous anterior uveitis, which can be differentiated from that observed in BS [29].

Scleroderma

Children with linear scleroderma, which is sometimes descriptively referred to as scleroderma *en coup de sabre*, typically have unilateral (90%) cerebral lesions underlying the cutaneous lesions [30]. Skin lesions can be missed (subtle or hidden in the hair), but when they are detected, they are diagnostic. Thus, careful local skin examination is recommended in patients with unilateral brain lesions. Also, CNS lesions precede skin lesions in 16% of cases [30]. Patients can present with seizures (73%), uveitis or optic neuritis/atrophy (22%), headache (29%), and/or focal neurologic symptoms (11%). Neuropsychological symptoms are not uncommon (14%). ANA are positive in 26–66% of cases. The presence of anti-histone and anti-single stranded DNA antibodies may be more frequent with localized or linear scleroderma lesions than systemic disease [31]. CSF may show leukocytosis (64%) and positive oligoclonal bands or elevated IgG index (64%).

Primary or isolated CNS vasculitis

CNS vasculitis is difficult to diagnose because of the absence of cutaneous or systemic signs or symptoms. Abnormal cerebral arteriography and brain biopsy are frequently required to make this diagnosis and differentiate it from other disorders [32]. The prolonged and aggressive immune suppression required to effectively treat this disorder justifies the brain biopsy, despite its inherent risk.

Infections

Straightforward clinical presentations of bacterial or aseptic meningoencephalitis or enhancing focal mass lesions from brain abscesses or parasitic infestation are usually not difficult to differentiate from the relapsing–remitting acquired CNS demyelinating disorders. However, some CNS infections present in an insidious or atypical manner and can be difficult to separate diagnostically. This differentiation is critical, because the treatments for CNS infections and acquired CNS demyelinating disease are different and inaccurate diagnosis could lead to a treatment that might be contraindicated in another disorder (e.g. steroid treatment for demyelinating disease would be contraindicated in the setting of some CNS infections).

Tuberculosis

The lifetime rate of tuberculosis (TB) infection in developing countries is 2–5%. Risk factors for developing disease include young age and immune compromise (as with HIV infection) [33]. The combination of a persistent non-remitting cough for >2 weeks, documented failure to thrive in the preceding 3 months and fatigue had an 80–90% positive predictive value for the diagnosis of TB in children of various ages in endemic regions. Symptoms of TB meningitis include fever (91%), vomiting (87%), personality change (65%), seizure (62%), nuchal rigidity (59%), and headache (58%) [34]. The widespread exposure to tuberculosis and use of BCG vaccination makes the use of tuberculin skin tests less useful in predicting disease due to the TB bacillus [35]. Further, tuberculin skin testing has been demonstrated to be positive in less than 20% of HIV-infected children with tuberculosis, likely due to their immune-suppressed state [35]. CNS infections comprise 10–15% of all tuberculous disease. Tuberculous meningitis is the most frequent and recognizable form. However, approximately 10% of these patients develop tuberculoma that are intracerebral or intraspinal. Most of the intracerebral lesions are supratentorial, but children have been reported with cerebellar lesions. CSF examination in patients with TB meningitis frequently demonstrates an increased cell count (mean of 71 cells/mm^3 in one series with 90% of individuals having <500 cells/mm^3). Early during the clinical course, polymorphonuclear cells can predominate, but this switches to lymphocytic predominance within days, particularly with treatment. However, 21% of patients in one series had acellular CSF. CSF glucose levels were low compared to serum (64% had CSF levels a mean of 33% of blood glucose levels). CSF protein is usually elevated (85% had elevated protein with a mean of 2.1 mg/dl) [36]. Imaging of the brain in CNS tuberculous infection demonstrates hydrocephalus, basilar meningeal enhancement, tuberculomas and, occasionally infarction [34,37]. A retrospective pathologic series observed that only small fractions of patients had multiple tuberculomas or concomitant meningitis and lung involvement (4%

and 13%, respectively) [38]. However, an MRI series noted that the majority of patients (69%) with CNS TB had multiple lesions noted on brain MRI with lesions >1 cm in diameter demonstrating variable enhancement. On T2 sequences, tuberculomas most commonly demonstrated an isointense or hypointense core with hyperintense rim [39].

The setting of an isolated intracranial lesion in a patient without fever or obvious systemic signs is one in which differentiation of CNS TB infection from acquired CNS demyelinating disease is most important. Systemic signs of illness (e.g. weight loss, fever, cough, etc.) are usually present in patients with CNS TB and these or basilar meningeal enhancement would increase the possibility of a TB infection. The utility of TB skin tests declines if the patient lives in an endemic region for TB or has been immunized against BCG, in which case a positive skin test does not clarify if that is causally related to an identified lesion and declines if the child is immunocompromised as that may produce a false negative result [35].

Human immunodeficiency virus (HIV)

The incidence of CNS involvement with HIV is highest in the first two years of life. CNS involvement can occur before any other signs of immunosuppression and is frequently the first Acquired Immunodeficiency Syndrome (AIDS)-defining illness in children [40]. Therefore, in very young children, evidence should be sought for HIV infection or immunity, even without prior opportunistic infection. Primary HIV infection is rarely identified; however, a description of meningoencephalitis during HIV seroconversion in adults demonstrated normal CSF glucose (mean of 51 mg/dl), primarily lymphocytic elevation of CSF white cell count (mean of 52 cells/mm^3 with mean of 91% lymphs) and elevated CSF protein (mean of 139 mg/dl) [41]. Imaging abnormalities associated with CNS HIV infection have been detected in advanced disease or opportunistic infection. In more advanced disease, CNS imaging shows cortical atrophy and basal ganglia calcifications on CT scans and white matter lesions and central atrophy on MRI of the brain. Late stage myelitis due to HIV has shown tract pallor and vacuolar myelopathy with a marked cystic appearance [42]. These MRI changes are readily differentiated from those seen in demyelinating diseases. There is a single case report of a boy with known perinatally acquired HIV infection and no sign of opportunistic infection who had relapsing, remitting neurologic deficits felt to represent acquired MS (right anterior parietal CIS at age 8 years 9 months and a unilateral optic neuritis at 10 years 3 months) with stable HIV (CD4 count of 282/μl and an HIV viral load of 4148 copies/ml) [43].

HTLV

The human T-cell lymphotropic virus (HTLV) causes a chronic retroviral infection with increased incidence in the Caribbean, southern Japan, sub-Saharan Africa, and portions of South America. Carriers can remain asymptomatic. Clinical infection occurs less commonly in children (only 17 well-documented cases in children and adolescents in the literature) and these were observed to have a more rapidly progressive course than in adults [44]. In the majority of children, infection begins as a chronic relapsing infective dermatitis involving the scalp with a picture similar to eczema. This usually progresses to an inflammatory myelopathy termed HTLV-1 associated myelopathy/tropical spastic paraparesis [45]. Diagnosis is made when, in addition to a mild lymphocytosis and protein elevation, the CSF demonstrates HTLV antibody titers elevated above that in the serum. Patients are reported to develop uveitis, opportunistic infections and lymphoproliferative disease [44]. In adults, the presence of CSF IgG oligoclonal bands has been reported [46]. MRI of the spinal cord has been reported to be normal in most cases and to only rarely show atrophy [42]. Cerebral involvement has not been described in HTLV infection, so the differential diagnosis for these patients would include acquired demyelinating myelopathies which would show T2 hyperintensities on spine MRI.

Progressive multifocal leukoencephalopathy (PML)

PML is a progressive neurologic disorder with multifocal lesions caused by primary infection or reactivation of the JC virus, usually in immunocompromised patients such as those with an HIV infection. Clinical symptoms depend on the location of the multi-focal involvement, but frequently involves changes in cognition, personality and motor skills [47]. Individuals immunosuppressed from any cause are at increased risk of reactivation of the JC virus. Subclinical reactivation of the JC virus has been documented in MS

patients treated with natalizumab. Chen and colleagues recently demonstrated an increase in the presence of JC virus in the urine of MS patients from 19% at baseline to 63% after 12 months of treatment with natalizumab. After 18 months of treatment, 20% of these patients demonstrated evidence of JC virus in plasma and 60% in peripheral mononuclear cells [48]. To date, PML has not been reported in 24 children who have been treated with natalizumab for refractory CNS demyelinating disease (Yeh et al., personal communication). However, this does not exclude that it might happen in children in the future, since follow-up time was limited in the children treated with natalizumab and PML is thought to occur mostly after prolonged treatment in adults [47]. CSF has been reported to be normal in 70% of patients with PML. Increased CSF white blood cell count has been described in 20% of patients and increased CSF protein in 30% [49]. The diagnosis can now be established by positive CSF-PCR for the JC virus [42]. MRI lesions due to PML tend to be sub-cortical and patchy and then spread deeper and become confluent [50]. Boster and colleagues compared MRI findings in adult PML and MS and reported that crescentic cerebellar lesions were only observed in PML, that large, confluent T2 weighted lesions were seen more frequently in adult PML (74% vs. 2%), and that deep gray matter lesions occurred more frequently in PML (31% vs. 7%) [51]. They also noted that the magnetization transfer ratio (MTR) was low in both PML and MS, but higher in normal-appearing brain tissue in PML than in MS, suggesting that PML lesions were more sharply localized [51].

Herpesvirus/family

Viral encephalitis and cerebral thrombosis can both be initiated by infections with viruses from the Herpes family. On MRI, the nonenhancing cortical and sub-cortical signal enhancement can be difficult to differentiate from acute disseminated encephalomyelitis (ADEM). Involvement of medial temporal, inferior frontal, insular and cingulate gyrus regions, the presence of hemorrhage or diffusion abnormalities are more suggestive of herpes encephalitis. Ventriculoencephalitis is most suggestive of cytomegaloviral infections. Varicella-zoster infections are associated with post-infectious venous thrombosis which produces diffusion abnormalities on MRI (tropism of posterior fossa) [52].

Neuroborreliosis (Lyme disease)

Borrelia burgdorferi is transmitted to humans via tic bites. While it was first described in Connecticut, the endemic areas have spread from the northeastern USA through to the Midwest. There are large endemic areas throughout Canada and Europe as well. Experience has shown that only 40–50% of diagnosed patients recall a tick bite. Neurologic symptoms develop between 1 and 12 weeks post-exposure [53]. Lyme Disease involves the nervous system in 10–20% of infected children with neurologic symptoms which can occur in a relapsing–remitting fashion and are quite variable. Cranial nerve (particularly facial nerve) and peripheral nerve involvement is more frequent than central nervous system involvement (acute myelitis, hemiparesis, opsoclonus/myoclonus, and ataxia have been described as well as meningoencephalitis) [53]. Large series in adults have shown CSF protein elevated in 85% (mean 1.4 g/l), elevated CSF white cell count in 96% (mean of 90 cell/mm^3 with predominantly lymphocytes and plasma cells) and CSF oligoclonal bands present in 66% [54]. CSF cytology can be suggestive of a lymphoproliferative disorder [55]. CSF oligoclonal bands and elevated immunoglobulin synthesis tend to differentiate this from a non-Hodgkin's lymphoma (NHL). MRI abnormalities occur in nearly half of patients with neuroborreliosis and consist of variable numbers of small, nonenhancing T1 hypointense and T2 hyperintense lesions without mass effect [56]. Lesions are usually hyperintense on DWI imaging with decreased intensity on ADC mapping. Gadolinium enhancement of meninges and spinal roots has been described [42]. A case report of an adult with an ADEM picture, clinically and radiographically, has been described with autopsy confirmation of neuroborreliosis [57].

Mycoplasma

Mycoplasma pneumoniae is a common cause of encephalopathy and transverse myelitis in children. Clinical findings, CSF analysis and imaging in processes due to mycoplasma infection are not easily differentiated from viral infections. CSF demonstrates pleocytosis in 64% (mean of 49 cells/mm^3, range 8–339, primarily lymphocytes) and elevated protein in 41% (mean 80 mg/dl, range 40–1444) [58]. *Mycoplasma*-associated ADEM rarely includes ON. MRI demonstrates patchy, asymmetric FLAIR and T2 hyperintensities involving gray and white matter [59].

Whipple's disease

Whipple's disease is a chronic, relapsing illness caused by infection with the *Tropheryma whipplei* bacillus. It involves the gastrointestinal (GI) tract and joints most commonly, with primary or secondary CNS involvement being relatively uncommon. Neurologic symptoms can be quite variable and include cognitive changes, supranuclear gaze palsies, ataxia, syndrome of inappropriate anti-diuretic hormone and other focal deficits. Oculomasticatory myorhythmia, an uncommon involuntary movement, in which slow repetitive movements of masticatory muscles and mouth occur in synchrony with a pendular convergent/divergent nystagmus, is considered pathognomonic for Whipple's disease. Primary CNS Whipple's disease is particularly uncommon in children and adolescents [60,61]. A relapsing–remitting clinical course, mimicking clinical multiple sclerosis, has been described in an adolescent [62]. Early in the disease course, CSF has been reported as normal; however, later in the disease course a polymorphonuclear leukocytosis, the presence of oligoclonal bands and positive PCR for *Tropheryma whipplei* have been reported [63]. MRI changes are nonspecific and include T1 hypointense and T2 hyperintense lesions which may enhance with gadolinium. The enhancing lesions can serve as a target for the biopsy which is sometimes needed to confirm the diagnosis in the absence of positive CSF PCR [62]. In the setting of a GI illness with unexplained neurologic symptoms, such as supranuclear vertical gaze palsy, rhythmic palatal myoclonus and eye movements, dementia with psychiatric symptoms, and/or hypothalamic manifestations, a small bowel biopsy should be strongly considered if there are no low-risk CNS lesions to consider for diagnostic biopsy [64].

CNS fungal infections

CNS fungal infections occur most frequently in immunocompromised individuals. If the clinical presentation is that of either meningitis or a ring-enhancing localized lesion in an immunocompromised patient, recognition may not be difficult. However, localized abscesses have been reported in immunocompetent children [65], and some mycotic infections, particularly aspergillosis, can present with multi-focal involvement [66]. Steroid-responsive demyelinating lesions in the central and peripheral nervous systems have been caused by diffuse histoplasmosis in a child (personal observation, JS). CSF findings vary depending on the immune competence of the individual patient, with immunocompromised patients frequently demonstrating normal to low lymphocyte counts in the CSF and large numbers of yeast forms on microscopic analysis as well as higher probability of positive fungal culture [67].

Neurocysticercosis

Cysticercosis is a parasitic infection caused by a pork tapeworm. Endemic areas include Central and South America, Mexico, India, Indonesia, China, and sub-Saharan Africa. Clinical presentation is usually either with focal onset seizures or increased intracranial pressure. Diagnosis is frequently made from imaging with confirmation by serology on serum or CSF. Immunoblot assay for the c. cellulosae antigen of the *Taenia* parasite is 100% specific. If there are two or more CNS lesions, there is a 90% sensitivity with serum testing; however, the sensitivity in children is only 16% when there is a single CNS lesion [68]. CSF can be normal or show a lymphocytic pleocytosis, mild eosinophilia and mildly low glucose [69]. CNS imaging demonstrates cysts, primarily in the cerebral hemispheres, that can either be solitary, clustered or racemic. Gadolinium enhancement is in a "ring-like" pattern on MRI and the lesions tend to be hypointense on DWI imaging [42]. Intramedullary spinal cord lesions have been described as etiology of a chronic myelopathy [70]. The diagnosis frequently depends on a combination of clinical features, direct imaging of the parasite within the cyst on CT or MRI and/or immune markers. Diagnostic overlap with acquired CNS demyelinating disorders is possible when there is a single CNS lesion with negative serology and an unclear history of exposure.

Neoplasms
CNS lymphoma

A report describing a large series of children with Burkitt's lymphoma indicates that primary CNS lymphoma is uncommon. Seventeen percent of children had CNS involvement documented (neurologic abnormalities on examination and/or abnormal CSF findings) with primary sites for the lymphoma being abdomen or skeletal in the majority of cases [71]. Another large series demonstrated only 10/141

children with CNS involvement from NHL who had primary CNS lymphoma. Another 10 children had low-grade NHL with head and neck primaries. The rest of the 121 children with CNS involvement had high-grade NHL with abdominal or skeletal primaries [72]. CSF cytology has high specificity for leptomeningeal involvement (95%) but is not as sensitive (<50% of patients have abnormal findings) [73]. There is a dissociation between CSF cell count and cytology, with 29% of patients with positive CSF cytology demonstrating <4 cells/mm^3 in the CSF [74]. Imaging of CNS lymphomas, in immunocompromised patients, demonstrates ring-enhancing lesions. However, in immunocompetent patients, CNS lymphomas appear as single or multiple periventricular lesions with gadolinium enhancement. Atypical presentations in 10% of patients demonstrate infiltrative lesions without gadolinium enhancement. Fine aspirate cytology or open biopsy are required for definitive diagnosis [75]. Unlike acquired CNS demyelinating disease, a patient has been described with a clinical myelopathy due to a primary CNS lymphoma who was symptomatic prior to detection of changes on spinal MRI [76]. Diagnostic evaluation should be performed prior to pulse steroid therapy, as lymphomas are steroid-responsive and diagnostic tests performed post steroids may be false-negative [73].

Optic pathway gliomas

Most optic pathway gliomas in children involve neural pathways beyond the optic nerve itself (chiasm, hypothalamus, etc.). The presenting symptoms are variable and include such symptoms as hypothalamic dysfunction, nystagmus, headache, and vomiting, as well as decreased visual acuity. A large fraction of children with optic pathway gliomas have recognizable stigmata of neurofibromatosis. In the above circumstances, the likelihood of misdiagnosing optic neuritis is very small. However, 22% of a recent large series of childhood optic pathway gliomas reported by the Hospital for Sick Kids in Toronto presented with unilateral optic nerve involvement only and over half of these had decreased visual acuity as the primary presenting complaint. If the glioma is limited to the optic nerve and does not demonstrate a globular silhouette and/or tortuosity, the imaging might suggest ON. In that circumstance, additional clinical evaluation would be useful. A history of eye pain with movement would be more suggestive of ON. Signs or symptoms consistent with a diagnosis of neurofibromatosis would be more suggestive of an optic nerve glioma [77].

Leukodystrophies

Leukodystrophies are a group of inherited disorders affecting myelin development. Pathologically they can be dysmyelinating, hypomyelinating, or cause spongiform degeneration. They can also be classified by their underlying etiology, either metabolic with abnormal metabolism of lipid or organic acid, a defect of energy production, a disorder of myelin protein or other, less common causes. These are usually slowly progressive degenerative disorders making the history key in differentiating these conditions from MS. Occasionally these disorders can present with episodic decline and, while they often present with symmetric changes on MRI, more patchy CNS involvement has been reported. Finally, while most of these diseases do not currently have proven treatments, some patients seemingly respond to steroid therapy, making it even more difficult to separate these conditions from MS.

Adrenoleukodystrophy (ALD)

This is an X-linked disorder due to abnormal lipid metabolism. Almost half of the cases present in childhood with cerebral dysfunction [78], while the other half present as either a cerebellar form or as adrenomyeloneuropathy. The latter is more common in female carriers, who typically present in their 20s to 40s. ALD tends to affect the parieto-occipital white matter symmetrically, helping to differentiate it from MS. The disorder can be diagnosed by finding elevated very long chain fatty acids (VLCFA) in plasma, which would be normal in cases that mimic MS [79]. It is caused by a mutation in ALD protein which is needed to localize VLCFA-CoA synthetase to the peroxisome.

Krabbe's disease

Also known as globoid cell leukodystrophy, Krabbe's is a disorder of glycosphingolipid storage. Most children present before 6 months of age with extreme irritability followed by rigidity and tonic spasms. The peripheral nervous system is affected early in the course and CSF protein is usually elevated. MRI shows symmetric plaque-like areas in the centrum semiovale on T1 and T2 [80]. However, the juvenile form usually begins between the ages of 4 and 20 years. These patients frequently have normal cognitive abilities and signs of a sensorimotor demyelinating polyneuropathy. CSF protein is usually normal and the parieto-occipital white matter is often affected in a symmetric manner. Diagnosis is made by measuring the deficient enzyme, galactocerebrosidase, in leukocytes or cultured fibroblasts.

Metachromatic leukodystrophy (MLD)

This is another lysosomal storage disease of glycosphingolipids causing white matter disease. It is due to a deficiency of arylsulfatase A, which can be measured in serum. Sulfatides can be measured in the urine as a screening test. Again, the peripheral nervous system can be involved, more commonly in younger children, while those presenting later in childhood through adulthood often present with behavioral or psychiatric changes [81].

Pelizaeus–Merzbacher disease (PMD)

PMD is a disorder of myelin formation, most often due to a mutation in proteolipid protein (PLP), which is located on the X chromosome. The majority of patients present early in life with nystagmus, developmental delay and progressive spastic paraparesis. Case reports have been published on adults and children with PMD whose clinical findings satisfy criteria for MS and who clinically respond to treatment with steroids [82,83]. In the cases presenting earlier in life, MRI shows diffuse T2 signal in the white matter and rarely shows more discrete lesions. The peripheral nervous system may also be involved.

Childhood ataxia with diffuse CNS hypomyelination (vanishing white matter disease)

Patients with this disorder typically present with a chronic progressive disease with episodic deterioration brought on by injury or intercurrent illness [84]. Older patients tend to present with spasticity and ataxia with fairly well preserved cognitive function. As with the other leukodystrophies, MRI most often shows symmetric involvement of the cerebral hemispheric white matter. In addition, part or all of the white matter has a signal intensity close to, or the same as, CSF on proton density scans.

Alexander's disease

Juvenile-onset Alexander's disease typically begins between 6 and 15 years of age with bulbar dysfunction and a slowly progressive ataxia and spastic diplegia [78]. It has been reported that the adult form mimics MS [85]. Unlike those presenting earlier, macrocephaly is not usually seen. On MRI, the bilateral frontal regions are usually affected and show cystic changes [85].

Mitochondrial disorders

Mitochondrial disorders are a heterogeneous group of diseases where the ultimate problem is a decrease in energy production. They are inherited both autosomally and through mitochondrial DNA (mtDNA) mutations, a significant reason for the diverse nature of these conditions. Muscle and brain utilize the largest amount of oxidative phosphorylation (OXPHOS), and therefore most of these conditions present with failure of one or both of these organs, although any organ system can be affected.

In the CNS, several patterns of injury can be seen in mitochondrial disorders, from neuronal loss to demyelination [86]. White matter lesions have been reported in several mitochondrial syndromes, which are often associated with less severe lesions of gray matter [86]. Therefore, these conditions can be misdiagnosed as MS, and vice versa. To complicate matters, mitochondrial dysfunction can lead to mitochondrial hyperpolarization, which in turn predisposes to pro-inflammatory necrosis instead of apoptosis [87], blurring the distinction between the two disorders. Unfortunately, additional imaging techniques may not help differentiate the two conditions, since lactate, a marker of OXPHOS failure and inflammation, has been reported in both types of disorders [88,89].

Brain biopsy can help differentiate the two conditions, since spongy degeneration of the white matter is more commonly described in mitochondrial disorders such as Kearn–Sayre syndrome, infantile hepato-cerebral syndrome due to mutations in deoxyguanosine kinase, and mtDNA depletion syndromes [86]. Focal white matter lesions have also been reported in individual as well as multiple defects in complexes within the electron transport chain (ETC) [88]. Conversely, complex I activity has been found to be reduced in tissue from chronic active MS plaques [90], and activity of complexes I and III were found to be reduced in the motor cortex of patients with MS [91], further blurring the distinction between these two entities.

Apart from white matter lesions, mitochondrial disorders can present with an optic neuropathy. The most common of these conditions is Leber's hereditary optic neuropathy (LHON), which typically affects males and is most often due to an mtDNA mutation affecting complex I of the ETC [92]. Suppression of complex I in mice using a ribozyme inserted into an adenoviral vector caused mild swelling of the optic nerve head in some animals [93]. More importantly, the retrobulbar optic nerve was found to have axonal loss accompanied by MS-like demyelination. In fact, there are a group of mostly female patients with MS-like ovoid white mater lesions, CSF oligoclonal bands and LHON mtDNA mutations [94]. Often, these patients do not typically respond to routine MS treatments.

Given the significant overlap between MS and mitochondrial disorders, patients undergoing a work-up for MS should be evaluated for mitochondrial disorders. This is often difficult to accomplish, since serologic and CSF studies looking for metabolic markers of energy production failure, such as lactate, pyruvate, and alanine, can often be normal in patients with confirmed mitochondrial disorders. One can look for mtDNA mutations in the blood, which would help pick up those patients with LHON mutations, but mtDNA mutations can be negative in the blood while found in the affected tissue. This screen would also not pick up those patients with mitochondrial dysfunction due to autosomal mutations. If a mitochondrial disorder is suspected, a muscle biopsy is often required to be able to measure ETC complex activity and perform mtDNA sequencing and quantification.

Vascular disorders
CADASIL

Cerebral autosomal dominant arteriopathy with subcortical infarcts and leukoencephalopathy (CADASIL) usually presents in middle age with migraine-like vascular episodes and resultant MRI brain abnormalities. Mutations in the NOTCH-3 gene have been identified in these patients. Asymptomatic children, whose parents have been diagnosed with CADASIL, have been noted to have MRI abnormalities (small T2-hyperintense lesions in periventricular and subcortical white matter) and a *NOTCH-3* mutation, which confirmed their diagnosis [95].

SUSAC syndrome

Susac syndrome is a rare microangiopathy characterized by recurrent attacks with deficits due to lesions in the brain, inner ear, and retina. It is more frequent in adults, but has been reported in school-aged children [96]. The characteristic triad of encephalopathy, hearing loss, and branch retinal artery occlusion is easier to recognize; however, patients frequently present with only some of the symptoms, making this more difficult to differentiate from MS [96]. MRI findings include gray and white matter lesions with corpus callosal lesions, including T1 holes that are due to rapid cystic transformation and considered pathognomonic [97].

Migraine and hemoglobinopathies

Migraine headaches are familial and are diagnosed clinically with no biomarkers to confirm the diagnosis. Classical migraines are easy to recognize; however, aura sine migraine and/or atypical presentations are less easily diagnosed. MRI can demonstrate one or more small T2 hyperintensities and, as compared to pediatric MS, these occur in far fewer numbers, particularly infrequent in deep or periventricular white matter or in infratentorial, cerebellar, or brainstem locations [98]. Asymptomatic children with sickle cell disease who have MRI changes consistent with small cerebral infarcts have been shown to have greater likelihood of experiencing clinically apparent strokes on follow-up [99]. The incidence of asymptomatic small cerebral infarcts is twice as high in adolescents and young adults with beta thalassemia/Hemoglobin E (HbE) disease [100]. This emphasizes that most disorders with either a hypercoagulable state or potential for vasospasm may be associated with transient or episodic clinical events and abnormalities on MRI of the brain that will need to be differentiated from acquired CNS demyelinating disorders.

Other rare vasculitides involving the CNS in children

Other types of systemic vasculitis are infrequent in children but can affect the CNS and be difficult to differentiate by clinical and imaging findings from acquired CNS demyelinating disorders. Polyarteritis nodosa may be suspected when there is renal, joint and peripheral nerve involvement, and Wegener's granulomatosis when there is sinus, pulmonary, and renal involvement. Sjögren's syndrome should be suspected when sicca symptoms are prominent [5,6]. Sjögren's syndrome can affect both the brain and spinal cord. Primary Sjögren's syndrome does not present significantly differently in children than in adults [101]. Henoch–Schoenlein syndrome is a common vasculitis in children presenting with GI, renal, and cutaneous involvement (purpura). Neurologic involvement is not uncommon [6]. Kawasaki syndrome is a vasculitis leading to thrombosis and aneurysm formation in cardiac and cutaneous vessels which is recognized by its fever, conjunctivitis, lymphadenopathy, and mucosal involvement. Multi-focal neurologic lesions are common accompaniments [6].

Other disorders leading to MRI brain abnormalities
Celiac disease

Celiac disease is caused by intolerance to dietary gluten and in children is frequently associated with abdominal bloating, chronic diarrhea, and failure to thrive [102]. The most common neurologic symptoms are ataxia and seizures or CEC (a syndrome of Cerebral calcifications, Epilepsy, and Celiac Disease with calcifications observed on CT imaging but not on MRI) [103]. In the setting of diagnosed or classical phenotype of celiac disease, neurologic signs and symptoms may be easy to ascribe to an immunologic process. However, patients have been reported with relapsing symptoms, MRIs with multiple enhancing and nonenhancing inflammatory lesions in the brain and positive oligoclonal bands noted in CSF. In this circumstance, heightened clinical suspicion leading to testing for tissue transglutaminase antibodies is necessary to diagnose or exclude celiac disease [104].

Histiocytosis

Langerhans cell histiocytosis (LCH) is a disorder created by excessive numbers of tissue macrophages which attack multiple organs including the nervous system [6]. Onset is usually in childhood and organ involvement can include skin, bone, muscles, liver, lung, spleen, and bone marrow. The most common CNS lesion occurs in the hypothalamic pituitary region (with resultant diabetes insipidus). The next most frequent phenotype is a cerebellar syndrome associated with bilateral symmetric lesions in the dentate nucleus and/or basal ganglia. Symptoms are usually progressive although a relapsing–progressive course has been described [105]. Early in a disease process, it can be difficult to differentiate between CNS lesions caused by this and other inflammatory, immune-mediated processes [105]. A non-Langerhans cell histiocytosis, hemophagocytic lymphohistiocytosis (HLH), can be acquired or familial due to a *Munc 13–4* mutation. Disease is caused by excessive activation of antigen-presenting cells. Cytopenias, fever, splenomegaly, hypofibrinogenemia, low or absent natural killer cell function, and/or elevated soluble IL-2 receptor, ferritin, or triglycerides can be observed in addition to neurologic symptoms. MRI findings include multiple nodular or ring-enhancing as well as confluent parenchymal lesions [106]. Individual cases have been confused with acute disseminated encephalomyelitis (ADEM) [107].

Toxic/medication-related

Recently developed medications used to treat autoimmune diseases such as inflammatory bowel disease and arthritis block tumor necrosis factor (TNF) alpha receptors and have been associated with development of white matter changes on MRI and neurologic symptoms similar to an exacerbation of MS. Infliximab [108], adalimumab [109], and etanercept [110] are among the medications reported to induce MS-like episodes in patients.

Summary

Careful clinical documentation, serum and CSF testing and neuroimaging (at presentation and longitudinally) will likely provide the diagnostic specificity desired to differentiate between acquired demyelinating disorders of the CNS in children and the other disorders outlined in this chapter. However, prognosis, for anxious patients and families, and treatment decisions often hang in the balance before enough of the above datapoints are available to clarify diagnosis.

Careful but preliminary studies looking at MRI characteristics are attempting to identify reliable findings to differentiate between pediatric MS and other, clinically relapsing neurologic disorders [18]. Validation of these early findings as well as studies to define additional risk factors, clinical features and biomarkers are needed to further improve our ability to recognize acquired CNS demyelinating disease

and to differentiate it from other types of CNS lesions in children. Newer imaging modalities such as diffusion tensor imaging, magnetization transfer ratios, and volumetric analysis will likely play a future role.

Differential diagnosis key points

- Obtain precise disease history (onset, course, response to treatments, especially steroids).
- Obtain history of other medical illness and medication use (e.g. TNF alpha blocker, etc.).
- Obtain family history (e.g. CADASIL, familial hemophagocytic lymphohistiocytosis (HLH)).
- Look for systemic signs and symptoms (fever, meningismus).
- Look for clues from other organ involvement:
  - hearing loss and branch retinal artery occlusion in Susac syndrome;
  - joints/kidneys/skin in SLE;
  - GI symptoms for celiac or Whipple's diseases;
  - diabetes insipidus for histiocytosis;
  - uveitis/mucosal ulcers for Behçet syndrome;
  - facial neuropathy for sarcoidosis, neuroborreliosis;
  - oculomasticatory myorhythmia for Whipple's disease;
  - eczema-like scalp lesion for HTLV;
  - lymph nodes, splenomegaly, hilar adenopathy for sarcoidosis;
  - ON, short stature, hearing loss, strokes, fatigue for mitochondrial disease.
- Consider obtaining non-routine CSF studies such as cytology, PCR, stains, AFB, and fungal cultures.
- Consider MRI findings:
  - calcifications: celiac disease, CADASIL, sarcoid;
  - lesion shape, number, type of enhancement;
  - temporal relationship of findings and treatments (e.g. steroids may mask disease activity).
  - specific localization
    - gray/white junction: SLE;
    - insular, cingulate gyrus, med. temporal/inf. frontal: HSV;
    - periventricular: CMV;
    - symmetric involvement: leukodystrophies;
    - sub-cortical: CADASIL;
    - multi-focal small infarcts: migraine, hemoglobinopathies;
    - involvement of meninges.

References

1. Belman DC, Chitnis T, Gorman M, *et al*. Clinical spectrum of diagnoses in children referred for acquired CNS demyelinating disorders including pediatric multiple sclerosis. *Ann Neurol* 2007; **62**(S11):S115.

2. Hahn JS, Pohl D, Rensel M, Rao S. Neurology Supplement. Differential diagnosis and evaluation in childhood multiple sclerosis. *Neurology* 2007;**68** (16 Suppl 2):S13–22.

3. Mina R, Brunner HI. Pediatric systemic lupus erythematosis. *Rheum Dis Clin N Am* 2010;**36**: 53–80.

4. Petri M. Review of classification criteria for systemic lupus erythematosus. *Rheum Dis Clin N Am* 2005;**31**: 245–254.

5. Warnatz K, Peter H, Schumacher M, *et al*. Infectious CNS disease as a differential diagnosis in systemic rheumatic diseases: Tthree case reports and a review of the literature. *Ann Rheum Dis* 2003; **62**:50–57.

6. Duzova A, Bakkaloglu A. Central nervous system involvement in pediatric rheumatic diseases: Current concepts in treatment. *Current Pharmaceut Design* 2008;**14**:1295–1301.

7. Sanna G, Piga M, Terryberry JW, *et al*. Central nervous system involvement in systemic lupus erythematosus: Cerebral imaging and serological profile in patients with and without overt neuropsychiatric manifestations. *Lupus* 2000;**9**: 573–583.

8. Espinosa G, Mendizabal A, Minguez S, *et al*. Transverse myelitis affecting more than 4 spinal segments associated with systemic lupus erythematosus: Clinical, immunological and radiological characteristics of 22 patients. *Semin Arthritis Rheum* 2010;**39**:246–256.

9. Birnbaum J, Petri M, Thompson, Izbudak I, Kerr D. Distinct subtypes of myelitis in systemic lupus erythematosus. *Arthritis & Rheum* 2009;**60**:3378–3387.

10. Kurne A, Isikay IC, Karlioguz K, *et al*. A clinically isolated syndrome: a A challenging entity. Multiple sclerosis or collagen tissue disorders: Clues for differentiation. *J. Neurol* 2008;**244**: 1625–1635.

11. Scolding N, Mottershead J. The differential diagnosis of multiple sclerosis. *J Neurol Neurosurg Psychiat* 2001;**71**(Suppl 2):ii9–ii15.

12. Avcin T, Sinernan ED. Antiphospholipid antibodies in pediatric SLE and the antiphospholipid syndrome. *Lupus* 2007;**16**:627–633.

13. Lee T, von Scheven E, Sanborg C. Systemic lupus ery; thematosis and antiphospholipid syndrome in children and adolescents. *Curr Opin Rheumatol* 2001;**13**:415–421.

14. Birnbaum J, Kerr D. Devic's syndrome in a woman with systemic lupus erythematosus: Ddiagnostic and therapeutic implications of testing for the neuromyelitis optica IgG autoantibody. *Arthritis Rheum* 2007;**57**:347–351.

15. Karussis D, Leker RR, Ashkenazi A, Abramsky O. A subgroup of multiple sclerosis patients with anticardiolipin antibodies and unusual clinical manifestations: do Do they represent a new nosological entity? *Ann Neurol* 1998;**44**:629–634.

16. Smeenk RJ, van den Brink HG, Brinkman J, Termaat RM, Berden JA, Swaak AJ. Anti-dsDNA: Choice of assay in relation to clinical value. *Rheumatol Int* 1991;**11**:101–107.

17. Kone-Paut I, Yurdakul S, Bahabri SA, *et al*. Clinical features of Behçet's disease in children: An international collaborative study of 86 cases *J Peds* 1998;**132**: 721–725.

18. Bauman RJ, Robertson WC Jr. Neurosarcoidosis presents differently in children than in adults. *Pediatr* 2003;**112**:480–486.

19. Beneteau-Burnet B, Baudin B, Morgant G, Bauman FCH, Gibodeau I. Serum angiotensin-converting enzyme in healthy and sarcoidotic children with the reference interval for adults. *Clin Chem* 1990;**36**:344–346.

20. Tahmoush AJ, Amir MS, Connor WW, *et al*. CSF-ACE Activity activity in probable CNS neurosarcoidosis. *Sarcoidosis Vasc Diffuse Lung Dis* 2002;**19**:191–197.

21. Cikes N, Bosnic D, Sentic M. Non-MS autoimmune demyelination. *Clin Neurol Neurosurg* 2008;**110**: 905–912.

22. Zajicek JP, Scolding NH, Foster O, *et al*. Central nervous system sarcoidosis – diagnosis and management. *Q J Med* 1999;**92**:103–117.

23. Vrielynck S, Mamou-Mani T, Emond S, Scheinmann P, Brunelle F, deBlic J. Diagnostic value of high-resolution CT in the evaluation of chronic infiltrative lung disease in children. *Am J Roentgenol* 2008;**191**:914–920.

24. Wurzel DF, Steinfort DP, Massie J, Ryan MM, Irving LB, Ranganathan SC. Paralysis and a perihilar protuberance: Aan unusual presentation of sarcoidosis in a child. *Pediatr Pulmonol* 2009;**44**:410–414.

25. Karfis EA, Roustanis E, Beis J, Kakadellis J. Video-assisted cervical mediastinoscopy: our Our seven-year

experience. *Interact Cardiovasc Thorac Surg* 2008;7:1015–1018.

26. Bolat S, Berding G, Dengler R, Stangel M, Trebst C. Fluorodeoxyglucose positron emission tomography (PDG-PET) is useful in the diagnosis of neurosarcoidosis. *J Neurol Sci* 2009;**287**:257–259.

27. Siva A, Saip S. The spectrum of nervous system involvement in Behçet syndrome and its differential diagnosis. *J Neurol* 2009;**256**:513–529.

28. Varol A, Seifert O, Anderson CD. The skin pathergy test: Iinnately useful? *Arch Dermatol Rev* 2010;**302**:155–168.

29. Acar MA, Birch MK, Abbott R, Rosenthal AR. Chronic granulomatous anterior uveitis associated with multiple sclerosis. *Clin Exp Ophthalmol* 1993;**231**: 186–188.

30. Kister I, Inglese M, Laxer RM, Herbert J. Neurologic manifestations of localized scleroderma: A case report and literature review. *Neurology* 2008;**71**: 1538–1545.

31. Arkachaisri T, Fertig N, Pino S, Medsgene TA Jr. Serum autoantibodies and their clinical association in patients with childhood and adult onset linear scleroderma: A single center study. *J Rheumatol* 2008;**12**:2439–2444.

32. Elbers J, Benseler SM. Central nervous system vasculitis in children. *Curr Opin Rheumatol* 2008;**20**:47–54.

33. Kabra SK, Lodha R, Seth V. Some current concepts on childhood tuberculosis. *Indian J Med Res* 2004;**120**:387–397.

34. Wasay M, Ajmal S, Taqui AM, *et al*. Impact of Bacille Calmette–Guerin vaccination on neuroradiologic manifestations of pediatric tuberculous meningitis. *J Child Neurol* 2010;**25**:581–586. Epub 30 Sep 2009.

35. Marais BJ, Gier P, Hessling AC, *et al*. A refined symptom-based approach to diagnosing pulmonary tuberculosis in children. *Pediatrics* 2006;**118**:e1350–e1359.

36. Hooker JAB, Muhindi DW, Amayo EO, Mcligeyo SO, Bhatt KM, Odhiambo JA. Diagnostic utility of CSF studies in patients with clinical suspicion of tuberculous meningitis. *Int J Tuberc Lung Dis* 2003;7:787–796.

37. Tinsa F, Epsaddam L, Fitouri Z, Bousetta K, Becher SB, Bousuina S. CNS tuberculosis in infants. *J Child Neurol* 2010;**25**:102–106.

38. Bayindir C, Mete O, Bilgic B. Retrospective study of 23 pathologically proven cases of central nervous system tuberculomas. *Clin Neurol Neurosurg* 2006;**108**:353–357.

39. Wasay M, Kheleani BA, Moolani MK, *et al*. Brain CT and MRI findings in 100 consecutive patients with intracranial tuberculoma. *J Neuroimaging* 2003;**13**:240–247.

40. van Riea A, Harringtonb PR, Dowa A, Robertson K. Neurologic and neurodevelopmental manifestations of pediatric HIV/AIDS: A global perspective. *Eur J of Paediatric Neurol* 2007;**11**:1–9.

41. Villar del Saz S, Sued O, Falco V, *et al*. Acute meningoencephalitis due to HIV type 1 infection in 13 patients: Clinical description and follow-up. *J Neurovirol* 2008;**14**:474–479.

42. Kastrup O, Wanke I, Maschke M. Neuroimaging of infections of the central nervous system. *Semin Neurol* 2008;**28**:511–522.

43. Facchini SA, Harding SA, Waldron II RL. Human immunodeficiency virus-1 infection and multiple sclerosis-like illness in a child. *Ped Neurol* 2002;**26**:231–235.

44. Bittencourt A, Premo J, Oliveira MF. Manifestations of the human T cell lymphocytic virus type 1 infection in childhood and adolescence. *J Pediatr (Rio J)* 2006;**82**:411–420.

45. Verdonck K, Gonzalez E, Van Dooren S, Van Damme AM, Vanham G, Gotuzzo E. Human T-lymphotropic virus 1: Recent knowledge about an ancient infection. *Lancet Infect Dis* 2007;7:266–268.

46. Cruickshank JK, Rudge P, Dalgleish AG, *et al*. Tropical spastic paraparesis and human T cell lymphotropic virus type 1 in the United Kingdom. *Brain* 1989;**112**:1057–1090.

47. Clifford DB, Deluca A, Simpson DM, Arendt G, Giovannoni G, Nath A. Natalizumab-associated progressive multifocal leukoencephalopathy in patients with multiple sclerosis: Lessons from 28 cases. *Lancet Neurol* 2010;**9**:438–446.

48. Chen Y, Bord E, Tompkins T, Miller J, *et al*. Asymptomatic reactivation of JC virus in patients treated with natalizumab. *N Engl J Med* 2009; **361**:1067–1074.

50. Shah I, Chudgar P. Progressive multifocal leukoencephalopathy (PML) as intractable dystonia in an HIV-infected child. *J Tropical Ped* 2005;**51**:380–382.

51. Boster A, Hreha S, Berger JR, *et al*. Progressive multifocal leukoencephalopathy and relapsing-remitting multiple sclerosis: A comparative study. *Arch Neurol* 2009;**66**:593–599.

52. Baskin HJ, Hedlund G. Neuroimaging of herpes virus infections in children. *Pediatr Radiol* 2007;**37**:949–963.

53. Mygland A, Ljostad U, Fingerle V, Rupprecht T, Schmutzhard E, Steiner I. EFNS guidelines on

diagnosis and management of European Lyme neuroborreliosis. *Eur J Neurol* 2009;**17**:8–e4.

54. Oschmann P, Dorndorf W, Hornig C, Schefer C, Wellensilk HJ, Pflughaupt KW. Stages and syndromes of neuroborreliosis. *J Neurol* 1998;**245**: 262–272.

55. Kieslich M, Fiedler A, Driever PH, Weis R, Schwabe D, Jacobi G. Lyme borreliosis mimicking central nervous system malignancy: The diagnostic pitfall of cerebrospinal fluid cytology. *Brain & Dev* 2000;**22**:403–406.

56. Fernandez RE, Rothberg M, Ferencz G, Wujack D. Lyme disease of the CNS: MR imaging findings in 14 cases. *Am J Neuroradiol* 1990;**11**: 479–481.

57. van Assen S, Bosma F, Staals LME, *et al.* Acute disseminated encephalomyelitis associated with *Borrelia burgdorferi*. *J Neurol* 2004;**251**: 626–629.

58. Daxboeck F, Blacky I, Seidl R, Krause R, Assadian O. Diagnosis, treatment and prognosis of mycoplasma pneumonia in childhood encephalitis. *J Child Neurol* 2004;**19**:865–871.

59. Bitnun A, Ford-Jones E, Blaser S, Richardson S. *Mycoplasma pneumoniae* Encephalitis. *Semin Ped Infect Dis* 2003;**14**:96–107.

60. Tan TQ, Vogel H, Tharp BR, Carrol CL, Kaplan SL. Presumed central nervous system Whipple's disease in a child: Case report. *Clin Inf Dis* 1995;**20**:883–889.

61. Patel SJ, Huard RC, Keller C, Foca M. Possible case of CNS Shipple's Whipple's disease in an adolescent with AIDS. *J Int Assoc Physicians AIDS Care* 2008;**7**:69–73.

62. Duprez TPJ, Grandin CBG, Bonnier C, *et al.* Whipple disease confined to the central nervous system in childhood. *Am J Neuroradiol* 1996; **17**:1589–1591.

63. Panegyres PK, Edis R, Beaman M, Fallon M. Primary Whipple's disease of the brain: Characterization of the clinical syndrome and molecular diagnosis. *Q J Med* 2006;**99**:609–623.

64. Louis ED, Lynch T, Kaufmann P, Rahn S, Odel J. Diagnostic guidelines in CNS Whipple's disease. *Ann Neurol* 1996;**40**:561–568.

65. Gologorsky Y, DeLaMora P, Souweidane MM, Greenfield JP. Cerebellar cryptococcoma in an immunocompetent child. Case report. *J Neurosurg* 2007;**107**(4, Suppl):314–317.

66. Dotis J, Iosifidis E, Roilides E. Central nervous system aspergillosis in children: A systematic review of

reported cases. *Int J Infect Dis* 2007;**11**:381–393. Epub 2007 May 16.

67. Capoor MR, Nair D, Deb M, Gupta B, Aggarwal P. Clinical and mycological profile of cryptococcosis in a tertiary hospital. *Ind J Med Micro* 2007; **25**:401–406.

68. Singhi P, Paz M. Focal seizures with single small ring-enhancing lesion. *Semin Ped Neurol* 1999; **6**:196–201.

69. Wooten EW, Kochowiec A, Stiles S. Neurocysticercosis: A classic case and clinical overview. *Antimicrob Infect Dis Newsl* 1995;**14**(4):25–28.

70. Goncalves FG, Neves PO, Jovern CL, Caetano C, Mai LB. Chronic myelopathy associated with intramedullary cysticercosis. *Spine* 2010; **35**:E159–162.

71. Mwanda, O. Aspects of epidemiological and clinical features of patients with central nervous system Burkitt's lymphoma in Kenya. *East African Medical J* 2004;**8** (Suppl):S97–103.

72. Salzburg J, Burkhardt B, Zimmermann M, *et al.* Prevalence, clinical pattern, and outcome of CNS Involvement in childhood and adolescent non-Hodgkin's lymphoma differ by non-Hodgkin's lymphoma subtype: A Berlin-Frankfurt-Mueünster Group Report. *J Clin Oncol* 2007;**25**:3915.

73. Chamberlain MC, Gilant ZM, Groves MD, Wilson WH. Diagnostic tools for neoplastic meningitis: Detecting disease, identifying patient risk and determining benefit of treatment. *Semin Oncol* 2009; **36**(4, Suppl 2):S35–45.

74. Chamberlain MC, Nolan C, Abrege E. Leukemic and lymphomatous meningitis: Iincidence, prognosis and treatment. *J Neuro Oncol* 2005; **75**:81–83.

75. Soussain C, Hoang-Xuan K. Primary CNS lymphoma: An update. *Curr Opin Oncol* 2009;**21**:550–558.

76. Herrlinger U, Weller M, Kuker W. Primary CNS lymphoma in spinal cord: Clinical manifestations may preceed MRI detectability. *Neuroradiology* 2002;**44**:239–244.

77. Nicolin G, Parkin P, Mabbott D, *et al.* Natural history and outcome of optic pathway gliomas in children. *Pediatr Blood Cancer* 2009;**53**:1231–1237.

78. Kaye EM. Update on genetic disorders affecting white matter. *Pediatr Neurol* 2001;**24**:11–24.

79. Wilkins A, Ingram G, Brown A, Jardine P, Steward CG, Robertson NP, Scolding NJ. Very long chain fatty acid levels in patients diagnosed with multiple sclerosis. 2009. *Mult Scler.* 2009; **15**(12):1525.

80. Sasaki M, Sakuragawa N, Takashima S, Hanaoka S, Arima M. MRI and CT findings in Krabbe disease. *Pediatr Neurol* 1991;7(4):283–288.

81. Shapiro EG, Lockman LA, Knopman D, Krivit W. Characteristics of the dementia in late-onset metachromatic leukodystrophy. *Neurology* 1994;44:662–665.

82. Gorman MP, Golomb MR, Walsh LE, *et al.* Steroid-responsive neurologic relapses in a child with a proteolipid protein-1 mutation. *Neurology* 2007;68:1305–1307.

83. Warshawsky I, Rudick RA, Staugaitis SM, Natowicz MR. Primary progressive multiple sclerosis as a phenotype of a PLP1 gene mutation. *Ann Neurol* 2005;58:470–473.

84. van der Knaap MS, Kamphorst W, Barth PG, Kraaijeveld CL, Gut E, Valk J. Phenotypic variation in leukoencephalopathy with vanishing white matter. *Neurology* 1998;51:540–547.

85. Pridmore CL, Baraitser M, Harding B, Boyd SG, Kendall B, Brett EM. Alexander's disease: Clues to diagnosis. *J Child Neurol* 1993; 8:134–144.

86. Filosto M, Tomelleri G, Tonin P, *et al.* Neuropathology of mitochondrial diseases. *Biosci Rep* 2007; 27:23–30.

87. Perl A, Gergely P, Jr., Nagy G, Koncz A, Banki K. Mitochondrial hyperpolarization: A checkpoint of T cell life, death and autoimmunity. *Trends Immunol* 2004;25:360–367.

88. Saneto RP, Friedman SD, Shaw DW. Neuroimaging of mitochondrial disease. *Mitochondrion* 2008; 8:396–413.

89. Lutz NW, Viola A, Malikova I, *et al.* Inflammatory multiple-sclerosis plaques generate characteristic metabolic profiles in cerebrospinal fluid. *PLoS ONE* 2007;2:e595.

90. Mahad D, Lassmann H, Turnbull D. Review: Mitochondria and disease progression in multiple sclerosis. *Neuropathol Appl Neurobiol* 2008; 34:577–589.

91. Dutta R, McDonough J, Yin X, *et al.* Mitochondrial dysfunction as a cause of axonal degeneration in multiple sclerosis patients. *Ann Neurol* 2006;59: 478–489.

92. Wallace DC. Mitochondrial diseases in man and mouse. *Science* 1999;283:1482–1488.

93. Qi X, Lewin AS, Hauswirth WW, Guy J. Suppression of complex I gene expression induces optic neuropathy. *Ann Neurol* 2003;53:198–205.

94. Harding AE, Sweeney MG, Miller DH, *et al.* Occurrence of a multiple sclerosis-like illness in women who have a Leber's hereditary optic neuropathy mitochondrial DNA mutation. *Brain* 1992;115:979–989.

95. Fattapposta F, Restuccia R, Pirro C, *et al.* Early diagnosis in cerebral autosomal dominant arteriopathy with subcortical infarcts and leukoencephalopathy (CADASIL): The role of MRI. *Funct Neurol* 2004;19:239–242.

96. Saliba M, Pelosse B, Omtchilova M, Laroche L. Susac syndrome and ocular manifestation in a 14-year-old girl. *Fr Ophthalmol* 2007;30:1017–1022.

97. Eluvathingal Muttikkal TJ, Vattoth S, Keluth Chavan VN. Susac syndrome in a young child. *Pediatr Radiol* 2007;37:710–713.

99. Kugler S, Anderson B, Cross D, *et al.* Abnormal cranial magnetic resonance imaging scans in sickle cell disease. Neurological correlates and clinical implications. *Arch Neurol* 1993;50:629–635.

100. Metarugcheep P, Chanyawattiwongs S, Srisubat K, Pootrakul P. Clinical silent cerebral infarct (SCI) in patients with thalassemia diseases assessed by magnetic resonance imaging (MRI). *J Med Assoc Thai* 2008;91:889–894.

101. Takei S. Sjogrens syndrome (SS) in childhood: Is it essentially different from adult SS. *Nihon Rinsho Meneki Gakkai Konishi* 2010;33:8–14.

102. Jones R, Sleet S. Easily Missed? Coeliac disease. *Br Med J* 2009;338:a3058.

103. Hernandez MA, Colina G, Ortigosa L. Epilepsy, cerebral calcifications and clinical or subclinical coeliac disease. Course and follow-up with gluten-free diet. *Seizure* 1998;7:49–54.

104. Ghezzi A, Filippi M, Falini A, Zaffaroni M. Cerebral involvement in celiac disease: A serial MRI study in a patient with brainstem and cerebellar symptoms. *Neurology* 1997;49:1447–1450.

105. Wnorowski M, Prosch H, Prayer D, Janssen G, Gadner H, Grois N. Pattern and course of neurodegeneration in Langerhans cell histiocytosis. *J Pediatr* 2008;153:127–132.

106. Goo HW, Weon YC. A spectrum of neuroradiological findings in children with haemophagocytic lymphohistiocytosis. *Pediatr Radiol* 2007; 37:1110–1117.

107. Weisfeld-Adams JD, Frank Y, Havalad V, *et al.* Diagnostic challenges in a child with familial hemophagocytic lymphohistiocytosis type 3 (FHLH3) presenting with fulminant neurologic disease. *Childs Nerv Syst* 2009; 25:153–159.

108. Jarand J, Zochodne DW, Martin LO, Voll C. Neurologic complications of infliximab. *J Rheumatol* 2006;**33**:1018–1020.

109. Mansoor A, Luggen M, Herman JH, *et al.* Hypertrophic pachymeningitis in rheumatoid arthritis after adalimumab administration. *J Rheumatol* 2006;**33**:2344–2346.

110. Sicotte NL, Voskuhl RR. Onset of multiple sclerosis associated with anti-TNF therapy. *Neurology* 2001;**57** (10):1885–1888.

Pediatric multiple sclerosis course and predictive factors

Christel Renoux and Emmanuelle L. Waubant

Course of the disease

Methodological considerations

While the natural history of multiple sclerosis (MS) has been extensively studied and is now relatively well known, it actually describes mostly the disease course in patients with adult onset, as they represent the vast majority of individuals affected by MS. Efforts towards the description of the course of childhood-onset MS are more recent. This is in part due to the smaller number of patients affected before the age of 18 years, and thus the need for collaborative data collection, but also due to the overall lack of diagnostic criteria for MS in younger patients until the operational criteria were published [1]. Although the definition of what constitutes a childhood onset varies between studies, the cut-off has been set at 15 or 16 years in most studies. Recent consensus definitions propose to set the upper limit of age of onset to 17 years (e.g. exclude onset occurring at age 18) [1].

The literature on the natural history of MS with childhood onset has long been dominated by case reports or case series [2–9]. Few studies consist of more than a handful of cases [10–14]. Such studies are generally hospital-based from MS centers, even though some authors consider their cohort as population-based in a well-defined region [5]. More recently, larger cohorts have emerged as a result of collaboration between MS centers, generally within a country. Some cohorts are composed of patients followed in child neurology MS centers [15], or both in pediatric and adult MS centers [16]. Others include patients with onset of MS in childhood followed in adult MS centers at the time of the study [17–20]. In these MS cohorts from adult neurology departments, some patients had been previously diagnosed and followed in pediatric neurology departments.

Therefore, the diagnosis was not necessarily made retrospectively in adulthood. Information gathered from these two sources, child and adult neurology departments, are best seen as complementary. The former allows a more precise description of characteristics at onset, unusual presentations, and challenges with differential diagnoses, whereas the latter takes advantage of a substantial follow-up to describe the long-term evolution and prognosis. Of note, the latter does not include cases that deceased early in life either from MS or from other causes, such as suicide. Some differences may also exist in the age distribution in these cohorts, the child neurology cohorts tending to over-represent younger patients at onset and patients with more severe presentations, whereas teenagers may be more frequent in cohorts from adult centers. In addition, patients with milder diseases may come to the attention of neurologists later during disease course, e.g. by the time they are adults. Finally, the above-cited cohorts virtually all consist of patients from Western Europe and North America. However, the number of studies on childhood-onset MS from other regions is increasing, which will allow the study of potential geographical variations in the course of the disease [21–24].

Our knowledge of the course of childhood-onset MS has increased considerably in the past 5 years, although at the price of several limitations. Mainly, as noted above, the small number of patients in most series precludes any firm conclusion, and the mean follow-up is often relatively short (not exceeding a few years) for such a lifelong disease. Other issues arise when, in an effort to precisely describe the onset of disease, only patients seen from the beginning or shortly after the first symptoms are studied. This restriction may introduce a selection bias towards the more severe cases or patients with a better access to care.

Demyelinating Disorders of the Central Nervous System in Childhood, ed. Dorothée Chabas and Emmanuelle L. Waubant. Published by Cambridge University Press. © Cambridge University Press 2011.

There are also some epidemiological issues worth considering when dealing with cohorts of patients with various durations of disease and follow-up and sometimes substantial loss to follow-up. For instance, only the most recent works have taken advantage of survival analysis such as Kaplan–Meier survival curves to estimate accrual of disability over time, despite studying cohorts of patients with different follow-up durations and not having all patients encountering the outcome under study (e.g. time to develop limited ambulation). In spite of these limitations, a number of studies add valuable information about natural history of childhood-onset MS, in terms of clinical presentation, disease course, and prognosis.

Disease onset (clinical, biological, radiological)

Initial symptoms

There are overall no major differences in the clinical presentation between childhood- and adult-onset MS that suggest that the childhood form of the disease has a totally different biological underlying. There are, however, some particularities that need to be recognized.

In most series, the initial presentation is predominantly monosymptomatic (or monoregional depending on the classification of symptoms), with a frequency ranging from 56.2 to 87.9% of the patients [14,18,19,25]. In one study of juvenile patients with MS, the onset was monosymptomatic in 48.6% of the 72 patients included, but the age at onset was less than 21 years old instead of the usual cut-off of 15 or 16 [26].

The respective frequency of different neurological symptoms at onset is difficult to establish due to the various classification systems used and to different referral patterns (e.g. in centers where ophthalmologists refer patients to MS clinics, optic neuritis will be over-represented). For instance, motor symptoms were the most frequent in two series (53.6% and 36.1% of the patients) [5,14], whereas sensory disturbance were more common in two other cohorts (26.4% and 25.9%) [17,19]. Other reported brainstem dysfunction (25%), optic neuritis (52%), diplopia, and sensory symptoms (27.7%) as being the most common at onset [12,18,25]. Although few studies to date have compared pediatric- and adult-onset MS patients seen at the same institutions [14], taken together, the overall data suggest, however, an over-representation of optic neuritis and brainstem dysfunction as compared to the adult-onset presentation and an under-representation of long tracts or spinal cord dysfunction [12,14,17–20]. In patients with very early onset (e.g. before the age of 10 years), ataxia may be the initial feature in up to 60% of the patients [27–29].

In some cases of pediatric-onset MS, neurological symptoms can be accompanied by an encephalopathy with various degrees of impaired consciousness, behavior abnormalities, and seizures, sometimes in addition to nausea, vomiting, and fever which contrasts with adult-onset presentation [3,7–9,25,30,31]. These manifestations may be more frequent in very young children at onset [15,28]. In fact, in a multivariate analysis of the UCSF cohort of 77 children with childhood-onset, the proportion of patients with encephalopathy at the time of first clinical presentation decreased with increasing age at onset (Odds ratio 0.69 (95% confidence interval, CI, 0.52–0.9) for each additional year) [29]. The presence of an encephalopathy during demyelinating events contributes to the difficulty in differentiating a first episode of MS from acute disseminated encephalomyelitis (ADEM) in some cases [1]. Thus clinical and MRI follow-up are important to distinguish between the two entities (see Chapters 17 and 18). In fact, among 296 patients who experienced a first demyelinating event of the central nervous system (CNS) before the age of 16 recruited from French child neurology departments, 20% of the patients who were ultimately diagnosed with MS after a mean follow-up of 3 years had been initially diagnosed with ADEM. Other unusual presentations of MS in childhood have also been reported. For instance, a case report described a pseudo-tumoral presentation with intermittent headache, nausea, vomiting subsequently followed by head tilt, poor balance, and deteriorating handwriting. Imaging showed a right cerebellar mass and the pathology of the resected mass revealed an extensive demyelinating process [32]. Another report mentioned the occurrence of bilateral intermediate uveitis in an 8-year-old girl. She presented with three subsequent relapses of similar symptoms before the first neurological manifestations which occurred at the age of 21 [33].

Biological findings at onset

In childhood-onset MS, the cerebrospinal fluid (CSF) profile is not fundamentally different from the adult-onset MS. A mild pleiocytosis is frequent, but cell counts up to 60 or $100/mm^3$ have been reported [30,34]. The total protein concentration is within normal limits or slightly increased [9,34]. Using iso-electric focusing followed by immunoblotting, oligo-clonal bands (OCB) were found in 92% of a cohort of 136 patients with onset before age 16, who had lumbar puncture at first or second attack, supporting the diagnosis of MS with a sensitivity similar to adult onset MS [34]. In addition, in the sub-group of 25 children with a disease onset before age 10, all but one had OCB at first analysis [34]. However, several reports suggest that the presence of OCB and elevated IgG index may be less common at disease onset in very young patients [31,35]. In a group of 39 patients with disease onset before the age of 6, OCB were reported in 8% at the time of their first attack, although the method used for detection was not provided [31]. The US Pediatric MS Network has made similar observations in a larger cohort of patients with an onset before the age of 11 years evaluated within 3 months of clinical onset. In addition to lower frequency of OCB and elevated IgG index, this young cohort also demonstrated an increased proportion of polynuclear neutrophils and monocytes compared to patients whose onset occurred between 11 and 18 years [35]. In the multivariate analysis including race/ethnicity, gender, and symptoms at onset of the UCSF cohort, OCB or elevated IgG index were 22% more likely with each additional year of age at disease onset (OR = 1.22, 95% CI 1.04–1.43).

Magnetic resonance imaging (MRI) findings at onset

As for adult-onset MS, MRI is the best imaging technique to detect lesions suggestive of MS in children (see specific chapter). The extent to which MRI characteristics are similar in adult- and childhood-onset MS is uncertain. The new diagnostic criteria for MS proposed for adults in 2001 formally incorporated MRI findings into the diagnosis algorithm [36]. While the basis for diagnosis remains the demonstration of dissemination in space and time [1], MRI can replace clinical manifestations as evidence for this dissemination. However, these criteria were not validated in a population of children with MS, and their usefulness for the diagnosis in this population is an area of debate [37]. In a recent study, the authors applied the McDonald criteria for dissemination in space retrospectively to a cohort of 20 children with a clinically definite MS according to Poser's criteria [38]. Of these, 17 had had their MRI at the time of the first

neurological episode and 18 at the time of the second episode. The authors found that only 9 (53%) patients fulfilled the McDonald criteria for dissemination in space at the time of the first attack and 12 (67%) at the time of the second attack.

MRI may also help to differentiate between ADEM and MS after a first episode of CNS demyelination. In a recent cohort of 296 patients with a first demyelinating event before the age of 16, MRI features associated with conversion to definite MS included the presence of lesions perpendicular to the corpus callosum, and well-defined discrete lesions [39]. These criteria along with the Barkhof criteria were applied to a cohort of 117 children from 11 neuropediatric centers in the Netherlands with a first CNS demyelinating event before the age of 16 [40]. Both criteria shared a high specificity (96 and 92%, respectively) as well as a high positive predictive value (83 and 81%) and negative predictive value (81 and 83%) for the conversion to MS. The sensitivity was low, however, especially in the group of patients with onset before the age of 10. More recently, a report studying retrospectively initial MRI of 28 children diagnosed with MS and 20 children with ADEM revealed that absence of a diffuse bilateral lesion pattern, presence of black holes and presence of 2 or more periventricular lesions allowed the distinction between MS and ADEM with 81% sensitivity and 95% specificity [41]. Unfortunately no information was available about the presence of gadolinium enhancement, thereby limiting the value of black holes as predictors.

Even though these criteria are predictors at the population level, none can be conclusive at the individual level. Also, as for adult-onset MS, MRI should be used as an aid to diagnosis along with a carefully conducted interview and clinical examination of the patient and certainly not as the sole diagnostic tool.

Initial course

The initial clinical course in most patients with childhood-onset MS is relapsing–remitting, with a relapse as the first manifestation of the disease in 85.7–100% of cases [5,17,19,20]. Primary progressive forms, with or without superimposed relapses, are not present in some cohorts [9,14,25]. The rarity of progressive forms at onset is not surprising, as long-term natural history cohort studies have consistently shown that the proportion of progressive forms from onset increases with age [42].

Course of the disease

Symptom severity at disease onset

There is very little known in terms of severity of symptoms at disease onset in children. In the UCSF cohort, the initial MS event was moderate or severe (according to definitions published in [43]) in 86% of children compared with 56% of adult-onset MS ($p < 0.0001$) [29]. It is possible that children who experience mild symptoms during their first MS event are not brought to the attention of a neurologist, thus at least in part explaining those findings. However, one cannot rule out that younger children have more severe onsets than teenagers, as recently found in adult-onset patients. In this population, younger patients are more likely to experience a severe MS onset [43].

Symptom recovery at disease onset

There is a notion that recovery from the first MS events, mostly in adults, is to some extent correlated with the event severity [43]. The degree of recovery after the first attack in children is poorly documented, based on few studies indicating a good recovery, and in case of incomplete recovery mild disability seems to be the rule [4,9,17]. In the largest cohort reporting this information, 68% of the 102 patients had complete recovery, 24% had partial recovery, and 8% had no recovery [17]. In the UCSF pediatric-onset cohort, although children had a moderate or severe onset more frequently, complete recovery was seen in 66%, which was similar to adults seen at the same center, questioning whether children have less irreversible neuronal injury during their first event or/and have a better ability to repair [29].

Time from onset of MS to the second neurological episode (including predictors of a shorter time to second episode)

The time between the first and the second neurological episodes varies greatly between studies, with a mean time estimated between 11 and 71.3 months [9,13,15,19,28,44], and a median time of 3.1 years in one study. Of note, a second neurological episode was documented up to 25 or 27.5 years after the first neurological manifestations [5,14]. Variations between studies may be due partly to the small sample size and local referral patterns but also to different durations of follow-up, since short-term studies cannot have included patients with a long time to the second attack. Differences may also exist in the regularity of clinical assessment of the patients and the definition of a relapse. The number of patients who experienced a second neurological episode within one year after onset varied from 23.3 to 75% [4,5,9,18,19]. Some authors have suggested a slightly shorter mean time to the second episode in childhood-onset patients (mean 1.6 years) compared to older patients at onset (1.7, 2.0 and 1.8 years for onset between 16–30, 31–40, and over 40 years of age, respectively) [45], and others a shorter median time, although in the latest case 28% of adult patients had received disease-modifying drugs following the first neurological episode [46]. In the multicenter French and Belgian KIDMUS study, the estimated median time, using survival analysis, of 2 years was not different from the estimate of 2.2 years for the adult onset group with an exacerbating-remitting onset from the Lyon MS cohort [20].

Recently, age of onset and race/ethnicity were reported to be the main demographic contributors to a higher risk of a second event during the first year of onset in a cohort mostly made up of adult-onset patients [47]. In this prospective cohort, younger patients and non-whites had a substantially higher risk of a second event during the first year of onset. Similarly, focusing on pediatric-onset patients, non-whites were found to have a higher risk of a second event during the first year of onset, even after adjusting for age of onset [29]. In another cohort, African-American children with MS had a higher relapse rate during the first years of the disease than white children [48].

Relapses (including relapse rate, location, and recovery)

The annualized relapse rate has been estimated to be between 0.38 and 0.87 for the whole relapsing–remitting period in the few studies with mean disease duration of 10 years or more that provided this information [12,13,19,49]. A prospective cohort study of patients with MS onset seen at a large MS center in Boston between 2000 and 2007 showed that patients with an onset before 18 years had a higher relapse rate during the first few years of the disease than adults seen at the same institution [46]. As compared to the above-cited cohorts, this one had different entry criteria, as only patients with the first visit within 12 months from first symptoms were included. Also, none of the pediatric-onset patients were treated at the first neurological event, whereas 28% of adult-onset patients were, although the authors attempted to adjust for it in the analysis.

Similar to the recovery after the initial episode, the quality of recovery after subsequent relapses during the relapsing–remitting phase has been reported to be good, at least in the early stages [5,29]. The suggestion by some authors that the degree of recovery may be better than in adult-onset MS is based more on clinical experience than on formal comparison between the two populations. The severity and recovery from the first MS event in adults predict the severity and recovery of subsequent events [43]. This has been reproduced in pediatric MS [29]. In addition, as in adults, non-white patients and possibly Hispanics are at increased risk of more severe demyelinating events [43,29].

Evolution to the secondary progressive phase

Time to secondary progression

Comparing the proportion of patients reaching the secondary progressive phase among studies is of little interest as it varies with the duration of follow-up. Indeed, the proportion of patients entering the progressive phase increases in a quasi-linear manner with duration of the follow-up [42,50]. Therefore, the proportion of patients reaching the secondary progressive phase is highly variable, from zero in studies with the shortest follow-up to more than 50% [4,5,7,14,19,20,25,49].

The median time between onset of the disease (first neurological episode) and conversion to secondary progression is therefore more informative and is ideally estimated using survival analysis. Three cohort studies of patients with onset before the age of 16 from adult neurology centers, taking advantage of an adult-onset comparison group and a long follow-up for two of them, provided such information. In their cohort of 113 patients followed at the University of British Columbia MS clinic for a mean of 19.8 years, Boiko and colleagues found that 53.1% converted to secondary progression [19]. The estimated median time from onset of MS to the secondary progressive phase was 23 years (no confidence interval provided) compared to 10 years for the comparison cohort of 722 adult-onset MS patients. Among the Italian cohort of 83 patients from the MS center of Bari, 14.4% reached the secondary progressive phase during a median disease duration of 14 years. The estimated median time to reach this endpoint was 16 years (4.3–44.3) compared to 6.9 years (0.6–29) for the patients with adult-onset MS [14]. However,

patients with childhood-onset MS were younger when reaching this stage (median age 30.7 years (17.6–52.6) compared to 37.5 years (22.7–60.2); $p<0.002$). Among the 385 patients with a relapsing–remitting initial MS course from the KIDMUS study, 110 patients (28.6%) converted to secondary progression [20]. The estimated median time from onset of MS to secondary progression was 28.1 years (95% CI 25.0–32.1) as compared to 18.8 years (95% CI 17.1–21.1) for the comparison cohort of patients with adult-onset MS ($p<0.0001$). The corresponding median age at assignment of the secondary progressive phase, estimated by Kaplan–Meier method, was 41.4 years (95% CI 37.8–45.7) in the childhood-onset MS cohort as compared to 52.1 years (95% CI 51.0–54.1) in the adult-onset MS cohort ($p<0.0001$). In summary, patients with childhood-onset MS convert to secondary progression on average 10 years later than patients with adult onset, but they are on average 10 years younger when reaching this phase of the disease.

Prognostic factors of secondary progression (clinical, paraclinical)

Both the Canadian and Italian cohorts described above were also used to examine prognostic factors associated with conversion to secondary progression. In univariate analysis, a high number of relapses during the first year or the first two years of the disease as well as a shorter time to the second neurological episode were associated with a higher rate of secondary progression [14,19]. In multivariate analyses, only a higher number of relapses in the first two years (more than one) was a prognostic factor for conversion to the secondary progressive phase [14].

Influence of environmental and genetic factors on the course of the disease

MS is likely the result of a complex interplay between genes and environment. The study of migrant populations has suggested childhood as the period of exposition to putative MS risk factors. Recently, the study of a Sardinian population suggested, by means of a space–time cluster analysis, that the susceptibility period in MS may be the first three years of life, particularly for patients with an onset before the age of 30 [51]. A recent Canadian study found an unexpectedly high proportion of childhood-onset MS patients born in North America with parents originating from low-prevalence countries [52]. This may indicate the prevailing detrimental role of the environment in triggering MS, at least during childhood.

Several environmental factors have been hypothesized to increase the risk of MS and have been studied in adults as well as in children with MS compared to healthy controls (see Chapter 3). Among these factors, childhood infections have received the greatest attention with little convincing results to date, except for infection with Epstein–Barr virus (EBV) [16,53–55]. The potential risk associated with vaccination and in particular hepatitis B has been studied in a cohort of patients from French child neurology departments followed since their first CNS acute demyelinating event. Hepatitis B and tetanus vaccination were not associated with an increased risk of a second neurological episode (considered as conversion to MS) after a first episode of acute inflammatory demyelination of the CNS [56]. Similarly, hepatitis B vaccination did not increased the risk of a first episode of acute CNS inflammatory demyelination or the risk of incident MS [57,58]. Using the same cohort of patients, the authors showed that parental smoking increased the risk of MS in children and that the risk increased with duration of exposure [59]. The influence of these factors on the course of the disease in childhood-onset MS patients is unknown. More recently, it was demonstrated that low levels of 25(OH) vitamin D3 predicted a higher risk of subsequent exacerbations after controlling for age, disease duration, and use of disease-modifying therapies, which was in part independent of the higher risk conferred by non-white race and Hispanic ethnicity [60].

The identification of susceptibility genes to MS in the pediatric population has been rare to date, but the role of the major histocompatibility complex (MHC) has been suggested and is concordant with findings in adults with MS [61,62]. It is unclear whether these susceptibility factors are also associated with a more severe disease course.

Prognosis
Methodological considerations
Studying the prognosis in MS requires the standardized and long-term follow-up of many patients. For this reason, information on the long-term prognosis of MS with childhood onset is limited, due to the usually short follow-up duration in most studies. Moreover, as mentioned above, many studies used crude observed data only, instead of survival analysis,

with the inherent limitations associated with these data. However, a few cohort studies from adult neurology centers have added valuable information on the long-term course of childhood-onset MS. It is likely that this information remains unique, as most patients are now being treated early in the course of the disease and do not represent a natural history cohort.

Development of irreversible disability
Time to disability milestones (limitation of ambulation, use of assistive devices)
In most studies, disability has been measured using the Expanded Disability Status Scale (EDSS) [63]. The EDSS is an ordinal scale based on the results of the neurological examination and the patient's ability to walk. Scores range from 0 (no neurological abnormality) to 10 (death from MS), with increments of 0.5 points. To facilitate the retrospective assessment and ensure a better reliability, some chose to use a simplified version of the EDSS, the Disability Status Scale (DSS), a 10-point scale with 1-point steps, and to focus on specific key points easy to assess, even retrospectively. That was the case for the KIDMUS study, for example [20]. Despite some limitations and some criticism that the scale put too much weight on motor performances, EDSS has reasonable reliability and validity [64] and remains widely used and accepted to measure disability in MS patients in clinical practice and in epidemiological studies [65]. It does not account well for cognitive disability.

The following studies assessed disability in terms of number of patients reaching different EDSS scores at different points in time among those not lost to follow-up. These results are crude observed data, with inherent limitations in the estimation of the accrual of disability over time, as mentioned previously. Still, these studies are useful in that they help to delineate the variability of the disease course. For instance, among a Canadian cohort of 125 patients, 51 could be scored after 10 years: 60% had an EDSS score <3.0, 24% had a score between 3.0 and 6.5 and 16% had a score of 7.0 or more [17]. In a cohort of 149 patients with onset before the age of 16 originating from 4 MS centers in Italy, the distribution of EDSS scores among the 105 patients with more than 8 years of disease duration was not different from the adult-onset MS comparison group with 26.7 and 25.7% of patients with a score of 6 or more, respectively [18]. However, several studies also pointed out the possibility of an aggressive course even in this age group [6,7,25], which stresses the great inter-individual variability in the disease course regardless of the age at onset.

The same three studies that provided estimates of time from onset to secondary progression (cf. time to secondary progression) also used survival analyses to estimate the time from onset of MS to several disability landmarks using the same cohorts of patients with childhood onset drawn from adult neurology departments [14,19,20]. All of them included a comparison group of patients with adult-onset MS from the same neurology department(s). In the Canadian cohort of 113 patients with a relapsing–remitting onset, 58.6% reached an EDSS score of 3.0 and 38.8% a score of 6.0 during follow-up [19]. The estimated median time from MS onset to the assignment of a score of 3.0 was 23 years compared to 10 years in the adult-onset comparison group (722 patients). The median time to the assignment of a score of 6.0 was 28 years compared to 18 years for the adult group (no confidence intervals were provided). In the Italian cohort of 83 patients with a relapsing–remitting onset and a median follow-up of 14 years, the estimated median time to reach an EDSS score of 4.0 was 20.2 years (range 4.4–47.9) compared to 10.8 years (range 0.5–44) in the adult comparison group of 596 patients ($p<0.0001$) [14]. Despite a longer time to reach disability milestones, patients with childhood onset were disabled at a younger age (median 31.6 years, range 18.1–58.3) compared to adults (median 41.2, range 21.8–69.2). The KIDMUS study took advantage of both a long follow-up (median = 15 years) and a substantial number of patients ($n = 394$) gathered from 12 departments of adult neurology in France and one in Belgium to estimate with a greater precision the time to irreversible disability [20]. The estimated median times from the onset of MS to the assignment of DSS scores of 4, 6, and 7 were 20.0 years (95% CI 19.0–22.4), 28.9 years (95% CI 27.0–33.0), and 37.0 years (95% CI 34.0–42.2), respectively (Table 7.1). These estimated median times were approximately 10 years longer in patients with childhood-onset MS than in patients with adult-onset MS: 8.1 years (95% CI 7.3–9.4) for DSS 4, 19.7 years (95% CI 17.4–21.9) for DSS 6, and 30.1 years (95% CI 25.1–35.1) for DSS 7 ($p<0.001$ for all comparisons). However, patients with childhood-onset MS reached these disability scores at a younger age than patients with an adult onset. The estimated median ages at assignment of DSS scores 4, 6, and 7 were 34.6 years (95% CI 31.2–36.0), 42.2 years (95% CI 40.5–46.9), and 50.5 years (95% CI 47.1–64.8), respectively, for the childhood-onset MS cohort, whereas they were 44.6 years (95% CI 43.7–45.5), 54.8 years (95% CI 54.0–56.7) and 63.2 years (95% CI 61.2–64.8) for the adult-onset MS cohort ($p<0.0001$ for all comparisons).

It has to be noted that evidence for a slower accumulation of irreversible disability has been found whatever the definition of early onset MS and not only for childhood-onset MS, but the earlier the onset of the disease, the more pronounced this phenomenon. In the Lyon, France, natural history MS cohort, it has been shown repeatedly that a young age at onset as compared to an older one exerts a positive influence on the evolution of MS by slowing down evolution to disability [42,66–69]. In the KIDMUS study, we also found that once a certain threshold of irreversible disability was reached, subsequent accumulation of disability was similar in childhood and adult onset MS patients [20]. Once a DSS score of 4 was attained, the median time to reach a score of 6 and 7 did not differ for patients with childhood and adult onset, and after a score of 6 was reached, did not differ to reach a score of 7. This could indicate that the early phase of MS, clinically characterized by relapses and mild disability, seems longer in young patients because the clinical onset is closer to the true biological onset, whereas part of this phase remains clinically silent in adult MS onset [70]. The underlying rate of neuronal loss and therefore of accumulation of irreversible disability could be similar but with a variation in the clinical expression of focal inflammatory lesions with age at onset. In this scenario, age at onset would mainly influence the clinical expression of MS but not the underlying biological process, suggesting a similar pathophysiology of the disease [70].

In summary, patients with childhood-onset MS take on average 10 years longer than patients with adult-onset MS to reach similar disability milestones, but they do so 10 years younger (i.e. at the time they start a family and are young professionals), therefore contradicting the generally accepted notion of a more favorable prognosis in this age group. This finding is true at the population level, with a great variability between individuals. This variability is illustrated by the fact that while most patients will have slow accumulation of disability, few have severe and rapidly disabling forms of the disease and few others benign

Table 7.1 Kaplan–Meier estimates of the time to and the age at the conversion to secondary progression and the assignment of irreversible disability landmarks among 2169 patients with multiple sclerosis (the KIDMUS study). Adapted from [20]

	Childhood onset				Adult onset				
	Number of patients	% censored*	Median (years)	95% CI	Number of Patients	% censored*	Median (years)	95% CI	p value**
Time to secondary progression†			28.1	25.0–32.1			18.8	17.1–21.1	<0.0001
Age at secondary progression	385‡	71.4	41.4	37.8–45.7	1496‡	68.6	52.1	51.0–54.1	<0.0001
Time to DSS 4†			20.0	19.0–22.4			8.1	7.3–9.4	<0.0001
Age at DSS 4	394	59.3	34.6	31.2–36.0	1775	44.1	44.6	43.7–45.5	<0.0001
Time to DSS 6†			28.9	27.0–33.0			19.7	17.4–21.9	<0.0001
Age at DSS 6	394	71.6	42.2	40.5–46.9	1775	67.9	54.8	54.0–56.7	<0.0001
Time to DSS 7†			37.0	34.0–42.2			30.1	25.1–35.1	<0.0001
Age at DSS 7	394	81.7	50.5	47.1–64.8	1775	79.8	63.2	61.2–64.8	<0.0001

Notes:
DSS, Kurtzke Disability Status Scale (1983).
* Patients who did not reach the outcome under study were censored at the date of their last visit.
** p Values were calculated using the log-rank test.
† From onset of multiple sclerosis.
‡ Patients with exacerbating–remitting initial course of multiple sclerosis.

forms with virtually no disability after many years. The same individual variability in the disease course exists in adult-onset MS, leading to the same difficulties in individualized long-term prognosis.

Prognostic factors of disability (clinical, paraclinical)

Potential prognostics factors associated with the assignment of disability milestones have been examined in several cohort studies from adult centers and one cohort from child neurology centers [13–15,19,20]. In three of these studies, the use of survival techniques with a multivariate analysis allowed independent assessment of the potential role of individual clinical or paraclinical factors [14,15,20].

In a cohort of 54 patients with relapsing–remitting onset at the age of 15 years or less, seen at an MS clinic at onset or during the first year after MS onset, the authors examined the predictive factors of disability among the sub-group of 37 patients with 8 years of follow-up [13]. The EDSS score eight years after MS onset was positively correlated with the

EDSS score after one year of disease duration. A trend was also found towards an association with the number of relapses in the first two years of the disease, whereas no correlation was found with age, gender, and type of symptoms at onset or mono/polysymptomatic onset. The mean EDSS score eight years after onset was higher in the secondary progressive group than in the relapsing–remitting group (the number of patients in each group were not provided). In a cohort of 113 patients with a relapsing–remitting onset of MS before the age of 16 years followed for a mean time of 19.8 years, patients with fewer relapses during the first year of MS had a longer time to the assignment of an EDSS score of 3. Similarly, those with fewer relapses during the first year or the first five years of the disease had a longer time to the assignment of EDSS 6 [19]. There was no correlation between sex or age at onset and time to these EDSS scores. As in the previous study, no multivariate analysis was performed. Using a cohort of 83 patients with a relapsing–remitting onset of MS before the age of 16 and a median disease duration of 14.1 years, other authors aimed to identify factors associated with the assignment of an EDSS score of 4 [14]. An older age at onset (>14 years), an interval between onset and the second episode shorter than one year, and a secondary progressive course were associated with an increased risk of EDSS 4. In multivariate analysis, however, only sphincter symptoms at onset of the disease and a secondary progressive evolution were associated with a higher risk of EDSS 4. The French child neurology prospective cohort of 197 patients with MS onset before the age of 16 was used to identify predictive factors of the assignment of an irreversible EDSS of 4 or more, but also of the occurrence of a third neurological episode in the context of a short follow-up (median disease duration 4.8 years from the date of the second neurological episode) [15]. Time zero for the survival analysis was defined as the date of the second neurological episode, i.e. calculation of the time to the third neurological episode or to reach EDSS 4 or higher was measured from the date of the second neurological episode (as opposed to MS onset for all the other studies). Prognostic factors associated with a higher risk of one of the two endpoints were female gender, a short time between the onset of MS and the second neurological episode (<1 year), MRI criteria for childhood-onset MS fulfilled at onset, no severe mental state changes at onset, and a secondary progressive evolution of MS.

In the KIDMUS study, several potential prognostic factors of assignment to irreversible DSS scores of 4, 6, and 7 were assessed from three different time-points during the early course of the disease [20]. Hence, potential clinical characteristics associated with each of these disability milestones were examined at MS onset, at the time of the second neurological episode and, finally, two years after onset of MS. At MS onset, the nature of the initial course (either relapsing–remitting or progressive from onset) was the only statistically significant prognostic factor, a progressive onset being associated with shorter times to reach irreversible disability (DSS 4, 6, and 7). At the time of the second neurologic episode, the time interval between the first two neurologic episodes did not influence the time to reach irreversible disability. Two years after MS onset, a progressive course at onset remained the main prognostic factor associated with the highest increased risk of disability. The other significant prognostic factor was the number of relapses during the first 2 years

of the disease, each additional relapse increasing the rate of disability, although to a lesser extent that the initial course. Sex, age at onset, and initial symptoms were not associated with times to develop disability in any analysis. The authors also examined prognostic factors of age at assignment of irreversible disability (DSS 4, 6, and 7). The only significant prognostic factor was the initial course of the disease: a progressive initial course was associated with a younger age at development of disability.

In summary, very few clinical predictors of long-term disability have been identified from prognostic studies in childhood-onset MS, in mostly white non-Hispanic cohorts of patients. The most influential predictor is the nature of the initial course, but, given the rarity of primary progressive presentations, few pediatric patients are at risk. Therefore, it remains difficult to make a prognosis for the majority of patients based solely on demographic and early clinical characteristics, as no other strong predictor has emerged from studies.

Development of cognitive problems

Cognitive dysfunction is a common feature in MS, but its characteristics are yet to be fully described in childhood-onset MS (reviewed in Chapter 13). Some of the methodological difficulties in the rare studies available include the small sample size, the disparity in the methods of assessment and the absence of agreement on cut-off points to define cognitive impairment. The later issues have already been raised in studies of cognitive impairment in adults with MS [71].

The prevalence of cognitive dysfunction cannot be estimated with precision due to the issues raised above. In small studies available, up to one-third of children evaluated were affected to various degrees [72,73]. The commonly affected domains include complex attention, verbal and visuospatial memory, and executive functions [72–75]. Some authors also reported a repercussion on the intellectual quotient in some patients [73]. The extent of cognitive dysfunction may increase with duration of the disease [74], and some children may experience progressive cognitive decline over time [3,72,76]. It has also been proposed that a younger age at onset is associated with a more severe cognitive impairment. In these studies, however, the youngest patients at onset also tended to have the longest disease duration, and the independent effect of age at onset and disease duration was not estimated. Cognitive impairment can exist in the absence of major physical disability, but whether or not, at the population level, the extent of cognitive dysfunction is correlated with disability has lead to contradictory results [72,73]. The potential consequences of cognitive problems on school performances and, more importantly, on long-term professional achievements are not known.

Conclusion

In conclusion, childhood-onset MS is rare and its course and prognosis have remained largely unknown until recently. This is not true anymore, thanks to the various collaborative research efforts developed to delineate the course of the disease in this population. Overall, these results contradict the notion of a more favorable prognosis usually associated with pediatric versus adult onset. Indeed, the disease may be benign in terms of rate of progression of disability but not in terms of age at disability, and patients with pediatric onset will be disabled for a longer part of their life. However, as in adult-onset MS, there is an important inter-individual variability concerning the course of the disease and the long-term prognosis. Predicting which patients will face a more severe long-term course remains a challenge, and early clinical predictors are of limited value at the individual level, as in adult-onset patients. Fortunately, if assuming similar underlying biological processes, these patients should benefit from the ongoing advances in the treatment of MS, and efforts should be deployed towards the study of the safety and effectiveness of new disease-modifying therapies on the population with childhood-onset MS.

Acknowledgments

Part of this chapter has been initially developed for a previous review article [70].

Dr. Christel Renoux is the recipient of a postdoctoral fellowship from the Multiple Sclerosis Society of Canada.

References

1. Krupp LB, Banwell B, Tenembaum S. Consensus definitions proposed for pediatric multiple sclerosis and related disorders. *Neurology* 2007;**68**:S7–12.

2. Bejar JM, Ziegler DK. Onset of multiple sclerosis in a 24-month-old child. *Arch Neurol* 1984;**41**:881–882.

3. Bye AM, Kendall B, Wilson J. Multiple sclerosis in childhood: A new look. *Dev Med Child Neurol* 1985;**27**:215–222.

4. Boutin B, Esquivel E, Mayer M, Chaumet S, Ponsot G, Arthuis M. Multiple sclerosis in children: Report of clinical and paraclinical features of 19 cases. *Neuropediatrics* 1988;**19**:118–123.

5. Cole GF, Stuart CA. A long perspective on childhood multiple sclerosis. *Dev Med Child Neurol* 1995;**37**: 661–666.

6. Cole GF, Auchterlonie LA, Best PV. Very early onset multiple sclerosis. *Dev Med Child Neurol* 1995;**37**: 667–672.

7. Guilhoto LM, Osorio CA, Machado LR, *et al.* Pediatric multiple sclerosis report of 14 cases. *Brain Dev* 1995;**17**:9–12.

8. Hanefeld F, Bauer HJ, Christen HJ, Kruse B, Bruhn H, Frahm J. Multiple sclerosis in childhood: Report of 15 cases. *Brain Dev* 1991;**13**:410–416.

9. Selcen D, Anlar B, Renda Y. Multiple sclerosis in childhood: Report of 16 cases. *Eur Neurol* 1996;**36**: 79–84.

10. Muller R. Course and prognosis of disseminated sclerosis in relation to age of onset. *AMA Arch Neurol Psychiatry* 1951;**66**:561–570.

11. Gall JC Jr, Hayles AB, Siekert RG, Keith HM. Multiple sclerosis in children; a clinical study of 40 cases with onset in childhood. *Pediatrics* 1958;**21**:703–709.

12. Sindern E, Haas J, Stark E, Wurster U. Early onset MS under the age of 16: Clinical and paraclinical features. *Acta Neurol Scand* 1992;**86**:280–284.

13. Ghezzi A, Pozzilli C, Liguori M, *et al.* Prospective study of multiple sclerosis with early onset. *Mult Scler* 2002;**8**:115–118.

14. Simone IL, Carrara D, Tortorella C, *et al.* Course and prognosis in early-onset MS: Comparison with adult-onset forms. *Neurology* 2002;**59**:1922–1928.

15. Mikaeloff Y, Caridade G, Assi S, Suissa S, Tardieu M. Prognostic factors for early severity in a childhood multiple sclerosis cohort. *Pediatrics* 2006;**118**: 1133–1139.

16. Banwell B, Krupp L, Kennedy J, *et al.* Clinical features and viral serologies in children with multiple sclerosis: A multinational observational study. *Lancet Neurol* 2007;**6**:773–781.

17. Duquette P, Murray TJ, Pleines J, *et al.* Multiple sclerosis in childhood: Clinical profile in 125 patients. *J Pediatr* 1987;**111**:359–363.

18. Ghezzi A, Deplano V, Faroni J, *et al.* Multiple sclerosis in childhood: Clinical features of 149 cases. *Mult Scler* 1997;**3**:43–46.

19. Boiko A, Vorobeychik G, Paty D, Devonshire V, Sadovnick D. Early onset multiple sclerosis: a longitudinal study. *Neurology* 2002;**59**:1006–1010.

20. Renoux C, Vukusic S, Mikaeloff Y, *et al.* Natural history of multiple sclerosis with childhood onset. *N Engl J Med* 2007;**356**:2603–2613.

21. Shiraishi K, Higuchi Y, Ozawa K, Hao Q, Saida T. Clinical course and prognosis of 27 patients with childhood onset multiple sclerosis in Japan. *Brain Dev* 2005;**27**:224–227.

22. Weng WC, Yang CC, Yu TW, Shen YZ, Lee WT. Multiple sclerosis with childhood onset: Report of 21 cases in Taiwan. *Pediatr Neurol* 2006;**35**: 327–334.

23. El-Salem K, Khader Y. Comparison of the natural history and prognostic features of early onset and adult onset multiple sclerosis in Jordanian population. *Clin Neurol Neurosurg* 2007;**109**:32–37.

24. Etemadifar M, Nasr-Esfahani AH, Khodabandehlou R, Maghzi AH. Childhood-onset multiple sclerosis: Report of 82 patients from Isfahan, *Iran. Arch Iran Med* 2007;**10**:152–156.

25. Ozakbas S, Idiman E, Baklan B, Yulug B. Childhood and juvenile onset multiple sclerosis: Clinical and paraclinical features. *Brain Dev* 2003;**25**:233–236.

26. Pinhas-Hamiel O, Barak Y, Siev-Ner I, Achiron A. Juvenile multiple sclerosis: Clinical features and prognostic characteristics. *J Pediatr* 1998;**132**:735–737.

27. Ruggieri M, Iannetti P, Polizzi A, Pavone L, Grimaldi LM. Multiple sclerosis in children under 10 years of age. *Neurol Sci* 2004;**25**(Suppl 4):S326–S335.

28. Banwell B, Ghezzi A, Bar-Or A, Mikaeloff Y, Tardieu M. Multiple sclerosis in children: Clinical diagnosis, therapeutic strategies, and future directions. *Lancet Neurol* 2007;**6**:887–902.

29. Fay A, Mowry E, Chabas D, Strober J, Waubant E. Relapse severity and recovery in early pediatric multiple sclerosis. Under review.

30. van Lieshout HB, van Engelen BG, Sanders EA, Renier WO. Diagnosing multiple sclerosis in childhood. *Acta Neurol Scand* 1993;**88**:339–343.

31. Ruggieri M, Polizzi A, Pavone L, Grimaldi LM. Multiple sclerosis in children under 6 years of age. *Neurology* 1999;**53**:478–484.

32. Rusin JA, Vezina LG, Chadduck WM, Chandra RS. Tumoral multiple sclerosis of the cerebellum in a child. *Am J Neuroradiol* 1995;**16**:1164–1166.

33. Jordan JF, Walter P, Ayertey HD, Brunner R. Intermediate uveitis in childhood preceding the diagnosis of multiple sclerosis: A 13-year follow-up. *Am J Ophthalmol* 2003;**135**:885–886.

34. Pohl D, Rostasy K, Reiber H, Hanefeld F. CSF characteristics in early-onset multiple sclerosis. *Neurology* 2004;**63**:1966–1967.

35. Chabas D, Ness J, Belman A, *et al.* Younger children with pediatric MS have a distinct CSF inflammatory profile at disease onset. *Neurology* 2010;**74**: 399–405.

36. McDonald WI, Compston A, Edan G, *et al.* Recommended diagnostic criteria for multiple sclerosis: Guidelines from the International Panel on the diagnosis of multiple sclerosis. *Ann Neurol* 2001;**50**:121–127.

37. Callen DJ, Shroff MM, Branson HM, *et al.* MRI in the diagnosis of pediatric multiple sclerosis. *Neurology* 2009;**72**:961–967.

38. Hahn CD, Shroff MM, Blaser SI, Banwell BL. MRI criteria for multiple sclerosis: Evaluation in a pediatric cohort. *Neurology* 2004;**62**:806–808.

39. Mikaeloff Y, Adamsbaum C, Husson B, *et al.* MRI prognostic factors for relapse after acute CNS inflammatory demyelination in childhood. *Brain* 2004;**127**:1942–1947.

40. Neuteboom RF, Boon M, Catsman Berrevoets CE, *et al.* Prognostic factors after a first attack of inflammatory CNS demyelination in children. *Neurology* 2008;**71**:967–973.

41. Callen DJ, Shroff MM, Branson HM, *et al.* Role of MRI in the differentiation of ADEM from MS in children. *Neurology* 2009;**72**:968–973.

42. Confavreux C, Compston A. The natural history of multiple sclerosis. In *McAlpine's Multiple Sclerosis*, 4th edn, ed. A. Compston, I. MacDonald, J. Noseworthy *et al.* London: Churchill Livingstone Elsevier, 2006;183–272.

43. Mowry EM, Pesic M, Grimes B, Deen S, Bacchetti P, Waubant E. Demyelinating events in early multiple sclerosis have inherent severity and recovery. *Neurology* 2009;**72**:602–608.

44. Gusev E, Boiko A, Bikova O, *et al.* The natural history of early onset multiple sclerosis: Comparison of data from Moscow and Vancouver. *Clin Neurol Neurosurg* 2002;**104**:203–207.

45. Trojano M, Paolicelli D, Bellacosa A, Fuiani A, Cataldi S, Di ME. Atypical forms of multiple sclerosis or different phases of a same disease? *Neurol Sci* 2004;**25** (Suppl 4):S323–S325.

46. Gorman MP, Healy BC, Polgar-Turcsanyi M, Chitnis T. Increased relapse rate in pediatric-onset compared with adult-onset multiple sclerosis. *Arch Neurol* 2009;**66**:54–59.

47. Mowry EM, Pesic M, Grimes B, Deen SR, Bacchetti P, Waubant E. Clinical predictors of early second event in

patients with clinically isolated syndrome. *J Neurol* 2009;**256**:1061–1066.

48. Boster AL, Endress CF, Hreha SA, Caon C, Perumal JS, Khan OA. Pediatric-onset multiple sclerosis in African-American black and European-origin white patients. *Pediatr Neurol* 2009;**40**:31–33.

49. Deryck O, Ketelaer P, Dubois B. Clinical characteristics and long term prognosis in early onset multiple sclerosis. *J Neurol* 2006;**253**:720–723.

50. Vukusic S, Confavreux C. Prognostic factors for progression of disability in the secondary progressive phase of multiple sclerosis. *J Neurol Sci* 2003;**206**:135–137.

51. Pugliatti M, Riise T, Sotgiu MA, *et al*. Evidence of early childhood as the susceptibility period in multiple sclerosis: Space–time cluster analysis in a Sardinian population. *Am J Epidemiol* 2006;**164**:326–333.

52. Kennedy J, O'Connor P, Sadovnick AD, Perara M, Yee I, Banwell B. Age at onset of multiple sclerosis may be influenced by place of residence during childhood rather than ancestry. *Neuroepidemiology* 2006;**26**:162–167.

53. Alotaibi S, Kennedy J, Tellier R, Stephens D, Banwell B. Epstein–Barr virus in pediatric multiple sclerosis. *JAMA* 2004;**291**:1875–1879.

54. Pohl D, Krone B, Rostasy K, *et al*. High seroprevalence of Epstein–Barr virus in children with multiple sclerosis. *Neurology* 2006;**67**:2063–2065.

55. Waubant E, The US Network of Pediatric MS Centers, Mowry E, James J. Remote EBV, CMV, and HSV-1 and -2 infection status in children with pediatric-onset MS and age-matched healthy controls [Abstract]. *Mult Scler* 2009;**15**:in press.

56. Mikaeloff Y, Caridade G, Assi S, Tardieu M, Suissa S. Hepatitis B vaccine and risk of relapse after a first childhood episode of CNS inflammatory demyelination. *Brain* 2007;**130**:1105–1110.

57. Mikaeloff Y, Caridade G, Rossier M, Suissa S, Tardieu M. Hepatitis B vaccination and the risk of childhood-onset multiple sclerosis. *Arch Pediatr Adolesc Med* 2007;**161**:1176–1182.

58. Mikaeloff Y, Caridade G, Suissa S, Tardieu M. Hepatitis B vaccine and the risk of CNS inflammatory demyelination in childhood. *Neurology* 2009;**72**:873–880.

59. Mikaeloff Y, Caridade G, Tardieu M, Suissa S. Parental smoking at home and the risk of childhood-onset multiple sclerosis in children. *Brain* 2007;**130**:2589–2525.

60. Mowry EM, Krupp L, Milazzo M, *et al*. Lower vitamin D levels are associated with a higher risk of relapse in early pediatric-onset multiple sclerosis. *Ann Neurol* 2010;**67**:618–624.

61. Boiko AN, Gusev EI, Sudomoina MA, *et al*. Association and linkage of juvenile MS with HLA-DR2 (15) in Russians. *Neurology* 2002;**58**:658–660.

62. Waubant E, Chabas D. Pediatric multiple sclerosis. *Curr Treat Options Neurol* 2009;**11**:203–210.

63. Kurtzke JF. Rating neurologic impairment in multiple sclerosis: An expanded disability status scale (EDSS). *Neurology* 1983;**33**:1444–1152.

64. Sharrack B, Hughes RA, Soudain S, Dunn G. The psychometric properties of clinical rating scales used in multiple sclerosis. *Brain* 1999;**122**(Pt 1):141–159.

65. Kurtzke JF. Natural history and clinical outcome measures for multiple sclerosis studies. Why at the present time does EDSS scale remain a preferred outcome measure to evaluate disease evolution? *Neurol Sci* 2000;**21**:339–341.

66. Confavreux C, Aimard G, Devic M. Course and prognosis of multiple sclerosis assessed by the computerized data processing of 349 patients. *Brain* 1980;**103**:281–300.

67. Confavreux C, Vukusic S, Adeleine P. Early clinical predictors and progression of irreversible disability in multiple sclerosis: An amnesic process. *Brain* 2003;**126**:770–782.

68. Confavreux C, Vukusic S. Natural history of multiple sclerosis: A unifying concept. *Brain* 2006;**129**:606–616.

69. Confavreux C, Vukusic S. Age at disability milestones in multiple sclerosis. *Brain* 2006;**129**:595–605.

70. Renoux C, Vukusic S, Confavreux C. The natural history of multiple sclerosis with childhood onset. *Clin Neurol Neurosurg* 2008;**110**:897–904.

71. Hoffmann S, Tittgemeyer M, von Cramon DY. Cognitive impairment in multiple sclerosis. *Curr Opin Neurol* 2007;**20**:275–280.

72. MacAllister WS, Belman AL, Milazzo M, *et al*. Cognitive functioning in children and adolescents with multiple sclerosis. *Neurology* 2005;**64**:1422–1425.

73. Amato MP, Goretti B, Ghezzi A, *et al*. Cognitive and psychosocial features of childhood and juvenile MS. *Neurology* 2008;**70**:1891–1897.

74. Banwell BL, Anderson PE. The cognitive burden of multiple sclerosis in children. *Neurology* 2005;**64**:891–894.

75. Montiel-Nava C, Pena J, Gonzalez-Pernia S, Mora-La CE. Cognitive functioning in children with multiple sclerosis. *Mult Scler* 2009;**15**:266–268.

76. MacAllister WS, Christodoulou C, Milazzo M, Krupp LB. Longitudinal neuropsychological assessment in pediatric multiple sclerosis. *Dev Neuropsychol* 2007;**32**:625–644.

Plasma exchange and IV immunoglobulin for acute demyelinating relapses

Khurram Bashir

The studies exploring the use of plasma exchange (PE) for severe MS-associated relapses that recover poorly following treatment with high-dose steroid therapy (or in rare instances where high-dose gluco-corticosteroids are contraindicated) has demonstrated conflicting results. Plasma exchange involves non-selectively removing plasma components that are potentially pathogenic in immune-mediated diseases from a patient's blood [1]. Some of these components are antibodies, immune complexes, and complement, while others are currently unknown. Vascular access is usually obtained by inserting a central venous catheter into the subclavian or internal jugular veins. Alternatively, vascular access may be obtained by inserting two needles in two peripheral veins. Plasma exchange is usually performed using a membrane filtration technique and the plasma is exchanged with 5% albumin solution. A total volume of 2000–3000 ml is typically exchanged during each treatment and the patients typically undergo 5–7 treatments, usually on every other day.

The results of several small, uncontrolled trials have been difficult to interpret because of the use of concomitant immunosuppressive therapy and poor trial design. A double-blind crossover trial showed that two-week alternate-day PE treatment resulted in appreciable clinical improvement in about 42% of the patients with acute inflammatory demyelination who had been unresponsive to intravenous glucocorticoid therapy (a minimum of 500 mg of intravenous methylprednisolone for 5 days) [2]. In this study, 22 patients with severe steroid-refractory demyelinating relapses (secondary to MS, neuromyelitis optica, acute disseminated encephalomyelitis, acute transverse myelitis, Marburg's variant, and focal cerebral demyelinating disease), were initially randomized to either an average exchange volume of 54 ml/kg (1.1 plasma

volume) by continuous flow centrifugation or alternatively to a sham exchange. The PE treatment was initiated within three months of the onset of symptoms. After 14 days of treatment (7 exchanges), patients were evaluated by masked evaluating physicians and those determined to have no recovery or minimal recovery underwent the alternate treatment. The results of the study showed that "in patients with acute severe attacks who failed to improve after high-dose corticosteroid treatment" PE was an acceptable therapeutic option to consider. Another study of 10 patients with acute severe optic neuritis reported a beneficial response in 7 of the 10 (70%) patients treated with PE [3]. All patients had previously received at least two courses of intravenous glucocorticoid therapy and, additionally, two patients were treated with intravenous immunoglobulins (IVIg) three weeks prior to PE. The median time interval from the onset of symptoms to initiation of PE was 34.5 days (range: 11–73 days), and the median interval from the last course of glucocorticoids to the start of PE was 2.5 days (range: 0–19 days). In this study a median of 5 exchanges (range 2–5) per patient were carried out using continuous-flow centrifugation exchanging a mean of 40.3 ml/kg of plasma. A small study of 6 patients with acute steroid-unresponsive episodes of severe inflammatory central nervous system demyelination reported improvement in 5 of the treated patients following a course of 3–5 exchanges within 6 months of the onset of the relapse symptoms [4]. Schilling et al., in a 16-patient (13 adult and 3 pediatric) observational study, reported a good or better response to 14 courses of PE in 71% of adult and 67% of pediatric patients with steroid-unresponsive MS relapses [5]. In another retrospective study of PE treatment in 18 patients with relapsing–remitting (RR) MS or clinically isolated syndrome (CIS)

Demyelinating Disorders of the Central Nervous System in Childhood, ed. Dorothée Chabas and Emmanuelle L. Waubant. Published by Cambridge University Press. © Cambridge University Press 2011.

and 2 patients with neuromyelitis optica (NMO), who experienced a total of 21 relapses that were unresponsive to 3–5-day course of intravenous methylprednisolone (IVMP), a moderate or marked clinical response was reported in greater than three-quarters of the study subjects [6]. A good clinical response was seen in 76% of acute optic neuritis and in 87% of all other types of relapses combined. Even in two patients with secondary progressive (SP) MS, PE therapy has been reported as an effective treatment for severe steroid-refractory relapses [7].

The experience with PE in the pediatric MS population is very limited. The initial report on the use of PE in pediatric MS was a 7-year-old MS patient with high titers of anti-nuclear antibodies, who experienced three relapses over an eight-month period, each time requiring high-dose intravenous steroids. Plasma exchange was substituted for steroids to avoid glucocorticoid-associated adverse effects and resulted in a marked reduction in relapse frequency. The patient was initially treated with a daily PE for three days and then every two to three weeks depending on the values of anti-nuclear antibody. The patient's clinical status improved and he remained relapse-free over the 18-month follow-up period. The authors suggested that PE should be considered as a potential therapy for severe childhood MS [8]. Recently, the network of Pediatric Multiple Sclerosis Centers in the United States reported their experience with use of PE as a promoter of relapse recovery in pediatric MS [9]. A total of 31 pediatric patients (80% female, 52% Caucasian) with MS ($n = 16$) and a variety of other demyelinating diseases were treated with PE 29 ± 5 days (range 1–64 days), following failure of initial relapse therapy with IVMP with or without IVIg. Patients received a mean of 7.9 ± 1.1 exchanges (mode: 5 exchanges; range: 2–24 exchanges) on average 29 ± 5 days (range: 1–64 days) after the onset of initial symptoms. Of the patients, 16% recovered completely; 48% had partial recovery; and 35% demonstrated no clinical improvement as determined by the treating physician. Complications related to the procedure or central lines were seen in 13% (4/31) of the patients (3 line infections, 2 adverse reactions to treatment with midazolam and fresh frozen plasma, 1 vessel perforation during central venous line placement). The authors concluded that PE "benefited a sub-group of pediatric patients with severe demyelinating episodes unresponsive to high-dose steroids and/or IVIG".

Although there are no definite randomized, placebo-controlled studies of PE in acute MS relapses, the accumulating evidence and consensus of experts favors the use of PE for acute, severe demyelinating relapses that are not responsive to high-dose intravenous steroids. The timing of PE in relation to the onset of symptoms and treatment with steroids is not entirely clear. While it has been suggested that early initiation (less than 20 days after onset of symptoms) of PE therapy potentially has a better predictive value for favorable outcome [10], other studies have reported a fairly robust response even when the PE treatment is initiated more than six weeks after the onset of symptoms [6]. Given that some patients respond to PE even when the treatment is initiated more than 60 days after the onset of an acute relapse [10], this treatment should probably not be withheld in patients who are seen late in the course of their relapse.

The PE procedure has been generally well tolerated by MS patients. The most common complications, especially in the pediatric group, are related to the placement and maintenance of the central line. However, there are a couple of cautionary notes. (1) In one study of 10 progressive MS patients who were treated with PE on a scheduled basis, two patients experienced a relapse following an acute allergic reaction to plasma [11]; (2) plasma exchange, alone or in combination with steroids, has not been shown be to be an effective therapy to alter the long-term disease course in relapsing–remitting or progressive forms of MS [12,13]. The underlying mechanism explaining the beneficial effect of PE in steroid-unresponsive MS relapses in not known. Plasma exchange works by removing putative pathogenic agent, such as auto-antibodies, immune complexes or complement, from the plasma. Whether this or another effect on the immunological system is responsible for the therapeutic effectiveness of PE remains to be found. The possible complications of PE include infection, damage to the vessel, pneumothorax, coagulopathies, bleeding, hypocalcemia, acid–base disturbances, arrhythmias, hemolysis, and hypotension [1]. A newer plasma immunoadsorption technique may represent an interesting and potentially more effective option for patients with very severe demyelinating relapses [14].

Initially developed as a treatment for immune deficiency states, IVIg are now widely used for a broad spectrum of immune-mediated disorders.

Intravenous immunoglobulin used for therapeutic purposes are pooled human immunoglobulins derived from the plasma of 10 000–100 000 healthy donors. The major component of IVIg preparations is IgG; very small amounts of other immunoglobulins, immunoglobulin fragments, and other smaller plasma proteins are also present. Single-donor IVIg contain only monomeric IgG fractions, while pooled IVIg contain both monomeric and dimeric IgG fractions that are maintained in a state of equilibrium by various factors [15]. Intravenous immunoglobulins affect several components of the immune system and have been used successfully in the treatment of several neuroimmunological disorders. Intravenous immunoglobulins are believed to cause down-regulation of the immune system through a number of mechanisms including inactivation of autoantibodies by administration of anti-idiotypes (anti-antibodies), reduction in absolute number of T-helper cells leading to a decreased T-helper:T-suppresser cell ratio, decreased antibody synthesis by direct inhibition of B-cell function, activation of T-suppressor cells which inhibit antibody production via T-cell-dependent mechanism, suppression of cells bearing Fc γ-receptors by antibodies to Fc γ-receptors present in the IVIg, possible stimulation of CNS remyelination, inhibition of the binding of activated complement components to their target cell, neutralization of viruses that provoke autoimmune disease, inhibition of cytokine (IL-1, TNF-α) production and release by lymphoid tissue, inhibition of lymphocyte proliferation, and decrease in antibody-dependent cellular toxicity [16–18]. Different preparations of IVIg vary in their content, specificity and composition, and these differences modify the tolerability and effectiveness of the various products currently available [19]. IVIg therapy is relatively safe and well tolerated in most patients and disease states. Aseptic meningitis, pulmonary edema secondary to fluid overload, acute tubular necrosis, thromboembolism, cerebral vasospasm leading to acute encephalopathy, and anaphylaxis in IgA-deficient individuals are some of the more serious complications associated with IVIg treatment [20]. The commonly used total dose of IVIg is 2 g/kg administered as an intravenous infusion divided over 2–5 days [21,22]. Small amounts of IgA are usually present in pooled IVIg and it is recommended that IgA levels be measured before the first infusion to reduce the risk of anaphylaxis in patients with IgA deficit.

IVIg therapy has been evaluated both as a treatment of acute demyelinating relapses as well as a maintenance therapy to alter the disease course in adult patients with MS. We will focus on studies pertaining to the treatment of acute relapses. In a phase II, double-blind, placebo-controlled study of 55 patients with acute optic neuritis (ON), subjects were treated with either IVIg 0.4 g/kg/day for five days followed by one infusion monthly for three months or comparable placebo. In this trial, IVIg treatment failed to demonstrate any therapeutic benefit on visual recovery after six months of follow-up [23]. In another study, 68 patients were treated with IVIg 0.4 g/kg/day for three days within 30 days of the onset of ON symptoms followed by a single dose of IVIg 0.4 g/kg at one month and two months after onset [24]. The primary endpoint in this study was measurement of contrast sensitivity at six months. The treatment with IVIg in this cohort did not result in any statistically significant improvement compared to placebo in the primary or any of the secondary endpoints. In a study of 76 adult MS patients presenting with acute relapses, IVIg 1 g/kg or placebo was administered 24 h before treatment with IVMP 1 g/day for three days within two weeks of the onset of symptoms [25]. At the end of 12 weeks, both groups demonstrated a similar degree of recovery from the neurological deficits related to the acute relapse. The authors found no benefit of IVIg in the treatment of acute MS relapses when administered prior to IVMP. In another study, Visser et al. studied combined IVIg and IVMP therapy compared to IVMP plus placebo in 19 adult patients with clinically definite MS experiencing an acute relapse [26]. Both treatment groups demonstrated similar improvement measured by expanded disability status scale (EDSS) at 4, 8, and 12 weeks of follow-up. In a recent open-label, non-randomized, prospective study, 47 adult RR MS patients with steroid-refractory severe visual loss (visual acuity of 20/400 or worse in the affected eye), secondary to ON, were treated with IVIg 0.4 g/kg/day for five days followed by once-monthly infusion of 0.4 g/kg for five months [27]. This treatment was administered 60–90 days after the onset of ON symptoms and was shown to result in normal or near-normal visual acuity in 78% of the patients compared to similar improvement in only 12.5% of patients who did not receive IVIg. Contrary to previous studies, the study by Tselis et al. suggests that treatment with IVIg within 90 days of onset of symptoms followed by monthly infusions for 5 months in steroid-refractory severe ON may be a beneficial therapeutic approach. The conclusions from this study are obviously limited by the small sample size, open-label non-randomized study design in a selected patient population introducing bias, and use of a relatively poorly sensitive outcome measure (visual acuity). A few case reports and small case series also suggest a beneficial effect of IVIg on severe acute demyelinating relapses that are unresponsive to steroids [28–33]. In a case report published in 1998, Finsterer *et al.* report the salutary effects of IVIg in an adult case of acute disseminated encephalomyelitis (ADEM) treated within a week of the onset of symptoms [28]. Apak and Anlar have reported a case of a 16-month-old child with ADEM who relapsed after initial treatment with IVMP and responded to IVIg treatment [30]. Similarly, Nishikawa *et al.* have reported excellent recovery in three 2–5-year-old patients with ADEM following a course of IVIg 0.4 g/kg/day for 5 days [29]. Pradhan and colleagues reported remarkable recovery in 4 adult patients with ADEM who were initially refractory to a 3–5-day course of IVMP [31]. Sahlas *et al.* describe two adult cases of ADEM who initially deteriorated while receiving IVMP treatment and then demonstrated a good therapeutic response to IVIg [32]. Similarly, Murthy *et al.* also reported clinical improvement in two patients with ADEM following IVIg treatment [33]. In all these case reports, IVIg appears to be most effective when the treatment is administered relatively early, within 1–2 weeks of the onset of symptoms. Whether the improvement reported is at least in part due to the natural history remains to be determined.

Conclusion

In conclusion, both IVIg and PE might have a beneficial effect and need to be considered for patients with severe demyelinating attacks that are refractory to steroids. Plasma exchange might be an effective and relatively well-tolerated treatment option for severe demyelinating relapses in MS patients, especially when the clinical improvement following high-dose glucocorticoids is not seen in a relatively short period of time. Similarly, IVIg may be a reasonable consideration for treatment in steroid-unresponsive acute severe relapses. The experience with these therapies in childhood MS is very limited. It is also unknown whether one is more beneficial than the other. There are no randomized controlled trials in childhood acute MS relapses. Anecdotal report and personal experience regarding the use of steroids, PE and IVIg in children with MS have been reported. These reports demonstrate that both IVIg and PE are probably safe and well tolerated. The issues of appropriate treatment regimen, efficacy, effect(s) on growth and development, both physical and emotional, effect(s) on the immature central nervous system and the immune system, and long-term safety remain unresolved and need to be addressed in future clinical trials.

References

1. Lehmann HC, Hartung HP, Hetzel GR, Stuve O, Kieseier BC. Plasma exchange in neuroimmunological disorders: Part 1: Rationale and treatment of inflammatory central nervous system disorders. *Arch Neurol* 2006;**63**:930–935.

2. Weinshenker BG. Therapeutic plasma exchange for acute inflammatory demyelinating syndromes of the central nervous system. *J Clin Apher* 1999;**14**:144–148.

3. Ruprecht K, Klinker E, Dintelmann T, Rieckmann P, Gold R. Plasma exchange for severe optic neuritis: Treatment of 10 patients. *Neurology* 2004;**63**:1081–1083.

4. Bennetto L, Totham A, Healy P, Massey E, Scolding N. Plasma exchange in episodes of severe inflammatory demyelination of the central nervous system. A report of six cases. *J Neurol* 2004;**251**:1515–1521.

5. Schilling S, Linker RA, Konig FB, *et al.* [Plasma exchange therapy for steroid-unresponsive multiple sclerosis relapses: Clinical experience with 16 patients]. *Nervenarzt* 2006;**77**:430–438.

6. Trebst C, Reising A, Kielstein JT, Hafer C, Stangel M. Plasma exchange therapy in steroid-unresponsive relapses in patients with multiple sclerosis. *Blood Purif* 2009;**28**:108–115.

7. Linker RA, Chan A, Sommer M, *et al.* Plasma exchange therapy for steroid-refractory superimposed relapses in secondary progressive multiple sclerosis. *J Neurol* 2007;**254**:1288–1289.

8. Takahashi I, Sawaishi Y, Takeda O, Enoki M, Takada G. Childhood multiple sclerosis treated with plasmapheresis. *Pediatr Neurol* 1997;**17**:83–87.

9. Ness J, Chabas D, Kuntz M, Yeh E. NMSS Network of Pediatric MS Centers of Excellence. Use of plasmapharesis in pediatric demyelinating disease. In: *ACTRIMS*; 2009; Atlanta, GA, 2009.

10. Keegan M, Pineda AA, McClelland RL, Darby CH, Rodriguez M, Weinshenker BG. Plasma exchange for severe attacks of CNS demyelination: Predictors of response. *Neurology* 2002;**58**:143–146.

11. Wirguin I, Shinar E, Abramsky O. Relapse of multiple sclerosis following acute allergic reactions to plasma during plasmapheresis. *J Neurol* 1989;**236**: 62–63.

12. The Canadian Cooperative Multiple Sclerosis Study Group. The Canadian cooperative trial of cyclophosphamide and plasma exchange in progressive multiple sclerosis. *Lancet* 1991;**337**:441–446.

13. Grapsa E, Triantafyllou N, Rombos A, Lagouranis A, Dimopoulos MA. Therapeutic plasma exchange combined with immunomodulating agents in secondary progressive multiple sclerosis patients. *Ther Apher Dial* 2008;**12**:105–108.

14. de Andres C, Anaya F, Gimenez-Roldan S. [Plasma immunoadsorption treatment of malignant multiple sclerosis with severe and prolonged relapses]. *Rev Neurol* 2000;**30**:601–605.

15. Miescher SM, Schaub A, Ghielmetti M, *et al.* Comparative analysis of antigen specificities in the monomeric and dimeric fractions of intravenous immunoglobulin. *Ann NY Acad Sci* 2005;**1051**:582–590.

16. Gonsette RE. Introductory remarks: Immunosuppressive and immunomodulating drugs, where and how do they act? *Mult Scler* 1996;**1**:306–312.

17. Becker CC, Gidal BE, Fleming JO. Immunotherapy in multiple sclerosis, Part 2. *Am J Health Syst Pharm* 1995;**52**:2105–2120; quiz 2132–2104.

18. Thornton CA, Griggs RC. Plasma exchange and intravenous immunoglobulin treatment of neuromuscular disease. *Ann Neurol* 1994; **35**:260–268.

19. Lemm G. Composition and properties of IVIg preparations that affect tolerability and therapeutic efficacy. *Neurology* 2002;**59**(Suppl 6):S28–32.

20. Hafler DA, Brod SA, Weiner HL. Immunoregulation in multiple sclerosis. *Res Immunol* 1989;**140**:233–239; discussion 245–248.

21. Pohl D, Waubant E, Banwell B, *et al.* Treatment of pediatric multiple sclerosis and variants. *Neurology* 2007;**68**(Suppl 2):S54–65.

22. Krupp LB, Macallister WS. Treatment of pediatric multiple sclerosis. *Curr Treat Options Neurol* 2005;**7**:191–199.

23. Noseworthy JH, O'Brien PC, Petterson TM, *et al.* A randomized trial of intravenous immunoglobulin in inflammatory demyelinating optic neuritis. *Neurology* 2001;**56**:1514–1522.

24. Roed HG, Langkilde A, Sellebjerg F, *et al.* A double-blind, randomized trial of IV immunoglobulin treatment in acute optic neuritis. *Neurology* 2005;**64**:804–810.

25. Sorensen PS, Haas J, Sellebjerg F, Olsson T, Ravnborg M. IV immunoglobulins as add-on treatment to methylprednisolone for acute relapses in MS. *Neurology* 2004;**63**:2028–2033.

26. Visser LH, Beekman R, Tijssen CC, *et al.* A randomized, double-blind, placebo-controlled pilot study of i.v. immune globulins in combination with i.v. methylprednisolone in the treatment of relapses in patients with MS. *Mult Scler* 2004;**10**:89–91.

27. Tselis A, Perumal J, Caon C, *et al.* Treatment of corticosteroid refractory optic neuritis in multiple sclerosis patients with intravenous immunoglobulin. *Eur J Neurol* 2008;**15**:1163–1167.

28. Finsterer J, Grass R, Stollberger C, Mamoli B. Immunoglobulins in acute, parainfectious, disseminated encephalo-myelitis. *Clin Neuropharmacol* 1998;**21**:258–261.

29. Nishikawa M, Ichiyama T, Hayashi T, Ouchi K, Furukawa S. Intravenous immunoglobulin therapy in acute disseminated encephalomyelitis. *Pediatr Neurol* 1999;**21**:583–586.

30. Apak RA, Anlar B, Saatci I. A case of relapsing acute disseminated encephalomyelitis with high dose corticosteroid treatment. *Brain Dev* 1999;**21**: 279–282.

31. Pradhan S, Gupta RP, Shashank S, Pandey N. Intravenous immunoglobulin therapy in acute disseminated encephalomyelitis. *J Neurol Sci* 1999;**165**:56–61.

32. Sahlas DJ, Miller SP, Guerin M, Veilleux M, Francis G. Treatment of acute disseminated encephalomyelitis with intravenous immunoglobulin. *Neurology* 2000;**54**:1370–1372.

33. Murthy SN, Faden HS, Cohen ME, Bakshi R. Acute disseminated encephalomyelitis in children. *Pediatrics* 2002;**110**:e21.

Corticosteroids in pediatric multiple sclerosis relapses

Gregory S. Aaen

Multiple sclerosis (MS) is a chronic disease of the central nervous system (CNS) characterized by inflammatory attacks on oligodendroglia and axons. Clinical attacks can manifest as periods of acute muscle weakness or paralysis, sensory disturbances, and visual impairment. In adults, acute attacks with moderate physical impairment are commonly treated with corticosteroids [1], which have been found to decrease relapse duration [2] and shorten recovery time [3,4]. Corticosteroids are commonly used to treat acute attacks in children, although no clinical trials have been performed to evaluate their efficacy in this age group. This chapter will briefly review the use of corticosteroids for acute relapses in pediatric MS.

Mechanism of action

Corticosteroids are widely used to treat inflammatory conditions as they modulate the immune system through multiple mechanisms. Many of their effects are exerted by altering gene transcription via interaction with the glucocorticoid receptor (GCR). T cells are present in MS lesions and are felt to participate in the inflammatory reaction [5]. Activated T cells are differentiated into either a Th1 or Th2 population based upon the types of cytokines that are produced. Th1 cells secrete the pro-inflammatory cytokines IL-12, tumor necrosis factor (TNF)-α, and interferon (IFN)-γ. Activated Th2 cells have been found to modulate inflammation via production of IL-10 and transforming growth factor (TGF)-β. Corticosteroids reduce production of Th1 cytokines [6] while increasing the secretion of anti-inflammatory Th2 cytokines [7]. They also decrease immunoglobulin secretion and opsonization [8–10].

Endothelial cells in the CNS are connected with tight-junctions which comprise the blood–brain barrier, preventing easy diffusion of leukocytes into the CNS. The vascular endothelium does not normally express the cell adhesion molecules ICAM-1, VCAM-1, and E-selectin that leukocytes require for attachment and subsequent migration into the CNS. Activated T cells express α4 integrin which facilitates leukocyte adhesion to the endothelial surface via VCAM-1. Because activated T cells are also able to induce endothelial cell expression of VCAM-1, they are able to facilitate their own migration into the CNS [11]. Corticosteroids decrease the expression of various cell adhesion molecules including VCAM-1, thereby inhibiting migration of activated T cells into the CNS [12–14].

Some data suggest that corticosteroids inhibit demyelination [15] and prevent oligodendrocyte apoptosis [16]. They might also inhibit axonal loss by decreasing inflammation [17,18]. While axonal loss is present in lesions of all ages, it appears to be more prominent in the early stages of MS [19–21], suggesting that corticosteroid use for early relapses in childhood may be particularly beneficial [22].

Use in adults

Corticosteroids are considered type A drugs for treating MS relapses in adults [23]. In patients with optic neuritis (ON), high-dose intravenous methylprednisolone (IVMP) 1 g/day for 3 days has been shown to be effective at hastening recovery [24], and might delay the onset of MS, as defined by a second demyelinating event, by up to 2 years [25], although this effect was lost at follow-up beyond 2 years. Low doses of oral prednisone (15 mg/day) and oral prednisolone (8–12 mg/day) have not shown efficacy

Demyelinating Disorders of the Central Nervous System in Childhood, ed. Dorothée Chabas and Emmanuelle L. Waubant. Published by Cambridge University Press. © Cambridge University Press 2011.

in terms of relapse recovery [26,27]. One trial followed 23 patients with relapsing–remitting MS (RRMS) who had an acute exacerbation and were treated with IVMP, initially with a 15-day IV pulse starting at 15 mg/kg/day for 3 days and then tapered down every 3 days. The initial 15-day IV pulse was followed by oral prednisone, starting at 100 mg/day, and tapered over 120 days. Patients receiving IVMP recovered sooner than patients receiving placebo [28]. A 2-week IV pulse and 4-month oral taper is uncommon practice today and would expose the patient to risks associated with long-term steroid use. Another study showed that patients receiving IVMP (500 mg/day for 5 days) within 8 weeks of an acute relapse had lower mean Expanded Disability Scale Scores (EDSS) assessed at 1 and 4 weeks compared to placebo [29]. A meta-analysis of randomized controlled trials shows that steroids reduce the number of patients without functional improvement 8 and 30 days after receiving pulse therapy [30]. This same analysis revealed that in the long term, corticosteroids do not prevent relapses, nor do they prevent progression of disability.

High-dose IVMP (1 g/day for 10 days) produced a rapid reduction in contrast-enhancing lesions on T1-weighted magnetic resonance imaging (MRI) scans [31]. This effect began within 30 days of treatment and persisted for 60 days [32]. Short-term administration of IVMP has been associated with a decrease in brain parenchyma fractions, presumably secondary to reduction in edema associated with active inflammatory lesions [18]. Thus, scans obtained for research, and often for clinical purposes, are usually performed at least one month after discontinuation of high-dose steroids, to avoid underestimation of the presence of enhancing lesions and brain atrophy progression.

Considerable controversy surrounds the question of whether IVMP is superior to an oral steroid pulse in acute MS exacerbations. There are data to suggest that 1250 mg of oral prednisone has the same bioavailability as 1 g of IVMP [33]. Many studies have compared efficacy between high-dose intravenous and low-dose oral corticosteroids, with high-dose IVMP usually found to be more effective. However, only a few randomized trials have used equivalent doses when making comparisons. One study randomized 38 patients with clinically definite MS who had suffered a relapse within the previous 4 weeks to receive either 500 mg IVMP with placebo tablets for 5 days, or 500 mg oral MP with IV placebo for 5 days [34]. Patients were evaluated at days 5 and 28 with the EDSS. While both groups showed an improvement in EDSS, there was no statistical difference in EDSS scores between the oral and IVMP groups at days 5 and 28. Another study enrolled 80 patients with an acute relapse and randomly assigned them to receive either an oral or IVMP pulse [35]. Those randomized to receive oral steroids received 500 mg oral methylprednisolone daily (equivalent to 60 mg prednisolone) for 7 days, followed by 24 mg daily for 7 days and then 12 mg daily for 7 days. The intravenous regimen consisted of 1 g of IVMP daily for 3 consecutive days. EDSS scores were obtained at weeks 1, 4, 12, and 24. There was no statistical difference in EDSS scores at any stage of the trial. Analysis of these and other trials suggests that there is no significant difference in efficacy between IVMP and high-dose oral steroids for acute relapse [36].

Dosing regimen

Most adult studies suggest that high-dose IVMP should be dosed at 500–1000 mg daily for 3–5 days. Recent data suggest that high-dose oral methylprednisolone (500 mg) every day for 5–21 days is equally effective as high-dose IVMP [4,36]. For children suffering a moderate to severe clinical attack, current practice usually consists of a pulse of IV methylprednisolone at 20–30 mg/kg/dose every day (up to 1 g/day) for 3–5 days [22]. However, the high cost of inpatient care, and the unique stresses placed on a family with a child in the hospital, makes an outpatient steroid pulse an attractive alternative. Future studies are needed to determine if there is similar efficacy between high-dose IVMP and high-dose oral steroids for acute MS relapse in children.

There is no consensus on whether pulse therapy should be followed by an oral steroid taper. Some practitioners always use a steroid taper of 1 mg/kg/day in a single daily dose for 3 days, followed by progressive tapering by 5 mg every 2–3 days [22]. Others only use a taper for particularly severe attacks or if symptoms have not significantly improved after the initial pulse therapy. There are no data in children to suggest that tapering is beneficial. Retrospective data in adults suggest that an oral taper provides no benefit in relapse recovery [37].

Side effects

Long-term use of corticosteroids is associated with numerous and substantial adverse effects. Fortunately, few severe adverse events have been reported with the short, high-dose pulses typical of regimens used to treat MS exacerbations [38], even if prolonged (3–4 week) tapers are employed. The most common complaints are mood irritability, facial flushing, sleep disturbance, acne, and weight gain. Risks of gastric upset can be reduced by administering gastric protection such as an H2 blocker or proton pump inhibitor during the steroid pulse. Monitoring of blood pressure, serum glucose and potassium should be initiated during pulse therapy. Severe adverse events are associated with prolonged and repeated exposure to corticosteroids. The side effects of prolonged exposure include osteoporosis, neutropenia, weight gain, adrenal suppression, acne, increased skin fragility, hypertension, and psychosis. Growth suppression in children is an additional concern.

Conclusions

Many years of corticosteroid use have shown that it is an effective therapy in shortening recovery and ameliorating disability during acute MS attacks. They have also been found to be safe and well tolerated when used for short durations. As short-term steroid pulses have not been found to alter the long-term course of the disease, they are typically only used for moderate to severe exacerbations, when the level of physical disability interferes with activities of daily living. Mild exacerbations, with only minimal impact on functioning, are frequently not treated.

Typical treatment regimens consist of high dose IVMP in doses of 20–30 mg/kg/day (up to 1 g/day) for 3–5 days, although recent data in adults suggest that high-dose oral prednisone is equally effective. There is no consensus on whether a taper should be employed, although many practitioners use a taper after the initial pulse. Experience with high-dose corticosteroids in children suggest that it is well tolerated and that adverse effects such as hyperglycemia and hypertension are rare. There are some data to suggest that aggressive corticosteroid treatment in early relapses may prevent axon loss, making this therapy especially beneficial to patients suffering from early onset MS.

References

1. Griffiths TD, Newman PK. Steroids in multiple sclerosis. *J Clin Pharm Ther* 1994;**19**:219–222.

2. Optic Neuritis Study Group. The 5-year risk of MS after optic neuritis. Experience of the optic neuritis treatment trial. *Neurology* 1997;**49**:1404–1413.

3. Oliveri RL, Valentino P, Russo C, *et al.* Randomized trial comparing two different high doses of methylprednisolone in MS: A clinical and MRI study. *Neurology* 1998;**50**:1833–1836.

4. Miller DM, Weinstock-Guttman B, Bethoux F, *et al.* A meta-analysis of methylprednisolone in recovery from multiple sclerosis exacerbations. *Mult Scler* 2000;**6**:267–273.

5. Sloka JS, Stefanelli M. The mechanism of action of methylprednisolone in the treatment of multiple sclerosis. *Mult Scler* 2005;**11**:425–432.

6. Almawi WY, Beyhum HN, Rahme AA, Rieder MJ. Regulation of cytokine and cytokine receptor expression by glucocorticoids. *J Leukoc Biol* 1996;**60**:563–572.

7. Ossege LM, Sindern E, Voss B, Malin JP. Corticosteroids induce expression of transforming-growth-factor-beta1 mRNA in peripheral blood mononuclear cells of patients with multiple sclerosis. *J Neuroimmunol* 1998;**84**:1–6.

8. Loughlin AJ, Woodroofe MN, Cuzner ML. Modulation of interferon-gamma-induced major histocompatibility complex class II and Fc receptor expression on isolated microglia by transforming growth factor-beta 1, interleukin-4, noradrenaline and glucocorticoids. *Immunology* 1993;**79**:125–130.

9. Ruiz P, Gomez F, King M, Lopez R, Darby C, Schreiber AD. In vivo glucocorticoid modulation of guinea pig splenic macrophage Fc gamma receptors. *J Clin Invest* 1991;**88**:149–157.

10. Cupps TR, Gerrard TL, Falkoff RJ, Whalen G, Fauci AS. Effects of in vitro corticosteroids on B cell activation, proliferation, and differentiation. *J Clin Invest* 1985;**75**:754–761.

11. Conlon P, Oksenberg JR, Zhang J, Steinman L. The immunobiology of multiple sclerosis: An autoimmune disease of the central nervous system. *Neurobiol Dis* 1999;**6**:149–166.

12. Gelati M, Corsini E, De Rossi M, *et al.* Methylprednisolone acts on peripheral blood mononuclear cells and endothelium in inhibiting migration phenomena in patients with multiple sclerosis. *Arch Neurol* 2002;**59**:774–780.

13. Pitzalis C, Sharrack B, Gray IA, Lee A, Hughes RA. Comparison of the effects of oral versus intravenous methylprednisolone regimens on peripheral blood T lymphocyte adhesion molecule expression, T cell subsets distribution and TNF alpha concentrations in multiple sclerosis. *J Neuroimmunol* 1997;**74**:62–68.

14. Elovaara I, Ukkonen M, Leppäkynnäs M, *et al.* Adhesion molecules in multiple sclerosis: Relation to subtypes of disease and methylprednisolone therapy. *Arch Neurol* 2000;**57**:546–551.

15. Barkhof F, Frequin ST, Hommed OR, *et al.* A correlative triad of gadolinium-DTPA MRI, EDSS, and CSF-MBP in relapsing multiple sclerosis patients treated with high-dose intravenous methylprednisolone. *Neurology* 1992;**42**:63–67.

16. Melcangi RC, Cavarretta I, Magnaghi V, Ciusani E, Salmaggi A. Corticosteroids protect oligodendrocytes from cytokine-induced cell death. *Neuroreport* 2000;**11**:3969–3972.

17. Medana I, Martinic MA, Wekerle H, Neumann H. Transection of major histocompatibility complex class I-induced neurites by cytotoxic T lymphocytes. *Am J Pathol* 2001;**159**:809–815.

18. Rao AB, Richert N, Howard T, *et al.* Methylprednisolone effect on brain volume and enhancing lesions in MS before and during IFNbeta-1b. *Neurology* 2002;**59**:688–694.

19. Kornek B, Storch MK, Weissert R, *et al.* Multiple sclerosis and chronic autoimmune encephalomyelitis: A comparative quantitative study of axonal injury in active, inactive, and remyelinated lesions. *Am J Pathol* 2000;**157**:267–276.

20. Bitsch A, Schuchardt J, Bunkowski S, Kuhlmann T, Brück W. Acute axonal injury in multiple sclerosis. Correlation with demyelination and inflammation. *Brain* 2000;**123**:1174–1183.

21. Kuhlmann T, Lingfeld G, Bitsch A, Schuchardt J, Brück W. Acute axonal damage in multiple sclerosis is most extensive in early disease stages and decreases over time. *Brain* 2002;**125**:2202–2212.

22. Kuntz NL, Chabas D, Weinstock-Guttman B, *et al.* Treatment of multiple sclerosis in children and adolescents. *Expert Opin Pharmacother* 2010;**11**: 505–520.

23. Goodin DS, Frohman EM, Garmany GP Jr, *et al.* Disease modifying therapies in multiple sclerosis: Report of the Therapeutics and Technology Assessment Subcommittee of the American Academy of Neurology and the MS Council for Clinical Practice Guidelines. *Neurology* 2002;**58**:169–178.

24. Beck RW, Cleary PA, Anderson MM Jr, *et al.* A randomized, controlled trial of corticosteroids in the treatment of acute optic neuritis. The Optic Neuritis Study Group. *N Engl J Med* 1992;**326**:581–588.

25. Beck RW. The optic neuritis treatment trial: three-year follow-up results. *Arch Ophthalmol* 1995;**113**:136–137.

26. Miller H, Newell DJ, Ridley A. Multiple sclerosis. Trials of maintenance treatment with prednisolone and soluble aspirin. *Lancet* 1961;**1**(7169):127–129.

27. Tourtellotte WW, Haerer AF. Use of an oral corticosteroid in the treatment of multiple sclerosis; a double-blind study. *Arch Neurol* 1965;**12**:536–545.

28. Durelli L, Cocito D, Riccio A, *et al.* High-dose intravenous methylprednisolone in the treatment of multiple sclerosis: Clinical–immunologic correlations. *Neurology* 1986;**36**:238–243.

29. Milligan NM, Newcombe R, Compston DA. A double-blind controlled trial of high dose methylprednisolone in patients with multiple sclerosis: 1. Clinical effects. *J Neurol Neurosurg Psychiatry* 1987;**50**:511–516.

30. Brusaferri F, Candelise L. Steroids for multiple sclerosis and optic neuritis: A meta-analysis of randomized controlled clinical trials. *J Neurol* 2000;**247**:435–442.

31. Barkhof F, Hommes OR, Scheltens P, Valk J. Quantitative MRI changes in gadolinium-DTPA enhancement after high-dose intravenous methylprednisolone in multiple sclerosis. *Neurology* 1991;**41**:1219–1222.

32. Miller DH, Thompson AJ, Morrissey SP, *et al.* High dose steroids in acute relapses of multiple sclerosis: MRI evidence for a possible mechanism of therapeutic effect. *J Neurol Neurosurg Psychiatry* 1992;**55**: 450–453.

33. Morrow SA, Stoian CA, Dmitrovic J, Chan SC, Metz LM. The bioavailability of IV methylprednisolone and oral prednisone in multiple sclerosis. *Neurology* 2004;**63**:1079–1080.

34. Alam SM, Kyriakides T, Lawden M, Newman PK. Methylprednisolone in multiple sclerosis: A comparison of oral with intravenous therapy at equivalent high dose. *J Neurol Neurosurg Psychiatry* 1993;**56**:1219–1220.

35. Barnes D, Hughes RA, Morris RW, *et al.* Randomised trial of oral and intravenous methylprednisolone in acute relapses of multiple sclerosis. *Lancet* 1997;**349**:902–906.

36. Burton JM, O'Connor PW, Hohol M, Beyene J. Oral versus intravenous steroids for treatment of relapses in multiple sclerosis. *Cochrane Database Syst Rev*, 2009 (3):CD006921.

37. Perumal JS, Caon C, Hreha S, *et al.* Oral prednisone taper following intravenous steroids fails to improve disability or recovery from relapses in multiple sclerosis. *Eur J Neurol* 2008;**15**:677–680.

38. Andersson PB, Goodkin DE. Glucocorticosteroid therapy for multiple sclerosis: A critical review. *J Neurol Sci* 1998;**160**:16–25.

Chapter 1

Disease-modifying therapy and response to first-line treatment in pediatric multiple sclerosis

E. Ann Yeh and Moses Rodriguez

Pediatric-onset multiple sclerosis (MS) may comprise up to 5% of cases of MS in North America. The natural history of the disease in children is unknown. Although multiple therapies have been developed and approved for the treatment of adult MS, data regarding these therapies in children are limited. Therefore, most treatment decisions are based in part on treatment studies performed in adults. In this chapter, we will review the current literature on disease-modifying therapies (DMT) for children with MS. The chapter will first focus on first-line therapies. We will then move to a discussion of treatment strategies for children experiencing breakthrough disease while on first-line therapies. Escalation therapies for breakthrough disease are discussed in Chapter 11.

First-line disease-modifying therapies in pediatric MS

Four first-line DMTs have been approved for treatment of relapsing–remitting MS in the adult population. They include glatiramer acetate, interferon beta-1a IM, interferon beta-1a SC, and interferon beta-1b SC.

Interferon beta

Interferon beta is thought to act in MS via inhibition of pro-inflammatory cytokines, induction of anti-inflammatory mediators, reduction of cellular migration, and inhibition of autoreactive T cells [1,2]. Large phase III studies showed that chronic administration of recombinant interferon beta (IFNB) reduced the number of relapses and slowed progression of physical disability in adult patients with RR MS. The randomized pivotal studies demonstrated an approximately 30% reduction in exacerbation (relapse) rate in patients treated for 2–4 years compared with placebo [3–9]. Most studies have presented their data in terms

of relative risk reduction. In terms of numbers needed to treat (NNT) to achieve the required outcome for these drugs, 7–9 patients must be treated for 2 years to prevent one patient from developing a clinically definite relapse [10].

Several retrospective case series have described the use of IFNB-1a in the pediatric population. Follow-up in these series has ranged from 12 to 48 months. Although the majority of reports described are of children over 10 years of age, Tenembaum and Segura [11] included eight children under the age of 10 at first injection in their series. Outside of four patients with SPMS reported in that paper, all patients had relapsing–remitting MS.

IFNB-1a and 1b appear to be safe and well tolerated in this population [12–16]. Many children on interferon (35–65%) report flu-like symptoms [11–13,15]. Other relatively frequently observed side effects include leukopenia (8–27%), thrombopenia (16%), anemia (12%), and transient elevation in transaminases (10–62%) [11–13,15].

Abnormalities in liver function tests (LFTs) may be more pronounced in younger children taking interferon. In one study, 25% of children (average age of initiation of medication 14.6 years, range 8.1–17.9 years) taking IFNB-1a SC were found to have elevated LFTs. None of these children required discontinuation of therapy. Over two-thirds of these elevations occurred in the first 6 months of therapy [15]. However, in another study evaluating IFNB-1b SC, 8 of 43 patients experienced elevation of LFTs (>two times the upper limit of normal). Importantly, the children with elevated LFTs were predominantly under 10 years of age. Five of 8 (62.5%) children under 10 years of age in this study experienced LFT elevations. Two of these children were on full adult doses (8 MIU every other day), two were on half

Demyelinating Disorders of the Central Nervous System in Childhood, ed. Dorothée Chabas and Emmanuelle L. Waubant. Published by Cambridge University Press. © Cambridge University Press 2011.

of the adult dose (4 MIU), and one on one-quarter of the adult dose (2 MIU). By contrast, only 10% (3/30) of older children in this study (over 10 years of age) suffered from elevated LFTs in the first six months of treatment with IFNB-1b SC [13,15]. Temporary interruption of interferon treatment appears to lead to normalization of LFTs in children and can be accompanied by safe reintroduction of therapy after a temporary withdrawal of medication [13,15].

Given these results, we recommend close LFT monitoring on all children on interferons, particularly in the first six months of treatment. In general, LFTs should be obtained on a monthly basis for three months, then every three months thereafter. Should the LFTs increase to greater than twofold higher than the upper limit of normal, we suggest that the medication be withheld, the LFTs rechecked within a month, and the medication reintroduced, initially at a lower dose, after normalization of the LFTs.

Over two-thirds of children taking the SC formulation of IFNB-1a have reported injection site reactions. The injection site reactions occur throughout the treatment course in equal proportions. Pohl et al. reported that after a mean follow-up of 1.8 years, children were equally likely to report injection site reactions early on (0–6 months) and later [14]. Six percent of children on IFNB-1a SC experienced abscess and 6% injection-site necrosis over an average follow-up of 1.8 years [14]. Of those on IFNB-1b, only 20% over 10 years of age and 25% under 10 years of age experienced mild injection site reactions (average follow-up of 33.8 months) that did not lead to discontinuation of therapy [13].

Dosing of IFNB is not established in this population. However, most patients tolerated doses titrated following adult protocols, or gradual titration to 30 μg once weekly for IFNB-1a IM and 22 μg TIW or 44 μg TIW for IFNB-1a SC. Children over the age of 10 tolerate full doses of IFNB-1b, although decreased tolerance may exist in the younger population. In one study, two of 8 children who initiated IFNB-1b at 25–50% of adult doses did not tolerate escalation to full adult doses. Both were under 10 years of age [13].

With respect to efficacy, there have been no randomized controlled trials (RCTs) evaluating the efficacy of IFNB in the pediatric population. However, in a prospective, open-label study, Ghezzi et al. [17] followed 52 patients with pediatric-onset MS that were treated with IFNB-1a IM and found a reduction in annualized relapse rate from 1.9 pre-treatment to 0.4 after an average of 42 months on therapy. Similarly, Mikaeloff et al., reporting on 197 children with RRMS on interferon followed for a mean of 5.5 years, found a reduction in risk of MS attack in both the first year of treatment with interferon (hazard ratio = 0.31, 95% confidence interval: 0.13–0.72) as well as over the first 2 years of treatment (hazard ratio = 0.40, 95% confidence interval: 0.20–0.83). After 4 years of follow-up, the annualized relapse rate remained lower, but the 95% confidence interval was broader due to the smaller sample size, as not all patients had such a long follow-up (hazard ratio = 0.57, 95% confidence interval 0.30–1.10) [18]. Since 25–30% of patients in the adult population will have a benign outcome [19,20], defined by most as EDSS<3.0 for greater than 10 years' duration, it is important to keep these natural history studies in mind when considering the effects of any treatment in children without placebo-controlled groups [21]. No data are available on whether IFNB slows down the progression of disability in children. Furthermore, no data on the MRI effect of these medications in children are available.

Neutralizing antibodies

It has been noted widely in the adult literature that neutralizing antibodies to interferon may appear after a patient has been treated with interferon. In the adult population, these antibodies are more likely to be seen with IFN preparations that are given SC multiple times a week [22]. The relationship between titers of neutralizing antibodies and efficacy has not been established in the adult population, although studies have shown an inverse relationship between sustained high titers of these antibodies and ancillary measures of disease activity in adult MS [23]. However, knowledge regarding the impact of IFN-neutralizing antibodies on the efficacy of medication in the pediatric population is even more limited. No studies have comprehensively evaluated the frequency and significance of neutralizing antibodies in the pediatric population.

Glatiramer acetate

Glatiramer acetate (GA, Copaxone®) is the acetate salt of a mixture of synthetic polypeptides composed of: L-alanine, L-glutamic acid, L-lysine, and L-tyrosine. The drug is designed to mimic human myelin basic protein and is postulated to induce the myelin-specific response of suppressor T-lymphocytes and to inhibit specific effector T-lymphocytes [24]. The treatment consists of daily SC injection of 20 mg. In a pivotal phase III trial of adult RRMS patients, GA showed a 29% reduction of number of relapses in the treated group versus placebo [22–24]. Reduction in MRI activity has been shown in an RCT of adults treated with GA vs. placebo [24]. For this drug, 14 adult patients need to be treated for 2 years to prevent one patient from having a relapse [10]. Recent studies in adults have suggested that GA and IFNB have similar efficacy on clinical and MRI activity [25].

Only 3 retrospective studies have been published regarding the use of GA in pediatrics [26–28]. Kornek *et al.* [28] followed 7 patients with pediatric-onset RRMS for 24 months and reported that the medication was well tolerated. Children were aged 9–16 years at the time of GA initiation. Only 2/7 patients were relapse-free over the 24-month treatment period, and EDSS was stable in only 3/7 of the children. In two separate papers, Ghezzi *et al.* described nine and 11 patients on GA. GA was found to be relatively well tolerated, with 3/11 patients experiencing side effects (injection site reactions in two and chest pain in one) [26]. The mean annualized relapse rate decreased from 2.8 to 0.25 [27]. Conclusions from these studies regarding the efficacy of this medication cannot be drawn, however, given the small numbers and the lack of a control group.

Breakthrough disease

Breakthrough disease is a concern in the pediatric MS population. Of 258 children on therapy for MS followed prospectively by the US Network of Pediatric MS Centers for an average of 2.7 years, therapies were switched for breakthrough disease in 27% of patients. Changes due to breakthrough disease for individual therapies were the following: IFNB-1a SC, 16% (12/76); IFNB-1a IM, 37% (34/92); IFNB-1b SC, 44%; GA, 21% (11/53) [29].

The definition of breakthrough disease is challenging: it is one that has undergone significant debate among practitioners treating adult-onset MS. Given the available data regarding the frequency of relapse in MS in the adult population, it is generally accepted that at least 6 months of observation on a given treatment is necessary prior to deeming that treatment suboptimal. At present, our practice is to follow these guidelines and observe all patients for at least 6 months after initiation of therapy before deciding to change

therapies. In addition, it is important to evaluate compliance to therapy, especially in teenagers, who are often in charge of their own injections.

Consensus criteria for breakthrough disease in pediatric MS do not exist. Proposed consensus criteria for breakthrough disease in adults include increase in relapse number, new or recurrent MRI lesions, and worsening of cognitive or motor disability [30]. Limitations of this particular approach include the lack of adequate observational time to gauge whether an individual's relapse rate has decreased. Some advocate clinical evaluation every 3–6 months and an annual MRI in the adult population in order to monitor response to therapy closely. Given the more frequent relapses seen in the pediatric population [31], our practice is to perform MRI scans of the brain on a semi-annual basis with clinical visits every three months for the first year after treatment initiation. All of the studies in adults have shown that disease course during the first 5 years is an excellent predictor of future deficits [32]. Therefore, more frequent follow-up in the early course of the disease is warranted.

There is no accepted algorithm for the management of breakthrough disease. However, the following steps may be considered.

1. Increase the frequency of IFNB therapy (i.e. switching from once a week (Avonex®) to three times a week (Rebif®) or every other day (Betaseron®) injections). While some data from adult randomized trials (Betaseron vs. Avonex, and Rebif vs. Avonex) support a short-term advantage of more frequent dosing on prevention of relapses, the magnitude of the advantage is small [33,34], and the effect of switching from one to the other not addressed. This small potential advantage must be weighed against the disadvantages associated with frequent subcutaneous doses vs. intramuscular once a week dose regimens, as more frequent dosing has been associated with high neutralizing antibodies (NABs) and decreased efficacy according to MRI and clinical parameters [35,36]. Several non-randomized studies of medication changes in adults have shown a decrease in annualized relapse rate when switching from interferon to interferon, suggesting improvement when performing this switch [37,38].

2. Switch from one first-line therapy to another. For example, adult patients with sustained positive

NAB titers $\geq$20 may be switched from IFNB to GA. Switching from GA to IFNB is also an option, particularly given the rapid and robust effect of IFNB on inflammatory activity as measured by MRI [22]. In the adult population, this has been shown to result in a reduction in annualized relapse rate [38].

3. Add agents to the "platform" IFNB or GA therapy, including other immunomodulatory or cytotoxic agents. These agents have not been studied in MS using RCTs. Therefore, their benefit and safety are unclear, especially in children.

The next chapter focuses on escalation therapies in patients with breakthrough disease.

References

1. IFNB Multiple Sclerosis Study Group. Interferon beta-1b is effective in relapsing–remitting multiple sclerosis. I Clinical results of a multicenter, randomized, double blind, placebo-controlled trial. *Neurology* 1993;**43**: 655–661.

2. Jacobs L, Cookfair DL, Rudick RA, *et al*. Intramuscular interferon beta-1a for disease progression in relapsing multiple sclerosis. *Ann Neurol* 1996;**39**:285–294.

3. PRISMS (Prevention of Relapses and Disability by Interferon β-1a subcutaneously in Multiple Sclerosis) Study Group. Randomized double-blind placebo-controlled study of interferon β-1a in relapsing/remitting multiple sclerosis. *Lancet* 1998;**352**: 1498–1504.

4. Weinstock-Guttman B, Ransohoff RRM, Kinkel RP, *et al*. The interferons: Biological effects mechanisms of action, and use in multiple sclerosis. *Ann Neurol* 1995;**37**:7–15.

5. Yong V, Chabot S, Stuve O, *et al*. Interferon beta in the treatment of multiple sclerosis. Mechanism of action. *Neurology* 1998;**51**:682–689.

6. European Study Group on interferon beta-1b in secondary progressive MS. Placebo-controlled multicentre randomised trial of interferon β-1b in treatment of secondary progressive multiple sclerosis. *Lancet* 1998;**352**:1491–1497.

7. Secondary Progressive Efficacy Clinical trial of Recombinant Interferon-beta-1a in MS (SPECTRIMS) Study Group. Randomized controlled trial of recombinant interferon beta-1a in secondary progressive MS. Clinical results. *Neurology* 2001;**56**:1496–1504.

8. Goodkin D. and The North American Study Group on Interferon Beta-1b in Secondary Progressive MS. Interferon beta-1b in secondary progressive MS: Clinical and MRI results of a 3-year randomized controlled trial [Abstract]. Late Breaking News. Presented at the 52nd annual meeting of the American Academy of Neurology, San Diego, 2000.

9. Cohen J, Cutter GR, Fischer JS, *et al*. Benefit of interferon beta-1a on MSFC progression in secondary progressive MS. *Neurology* 2002;**59**:679–687.

10. Pittock SJ, Rodriguez M. Benign MS: A distinct clinical entity with therapeutic implications. In: *Advances in Multiple Sclerosis*, ed. M. Rodriguez. Heidelberg: Springer-Verlag, 2008. (Current Topics in Microbiology and Immunology, vol. 318); pp. 1–18.

11. Tenembaum SN, Segura MJ. Interferon beta-1a treatment in childhood and juvenile-onset multiple sclerosis. *Neurology* 2006;**67**:511–513.

12. Mikaeloff Y, Moreau T, Debouverie M, *et al*. Interferon-beta treatment in patients with childhood-onset multiple sclerosis. *J Pediatr* 2001;**139**:443–446.

13. Banwell B, Reder AT, Krupp L, *et al*. Safety and tolerability of interferon beta-1b in pediatric multiple sclerosis. *Neurology* 2006;**66**:472–476.

14. Bykova OV, Kuzenkova LM, Maslova OI. [The use of beta-interferon-1b in children and adolescents with multiple sclerosis]. *Zh Nevrol Psikhiatr Im S S Korsakova* 2006;**106**:29–33.

15. Pohl D, Rostasy K, Gartner J, *et al*. Treatment of early onset multiple sclerosis with subcutaneous interferon beta-1a. *Neurology*, 2005. **64**(5): pp. 888–90.

16. Waubant E, Hietpas J, Stewart T, *et al*. Interferon beta-1a in children with multiple sclerosis is well tolerated. *Neuropediatrics*, 2001. **32**(4): pp. 211–3.

17. Ghezzi A, Amato MP, Capobianco M, *et al*. Treatment of early-onset multiple sclerosis with intramuscular interferonbeta-1a: Long-term results. *Neurol Sci* 2007;**28**:127–132.

18. Mikaeloff Y, Caridade G, Tardieu M, *et al*. Effectiveness of early beta interferon on the first attack after confirmed multiple sclerosis: A comparative cohort study. *Eur J Paediatr Neurol* 2008;**12**: 205–209.

19. Pittock SJ. Does benign multiple sclerosis today imply benign multiple sclerosis tomorrow? Implications for treatment. *Neurology* 2007;**68**:480–481.

20. Ramsaransing GS, De Keyser J. Benign course in multiple sclerosis: A review. *Acta Neurol Scand* 2006;**113**:359–369.

21. Pittock SJ, McClelland RL, Mayr WT, *et al*. Clinical implications of benign multiple sclerosis: A 20-year population-based follow-up study. *Ann Neurol* 2004;**56**:303–306.

22. Malucchi S, Sala A, Gilli F, *et al*. Neutralizing antibodies reduce the efficacy of betaIFN during

treatment of multiple sclerosis. *Neurology* 2004;**62**:2031–2037.

23. Perini P, Calabrese M, Biasi G, *et al.* The clinical impact of interferon beta antibodies in relapsing–remitting MS. *J Neurol* 2004;**251**:305–309.

24. Comi G, Filippi M, Wolinsky JS. European/Canadian multicenter, double-blind, randomized, placebo-controlled study of the effects of glatiramer acetate on magnetic resonance imaging – Measured disease activity and burden in patients with relapsing multiple sclerosis. European/Canadian Glatiramer Acetate Study Group. *Ann Neurol* 2001;**49**:290–297.

25. Cadavid D, Wolansky LJ, Skurnick J, *et al.* Efficacy of treatment of MS with IFNbeta-1b or glatiramer acetate by monthly brain MRI in the BECOME study. *Neurology* 2009;**72**:1976–1983.

26. Ghezzi A. Immunomodulatory treatment of early onset multiple sclerosis: Results of an Italian Co-operative Study. *Neurol Sci* 2005;**26**(Suppl 4): S183–186.

27. Ghezzi A, Amato MP, Capobianco M, *et al.* Disease-modifying drugs in childhood-juvenile multiple sclerosis: Results of an Italian co-operative study. *Mult Scler* 2005;**11**:420–424.

28. Kornek B, Bernert G, Balassy C, *et al.* Glatiramer acetate treatment in patients with childhood and juvenile onset multiple sclerosis. *Neuropediatrics* 2003;**34**:120–126.

29. Yeh E, Krupp L, Ness J, *et al.* Breakthrough disease in pediatric MS patients: a pediatric network experience. In Annual Meeting of the American Academy of Neurology. 2009: Seattle, WA.

30. Cohen BA, Khan O, Jeffery DR, *et al.* Identifying and treating patients with suboptimal responses. *Neurology* 2004;**63**(Suppl 6):S33–40.

31. Gorman MP, Healy BC, Polgar-Turcsanyi M, *et al.* Increased relapse rate in pediatric-onset compared with adult-onset multiple sclerosis. *Arch Neurol* 2009;**66**:54–59.

32. Binquet C, Quantin C, Le Teuff G, *et al.* The prognostic value of initial relapses on the evolution of disability in patients with relapsing–remitting multiple sclerosis. *Neuroepidemiology* 2006;**27**:45–54.

33. Panitch H, Goodin DS, Francis G, *et al.* Randomized, comparative study of interferon beta-1a treatment regimens in MS; The EVIDENCE Trial. *Neurology* 2002;**359**:1453–1460.

34. Durelli L, Verdun E, Barbero P, *et al.* Every other day interferon beta-1b versus once-weekly interferon beta-1a for multiple sclerosis; results of a 2-year prospective randomized multicenter study (INCOMIN). *Lancet* 2002;**359**:1453–1460.

35. IFNB Multiple Sclerosis Study Group and the University of British Columbia MS/MRI Analysis Group. Neutralizing antibodies during treatment of multiple sclerosis with interferon beta-1b: Experience during the first 3 years. *Neurology* 1996;**47**:889–894.

36. Sorensen P, Ross C, Clemmesen KM, *et al.* Clinical importance of neutralizing antibodies against interferon beta in patients with relapsing remitting multiple sclerosis. *Lancet* 2003;**302**:1184–1191.

37. Carra A, Onaha P, Luetic G, *et al.* Therapeutic outcome 3 years after switching of immunomodulatory therapies in patients with relapsing–remitting multiple sclerosis in Argentina. *Eur J Neurol* 2008;**15**:386–393.

38. Gajofatto A, Bacchetti P, Grimes B, *et al.* Switching first-line disease-modifying therapy after failure: Impact on the course of relapsing–remitting multiple sclerosis. *Mult Scler* 2009;**15**:50–58.

Treatment of breakthrough disease

Daniela Pohl and Emmanuelle L. Waubant

There is consensus that therapy in relapsing–remitting multiple sclerosis (MS) in the pediatric age group should be initiated with first-line treatments approved for adult MS, namely one of the three forms of interferon-beta (IFNB) or glatiramer acetate (GA) [1]. However, as in adults with MS, the disease remains clinically or radiologically active in some children despite first-line therapies even 6–12 months after initiation of an appropriate regimen (see Chapter 10). In adult breakthrough disease, treatment strategies include switching to another first-line agent [2], adding another agent to the on-going therapy (combination therapy) [3,4], or switching to a second-line drug such as natalizumab or immunosuppression [5].

Although very few data are available regarding tolerability and efficacy of these therapeutic strategies in pediatric MS, there is anecdotal evidence from several pediatric MS centers that a variety of treatments are being used for the treatment of breakthrough disease in this age group [1]. Most of the drugs considered are either approved for the treatment of MS in the adult age group (natalizumab, mitoxantrone) or approved for other indications than MS (e.g. cyclophosphamide, methotrexate, rituximab, daclizumab, alemtuzumab, mycophenolate mofetil).

Therapeutic strategies such as switch to a second-line agent or off-label drugs are typically associated with the possibility of more severe adverse events than those seen with first-line agents, including life-threatening conditions such as progressive multifocal leukoencephalopathy (PML), leukemia, secondary cancers, or infections. Therefore, the potential benefits of such escalation therapies have to be carefully weighed against the risk profile of each drug being considered. Due to the paucity of experience with breakthrough therapeutic strategies in the pediatric age group, the following overview is largely based on data derived from adult patients. The lack of age-specific tolerability data, e.g. with regard to growth, as well as the mostly undetermined long-term toxicity profile (such as secondary cancer), remains a major concern.

Goals of breakthrough therapy in pediatric MS

The primary goal of breakthrough therapy in pediatric MS is to prevent disease activity and disability progression in patients who have continued disease activity despite appropriate first-line therapy. If breakthrough therapies were very safe, they could all be used for the long term. However, some of these drugs have cumulative doses above which risks are substantially higher, thus limiting the period of time during which they are used. Alternatively, it is conceivable, although not properly tested, that breakthrough therapies associated with significant risks could be used as "induction therapies" to stabilize disease course, allowing for reintroduction of first-line agents such as IFNB or GA. The caveat, though, is that it is unclear whether "induction therapies" have the potential to reset the "immune dysfunction" that is thought to be associated with breakthrough on first-line agents (e.g. it is unlikely that a patient with breakthrough disease on interferon will become stable on interferon after having received second-line therapies for a while).

Definition of breakthrough disease

Because all available MS agents are only partially effective, the notion of breakthrough disease has been

---

Demyelinating Disorders of the Central Nervous System in Childhood, ed. Dorothée Chabas and Emmanuelle L. Waubant. Published by Cambridge University Press. © Cambridge University Press 2011.

a sore issue over the past decade [5]. Some refer to disease activity on a well-conducted treatment as poor response or partial response to therapy. However, it remains to be determined whether continued disease activity on first-line agents is related to a lack of a biological response to treatment itself or is largely related to the underlying disease processes. At this point there is no consensus on how to define breakthrough disease during well-conducted disease-modifying therapy (DMT). Some physicians consider one relapse per year is sufficient, while others require two [5]. Also, some consider that radiological activity despite clinical stability is sufficient to meet breakthrough criteria [5]. Again, the number of new MRI lesions occurring during therapy that would define breakthrough is not standard across studies or providers. In addition, the minimum time on first-line therapy acceptable to call breakthrough is unclear, but is likely to be at least 6–12 months of well-conducted first-line therapy in a patient compliant with treatment regimen. In case poor compliance to therapy is identified as a possible cause of breakthrough, especially in teenagers who tend to self-inject without parental supervision, it should be re-emphasized during follow-up visits that compliance is key to treatment benefit and all efforts should be directed at understanding the reasons for poor compliance, as some might be easy to address. Poor compliance should not prompt treatment switch unless non-tolerable side effects of the current therapy result in decreased compliance.

Breakthrough therapies

Second-line drugs approved in adult MS

Natalizumab

Natalizumab is a humanized monoclonal antibody directed against alpha-4-integrin, a component of very late antigen-4 (VLA-4) present on leukocytes. By binding to VLA-4, natalizumab blocks the interaction of VLA-4 with the vascular cell adhesion molecule (VCAM) on the surface of endothelial cells at the blood–brain barrier, thereby greatly reducing the passage of lymphocytes and monocytes into the central nervous system (CNS) [6]. Natalizumab is administered intravenously in adults once every 4 weeks over 1 h at a dose of 300 mg.

The efficacy of natalizumab in relapsing–remitting adult MS has been demonstrated in two large phase III

trials. It decreases relapse rate by up to 68% and progression of disability by 42% over two years compared to placebo [7,8]. Due to three cases of PML, two of which had a lethal outcome in natalizumab-treated patients with MS and Crohn's disease in two separate clinical trials, the drug was withdrawn temporarily from the market shortly after its approval. In 2006, it was reintroduced for use as a single drug under a strict pharmocovigilance and risk management program. Even under these restrictions, over 70 new PML cases have been reported including in patients naïve to any other immunomodulating or immunosuppressive agents (http://www.fda.gov/Drugs/DrugSafety). The estimated risk of PML is in the range of 1/10 000 patient years [9]. This risk seems to be low during the first year of treatment, and increases for longer exposures. However, although to date more than 50 000 patients have been treated with natalizumab, most have received therapy for a relatively short period of time (<2 years), thus limiting our understanding of safety in the long term (i.e. whether the risk of PML increases linearly with increased duration of exposure). Other side effects of concern with natalizumab include allergic reactions in 3–6% of recipients, mostly occurring with the second infusion. The long-term risk of opportunistic infections other than PML and the risk for secondary cancers are unclear. Natalizumab is used within a restricted program that requires visits every months during the first three months followed by every six months visits thereafter. There are no guidelines on how long one can be treated with this medication, and the decision of treatment discontinuation or of a therapeutic holiday should be made in agreement with the patient and family in light of updated pharmacovigilance data. Physicians often request yearly brain MRI scans to monitor for clinical efficacy, but also for potential subclinical changes suggestive of PML.

Although natalizumab was mostly tested in patients naïve to MS therapies, it is currently used most of the time as a second-line agent. Only a few studies have evaluated its effect in patients with breakthrough relapsing MS on first-line agents. However, these studies consistently suggest that natalizumab as a single agent has a beneficial effect in adult patients with breakthrough disease that might be similar to the effect reported in patients naïve to MS drugs [10,11].

Experience with the use of natalizumab in the pediatric age group is very limited. The four published adolescents treated with natalizumab did not show severe adverse events or unexpected side effects during a treatment duration of up to 24 months [12,13]. More data on safety and efficacy in this age range are warranted. Another study of 19 patients with pediatric MS reported good tolerability and substantial suppression of disease activity over a median follow-up of 15 months [14].

Mitoxantrone

Mitoxantrone is an immunosuppressive agent also used in hairy cell leukemia and breast cancer treatment. As a topoisomerase inhibitor, it disrupts DNA synthesis, thereby inhibiting the proliferation of immune cells and suppressing the inflammatory response in MS [13].

A phase III study in patients with worsening MS has demonstrated its efficacy with regard to disability progression, number of treated relapses, and number of new T2-weighted brain MRI lesions. Mitoxantrone decreased relapse rate over 2 years by 68% compared with placebo and significantly prolonged the time to confirmed progression [15]. Mitoxantrone was approved in 2002 for worsening relapsing or secondary progressive MS patients not requiring wheelchairs in case of failure or intolerance of a previous therapy with immunomodulators.

Mitoxantrone 12 mg/m^2 is usually administered intravenously every 3 months for up to 2 years. Side effects include leukopenia, cardiomyopathy (with acute heart failure in 0.1–5.8% of mitoxantrone-treated MS patients) [16,17]. secondary leukemias (in approximately 0.3% of mitoxantrone-treated MS patients at a median of 19 months following the treatment) [18], and increased susceptibility to infections and early menopause, especially after the age of 35 years. Above a cumulative dose of 100 mg/m^2 the risk of cardiotoxicity increases significantly.

Therefore, a restriction of the cumulative dose to 100 mg/m^2, maximally 140 mg/m^2, is recommended. Monitoring ventricular ejection fraction with cardiac echograms or multigated angiocardiography (MUGA) should be performed before each infusion in order to halt therapy if left ventricular fraction is compromised. Cell blood count should be obtained prior to each infusion to ensure the patient has recovered white blood cell counts within normal range.

Mitoxantrone has been used in a few pediatric MS patients with breakthrough disease on first-line treatments [1]. However, conclusive data with regard to tolerability and efficacy in the treatment of MS in the pediatric age group are not yet available.

Drugs approved in other indications
Cyclophosphamide

Cyclophosphamide is an alkylating agent that is used to treat various types of cancer as well as autoimmune diseases. The main effect of cyclophosphamide is attributed to its metabolite phosphoramide mustard, which forms DNA interstrand crosslinks in cells with low levels of aldehyde dehydrogenase, leading to cell death. For MS therapy, cyclophosphamide is administered intravenously on a monthly basis, sometimes preceded by an induction course over 5 days. Antiemetic therapy during the infusions is recommended, such as odansetron, as well as good hydration to decrease the risk of hemorrhagic cystitis.

The magnitude of the efficacy of cyclophosphamide in the treatment of MS is still under debate. There have been reports of reduced relapse rate and decreased MRI lesion accrual [19–21]. However, its efficacy with regard to delaying disease progression is less well established, especially in patients with advanced disease stages. There is some evidence that younger adult patients with relapsing MS and patients with earlier stages of the disease may derive most benefit of cyclophosphamide treatment [22,23].

Very recently, a retrospective review of 17 children with MS (15 with relapsing–remitting, two with secondary progressive MS) treated with cyclophosphamide was published. The children were treated with three different regimens, induction therapy (5 doses over 8 days) alone, induction plus monthly maintenance or only monthly maintenance therapy. Cyclophosphamide was administered at a dose of 600–1000 mg/m^2 once a month. The minimum dose required to achieve leukopenia (nadir total white blood cell count less than 3000/mm^3 or between 1500 and 2000/mm^3, depending on the institution) was used to guide dose adjustment for the subsequent maintenance pulses. Cyclophosphamide was overall relatively well tolerated in most patients. However, one patient developed bladder carcinoma after a total of 72.7 g of cyclophosphamide over a period of 8 years. The transitional cell carcinoma was successfully treated. Other adverse events included nausea and vomiting (in 88% of patients), transient alopecia, osteoporosis, and amenorrhea. In the majority of patients, treatment resulted in a reduced relapse rate and stabilization of disability scores assessed one year after treatment initiation. However, over 50% of patients with a follow-up of over one year after cessation of therapy experienced the return of frequent relapses and required additional second-line treatments [24].

Methotrexate

Methotrexate (MTX) is a dicarboxylic acid used in the treatment of various cancers and autoimmune diseases. It acts via the inhibition of dihydrofolate reductase and other enzymes involved in purine metabolism, DNA and RNA synthesis. High-dose MTX is toxic for rapidly dividing cells and is regarded as a potent immunosuppressive agent. At lower doses, MTX still inhibits T-cell activation and suppresses T-cell intercellular adhesion molecule expression [24].

In patients with chronic progressive MS (primary and secondary progressive), oral weekly low-dose MTX (7.5 mg) as compared to placebo was reported to have better outcome as measured with a composite score, including timed ambulation, hand function, and MRI changes [25,26]. However, in relapsing–remitting patients with disease activity on weekly IFNB-1a, the addition of oral weekly MTX (20 mg) did not appear to affect positively brain MRI changes [3,25].

MTX therapy can result in macrocytic anemia responding to folic acid supplement, and thus folic acid is often combined systematically. Other side effects include bone marrow depletion, gastrointestinal disturbances, liver toxicity (fibrosis), and interstitial pneumonitis. Liver function and cell blood count monitoring are thus recommended on treatment. There are no data published on the use of MTX in pediatric MS.

Mycophenolate mofetil

Mycophenolate mofetil is an immunosuppressant acting via the inhibition of inosine monophosphate dehydrogenase, thereby reducing purine synthesis required for the proliferation of B and T lymphocytes. It is mainly used to prevent rejection in organ transplantation in adults and children >2 years of age. More recently, it has been increasingly utilized in various autoimmune disorders, including MS and NMO.

Adverse drug reactions include PML as well as increased risk of infections in general. Furthermore, diarrhea, nausea, vomiting, fatigue, headache, leukopenia, and anemia have been reported as side effects. Thus it is common to initiate therapy progressively over the first 4 weeks of treatment up to 2 g per day depending on weight. Combination with stomach protection is recommended.

Mycophenolate mofetil has been used off-label in a number of MS and NMO patients. However, there are currently no randomized controlled trials demonstrating its efficacy in the treatment of MS. Whether the improved disease course reported in one retrospective study and one open-label, single-centre study with a combination therapy with IFNB-1a will be confirmed in large randomized MS studies remains to be seen [27,28]. There are currently no reports on the treatment of pediatric MS patients with mycophenolate mofetil.

Monoclonal antibodies

Rituximab

Rituximab is a chimeric monoclonal antibody specific for the B-lymphocyte surface protein CD20. Rituximab induces a very rapid and dramatic depletion of B cells via mechanisms including apoptosis and immune-mediated cytotoxicity. Plasma cells lack CD20 and are therefore not affected by rituximab. B cells are replenished from pre-B cells coming from the bone marrow within 6–12 months after treatment, sometimes longer [29].

In adults, rituximab is approved for the treatment of non-Hodgkin's B-cell lymphoma, and refractory rheumatoid arthritis. It is also used off-label for systemic lupus erythematosus and neuromyelitis optica. It is not approved for use in children.

The proof-of-concept of rituximab efficacy in the treatment of relapsing–remitting MS was recently made in a phase II randomized study. One course of rituximab (two 1000 mg infusions two weeks apart) dramatically reduced new brain lesions on MRI for up to 48 weeks and also decreased relapse rate. Frequent infusion-related adverse events included chills, headaches, nausea, pruritus, fever, fatigue, throat irritation, and pharyngeal pain. Most of these were mild or moderate and mostly occurred with the first infusion [29]. Severe adverse events observed with rituximab used for conditions other than MS include increased risk of infections. While used in combination with other immunosuppressive medications, several cases of PML have been reported [30].

There is one case report of a 16-year-old girl with highly active relapsing–remitting MS treated with rituximab. She had breakthrough disease while on interferon therapy, then received a cumulative dose of 120 mg/m^2 of mitoxantrone, and subsequently failed glatiramer acetate, methotrexate, and mycophenolate mofetil treatment. The patient finally received off-label treatment with 750 mg of intravenous rituximab twice in 4 weeks, leading to a complete depletion of CD20-positive B cells in the peripheral blood and CSF. After 10 months, reconstitution of B cells was detected and the patient received a second course of rituximab with the same regimen. During the reported follow-up of 2 years, the patient remained clinically stable without further relapses and did not experience any side effects [31].

Alemtuzumab

Alemtuzumab is a humanized monoclonal antibody targeting CD52, a cell surface glycoprotein present on mature lymphocytes, but not stem cells. Administration of alemtuzumab results in a dramatic and prolonged drop in the levels of circulating T cells, B cells and some monocytes. Reconstitution of cell populations is sequential, with initial recovery of monocytes followed by B cells and T cells [28]. Alemtuzumab is currently licensed for the treatment of chronic lymphocytic leukemia in adults.

There is class I evidence for its efficacy in patients with relapsing–remitting MS. In a randomized phase II trial, alemtuzumab reduced relapse rate, disability progression and MRI activity compared to thrice-weekly subcutaneous IFNB-1a 44 µg. Adverse events observed in the alemtuzumab-treated patients included the development of other autoimmune disorders: six cases of immune thrombocytopenic purpura (one of them fatal) were reported. In addition, 23% of alemtuzumab recipients developed autoimmune thyroid conditions, especially Grave's disease. Other side effects reported in the alemtuzumab-treated patients included three cancers with onset ranging from 22 to 64 months after the first annual cycle (non-EBV-associated Burkitt's lymphoma, breast cancer, and cervical cancer in situ), as compared to one case of colon cancer in the group of IFNB-1a treated patients. Furthermore, three patients treated with alemtuzumab developed serious infusion reactions. Minor side effects of alemtuzumab were mild-to-moderate infections, especially of the respiratory tract [32].

There are currently no reports of treatment of pediatric MS with alemtuzumab.

Daclizumab

Daclizumab is a humanized monoclonal antibody directed against CD25, the interleukin-2 receptor alpha sub-unit of the human high affinity receptor, present on activated T cells and B cells. The exact mechanisms of action are still unclear, but may include blockade of the IL-2 receptor, augmentation of NK cell function-regulating T cells, and inhibition of CD4+CD25+ effector T cells [28]. Daclizumab is FDA-approved for the prevention of renal transplant rejection in adults.

There are several off-label studies and an on-going randomized phase II trial demonstrating an effect of daclizumab on MRI or clinical activity, either as add-on therapy to IFNB or as monotherapy, in relapsing remitting or secondary progressive MS patients [33–36]. Adverse events include an increased risk of infections, cutaneous reactions, fever, and lymphadenopathy.

There are currently no reports of daclizumab use in pediatric MS.

Corticosteroids

Corticosteroids are commonly used to treat moderate to severe MS attacks, since they have been shown to hasten recovery. Long-term treatment with corticosteroids is associated with significant side effects and is not recommended for MS. Oral continuous prednisolone treatment (15 mg/day for 8 months, then 10 mg/day for 10 months) as compared to placebo did not show significant benefit with regard to acute exacerbations or accrual of disability in MS patients [37].

Pulses of methylprednisolone (1 g/day intravenously for 5 days with oral prednisone taper) administered every 4–6 months for 5 years has been reported to delay disability progression and whole-brain atrophy and to slow the development of T1 black holes in adult relapsing–remitting MS patients [38].

Methylprednisolone pulses may suppress the formation of neutralizing antibodies to IFNB, thereby enhancing IFNB biological effect and clinical benefit. A recent study therefore evaluated the effect of methylprednisolone in MS patients with breakthrough disease on IFNB therapy and positive IFNB neutralizing antibodies. All patients discontinued IFNB therapy, and 38 patients were treated with monthly pulsed methylprednisolone as compared to 35 control patients discontinuing any therapy or switching to glatiramer acetate. At the end of the study, 8 patients (21%) in the methylprednisolone group and 4 patients (11%) in the control group had regained in-vivo response to IFNB (as measured by Myxovirus Resistance Protein

A mRNA induction in whole blood using real-time PCR). This difference, however, was not statistically significant ($p = 0.35$) [39]. Of note, IFNB discontinuation ultimately results in decrease of neutralizing antibodies within a few months. Pulsed methylprednisolone has been associated with increased susceptibility to infections (urosepsis, peritoneal infection), psychiatric symptoms (insomnia, restlessness, psychosis), gastrointestinal symptoms (particularly dyspepsia, rare pancreatitis), and neurological symptoms (most commonly changes in taste) [4]. It has also been associated with osteoporosis, although some studies do not confirm this risk as compared to control patients [40,41]. Monthly intravenous methylprednisolone pulses (up to 1 g/day for 3 days) have been used in the management of pediatric MS patients who continued to present frequent attacks or new MRI lesions while on appropriate regimen of IFNB or GA [1]. However, no details with regard to tolerability or efficacy have been published to date. The main concern for children receiving such therapy in addition to possible side effects reported in adults entail the risk of short stature, as steroids can reduce growth.

Combination therapies

Combination therapy of either first-line drugs (IFNB and GA) or first-line drugs with a second-line agent is sometimes used as an approach to obtain better disease control in breakthrough MS. Similar treatment strategies combining drugs with different mechanisms of action have provided utility in other autoimmune diseases, such as rheumatoid arthritis where early, aggressive combination therapy is considered the best treatment paradigm for ensuring adequate disease control and optimizing long-term outcome [42]. The goal of combination therapy should be to improve disease control without aggravating adverse events. Very few studies have appropriately looked at the effect of combining therapies in adult MS patients with breakthrough disease on first-line agents, and none in children.

Interferon beta and glatiramer acetate

An obvious combination treatment would be GA and IFNB. The two first-line treatments have quite different mechanisms of action and thus could, in theory, have additive or synergistic effects. However, studies

on the mechanism of action of GA and IFNB have indicated that a combination of both might be contraindicated, since GA may require the entry of specific T cells into the CNS to exert its effect, whereas IFNB non-specifically prevents access of T cells to the nervous system [42].

There has been one small non-randomized study including 21 adult MS patients with breakthrough disease on monotherapy with GA or IFNB. These patients received combination therapy with GA and IFNB for a duration of 16–24 months. The combination was well tolerated. However, treatment effect is difficult to estimate since there was no control group with breakthrough disease remaining on monotherapy [43]. A large clinical trial including around 1000 patients is currently evaluating the efficacy and safety of a combination of GA and weekly IFNB-1a and will show if this combination is beneficial.

Interferon beta and methylprednisolone

In patients with breakthrough disease while on monotherapy with IFNB, add-on methylprednisolone pulses might provide additional disease control.

However, two recent large randomized placebo-controlled studies in patients with continued disease activity on IFNB monotherapy and add-on methylprednisolone were inconclusive. The NORdic trial included patients treated with subcutaneous IFNB-1a 44 μg thrice-weekly who suffered at least one relapse in the preceding 12 months. It showed that oral monthly add-on methylprednisolone (200 mg/day for 5 day) for at least 96 weeks significantly reduced yearly relapse rate by 62% as compared to IFNB-1a treatment alone [4]. This study was limited by the high drop-out rate, especially in the oral methylprednisolone group. The Avonex Combination Trial (ACT) included patients with at least one relapse or gadolinium-enhancing MRI lesion in the prior year on weekly intramuscular IFNB-1a monotherapy. Add-on therapy with pulsed intravenous methylprednisolone (every other month 1000 mg/day for 3 days) did not appear to slow down accumulation of T2-bright lesions during 12 months of treatment [3].

Interferon beta and azathioprine

Azathioprine is a long-established immunosuppressant drug used in organ transplantation and autoimmune disease such as rheumatoid arthritis, pemphigus, inflammatory bowel disease, and auto-immune hepatitis. The active metabolites of azathioprine, 6-mercaptopurine, and 6-thioinosinic acid, act as purine synthesis inhibitors, thereby unspecifically inhibiting proliferation of cells. Furthermore, azathioprine inhibits T-cell activation by blocking the CD28 signal transduction pathway. Due to a lack of phase III randomized, placebo-controlled studies with MRI outcomes, azathioprine is considered to be of unclear benefit in MS when used as monotherapy. However, it is widely used, especially in countries in which access to interferon or GA is limited. Since it suppresses the formation of anti-acetylcholine receptor antibodies in myasthenia, it was suggested as a potentially beneficial add-on therapy to IFNB to inhibit the synthesis of neutralizing IFNB antibodies in MS patients [42].

A number of small studies have evaluated azathioprine in combination with IFNB in MS. One study of 15 patients with breakthrough disease on IFNB-1b demonstrated that add-on azathioprine resulted in a 65% reduction in the number of gadolinium-enhancing lesions compared to the baseline value under IFNB-1b monotherapy. There was a highly significant correlation ($r = 0.61$; $p = 0.0002$) between the total leukocyte count and the number of active lesions, with a count less than 4800/mm^3 being associated with a loss of lesion activity on MRI. Add-on azathioprine therapy was also associated with a stabilization of neurological disability as measured with the Multiple Sclerosis Functional Composite score [44].

Another small study included 23 patients either previously untreated (eight patients), or with breakthrough therapy on monotherapy with subcutaneous IFNB-1a (seven patients) or azathioprine (eight patients). A combination treatment with IFNB-1a (6 MIU every other day) and azathioprine (dose adjustment throughout the two-year treatment period in order to achieve a lymphocyte count of 1000/μl or less) was associated with significant reduction in relapse rate, change in EDSS disability score and MRI measures of lesion activity compared to the pre-baseline observation period [45].

Long-term MS therapy with azathioprine has been associated with increased risk of malignancy, especially after a treatment duration of more than five years and cumulative doses of >600 g [46]. Less severe side effects of azathioprine therapy in MS include gastrointestinal complaints, allergic reactions, bone marrow suppression, and hepatic toxicity [47,48].

Interferon beta and mitoxantrone

Mitoxantrone has been almost exclusively used either as monotherapy in breakthrough disease or, off-label, as induction therapy followed by GA or IFNB. Currently there has been only one very small study with a combination therapy of mitoxantrone and IFNB-1b. In this study, 10 patients with worsening relapsing–remitting or secondary progressive MS with breakthrough disease on IFNB-1b monotherapy for at least 6 months were treated with an add-on therapy of mitoxantrone (12 mg/m^2 at induction, then two monthly pulses of 5 mg/m^2, then 5 mg/m^2 every third month). There were no serious adverse events on combination therapy and no drop-outs due to toxicity. Following the addition of mitoxantrone to IFNB-1b, mean enhancing lesion frequency decreased by 90% at month 7 and enhancing lesion volume decreased by 96%. Relapse rates decreased by 64%. However, since there has been no control group with mitoxantrone monotherapy, it is unclear whether these positive treatment effects are attributable to the combination therapy as opposed to mitoxantrone alone [49].

Interferon beta and natalizumab

Two large randomized, placebo-controlled trials have evaluated the efficacy and safety of natalizumab in patients with relapsing–remitting MS. One of these studies evaluated natalizumab in monotherapy, the other in combination with intramuscular IFNB-1a. The trial that combined natalizumab to IFNB-1a was the first large phase III trial testing the safety and efficacy of combination strategies. There was no evidence for a synergy between the two treatments, since the on-treatment relapse rate in the combination group (0.38 relapses/year) was not lower than in the natalizumab monotherapy group (0.27 relapses/year), although inclusion criteria were somewhat different. Similarly, gadolinium-enhancing lesions were almost completely abolished at the end of the first treatment year in both trials (mean 0.1 lesions per patient) [7,8].

Thus, the combination therapy of natalizumab with IFNB does not seem to bring any advantage over natalizumab alone. Moreover, it has been hypothesized that a combination of two agents that prevent access of immune cells to the CNS may increase the risk of PML. In an effort to minimize risk factors for the development of PML, combination

Table 11.1 Second-line agents used for breakthrough MS

Drug	Licensed for MS in adults	Dose (adults) and administration	Serious adverse events*
Natalizumab	Yes	300 mg IV monthly	PML, Infusion-associated reactions
Mitoxantrone	Yes	12 mg/m^2 IV every 3 months for $\leq$2 years	Cardiotoxicity, Acute leukemia, Infertility
Methylprednisolone	Off-label	1 g/d for 3–5 days IV every 1–6 months	Psychosis, Aseptic necrosis, Diabetes, Hypertension
Azathioprine	Off-label	~2.5–3 mg/kg PO daily	Secondary malignancies, Hepatotoxicity
Cyclophosphamide	Off-label	~600–1000 mg/m^2 IV monthly	Secondary malignancies, Infertility
Rituximab	Off-label	2×1000 mg IV 2 weeks apart ~ yearly	PML, Infusion-associated reactions
Mycophenolate mofetil	Off-label	$\leq$2 g PO daily	Secondary malignancies, PML
Methotrexate	Off-label	7.5–20 mg PO weekly	Secondary malignancies, Hepatotoxicity, Interstitial pneumonitis
Alemtuzumab	Off-label	12–24 mg IV yearly	Immune thrombocytopenic purpura, Thyroid autoimmune disease, Infusion-associated reactions
Daclizumab	Off-label	1 mg/kg IV monthly	Infusion-associated reactions

Note:
* This is not a complete list of all reported serious adverse events, e.g. all drugs listed may increase the risk of potentially life-threatening infections. Long-term immunosuppression increases the risks for malignancy. Furthermore, there are currently no conclusive safety data for the pediatric age group, especially with regard to long-term risks

of natalizumab with other immunomodulating or immunosuppressive agents is now regarded as strictly contraindicated.

Conclusions

Continuing disease activity in pediatric MS patients treated with first-line drugs presents a major challenge to the care provider. Even in adult MS patients, there is no general consensus on the definition of breakthrough disease and on the most appropriate treatment strategy and algorithm. However, since current first-line therapies are only partially effective, breakthrough disease activity will be seen in many patients at some point, in adults as well as in children and adolescents with MS. Breakthrough disease is associated with a worse prognosis [5]. Hence, detection of breakthrough disease and subsequent change of treatment strategy seems to be of the utmost importance. Appropriate strategies to identify breakthrough disease may include regular follow-up visits,

assessment of compliance, discussion and management of adverse events, and meticulous monitoring of relapses, disability, and MRI measures [5]. Although there is little evidence available to guide specific drug choice in breakthrough disease, changing from IFNB to GA or vice versa in patients with low disease activity might be an option, as these are relatively safe drugs. On the other hand, advancing treatment to natalizumab, mitoxantrone, or off-label immunosuppressive agents makes sense for patients with worrisome levels of disease activity [5]. Combination therapies may increase toxicity and it is unclear whether this risk is outweighed by improved efficacy. New immunomodulatory agents such as teriflunomide, fingolimod (FTY 720), laquinimod, fumaric acid, and cladribine may hold some promise for the future treatment of breakthrough disease [50–54]. However, it is to be anticipated that, once they have been approved for adult MS, safety concerns will delay their use in the pediatric population until there are sufficient long-term safety data. Experience has highlighted that some rare severe adverse events only become evident post-approval, when larger numbers of patients are exposed to the drug for longer periods of time. Since pediatric MS patients potentially have close to a century of lifetime before them, very long-term safety issues will remain a major concern with all MS treatments, but logically more so with relatively new drugs.

In conclusion, there is an urgent need not only for well-designed trials for the treatment of breakthrough disease in adult and pediatric-onset MS, but also for collaborative, multicenter studies analyzing the safety and efficacy of second-line treatments in children and adolescents with MS.

References

1. Pohl D, Waubant E, Banwell B, *et al.* Treatment of pediatric multiple sclerosis and variants. *Neurology* 2007;**68**:S54–S65.

2. Gajofatto A, Bacchetti P, Grimes B, High A, Waubant E. Switching first-line disease-modifying therapy after failure: Impact on the course of relapsing–remitting multiple sclerosis. *Mult Scler* 2009;**15**:50–58.

3. Cohen JA, Imrey PB, Calabresi PA, *et al.* Results of the Avonex Combination Trial (ACT) in relapsing–remitting MS. *Neurology* 2009;**72**:535–541.

4. Sorensen PS, Mellgren SI, Svenningsson A, *et al.* NORdic trial of oral Methylprednisolone as add-on therapy to Interferon beta-1a for treatment of relapsing–remitting Multiple Sclerosis (NORMIMS study): A randomised, placebo-controlled trial. *Lancet Neurol* 2009;**8**:519–529.

5. Rudick RA, Polman CH. Current approaches to the identification and management of breakthrough disease in patients with multiple sclerosis. *Lancet Neurol* 2009;**8**:545–559.

6. Yednock TA, Cannon C, Fritz LC, Sanchez-Madrid F, Steinman L, Karin N. Prevention of experimental autoimmune encephalomyelitis by antibodies against alpha 4 beta 1 integrin. *Nature* 1992;**356**:63–66.

7. Polman CH, O'Connor PW, Havrdova E, *et al.* A randomized, placebo-controlled trial of natalizumab for relapsing multiple sclerosis. *N Engl J Med* 2006;**354**:899–910.

8. Rudick RA, Stuart WH, Calabresi PA, *et al.* Natalizumab plus interferon beta-1a for relapsing multiple sclerosis. *N Engl J Med* 2006;**354**:911–923.

9. Hartung HP. New cases of progressive multifocal leukoencephalopathy after treatment with natalizumab. *Lancet Neurol* 2009;**8**:28–31.

10. Putzki N, Kollia K, Woods S, Igwe E, Diener HC, Limmroth V. Natalizumab is effective as second line

11. Oturai AB, Koch-Henriksen N, Petersen T, Jensen PE, Sellebjerg F, Sorensen PS. Efficacy of natalizumab in multiple sclerosis patients with high disease activity: A Danish nationwide study. *Eur J Neurol* 2009;**16**: 420–423.

12. Borriello G, Prosperini L, Luchetti A, Pozzilli C. Natalizumab treatment in pediatric multiple sclerosis: A case report. *Eur J Paediatr Neurol* 2009;**13**:67–71.

13. Huppke P, Stark W, Zurcher C, Huppke B, Bruck W, Gartner J. Natalizumab use in pediatric multiple sclerosis. *Arch Neurol* 2008;**65**:1655–1658.

14. Ghezzi A, Pozzilli C, Grimaldi LM, *et al.* Safety and efficacy of natalizumab in children with multiple sclerosis. *Neurology* 2010;**75**:912–917.

15. Hartung HP, Gonsette R, Konig N, *et al.* Mitoxantrone in progressive multiple sclerosis: A placebo-controlled, double-blind, randomised, multicentre trial. *Lancet* 2002;**360**:2018–2025.

16. Feuillet L, Guedj E, Eusebio A, *et al.* [Acute heart failure in a patient treated by mitoxantrone for multiple sclerosis]. *Rev Neurol (Paris)* 2003;**159**: 1169–1172.

17. Goffette S, Van Pesch V, Vanoverschelde JL, Morandini E, Sindic CJ. Severe delayed heart failure in three multiple sclerosis patients previously treated with mitoxantrone. *J Neurol* 2005;**252**:1217–1222.

18. Ellis R, Boggild M. Therapy-related acute leukaemia with Mitoxantrone: What is the risk and can we minimise it? *Mult Scler* 2009;**15**:505–508.

19. Smith DR, Weinstock-Guttman B, Cohen JA, *et al.* A randomized blinded trial of combination therapy with cyclophosphamide in patients with active multiple sclerosis on interferon beta. *Mult Scler* 2005;**11**:573–582.

20. Reggio E, Nicoletti A, Fiorilla T, Politi G, Reggio A, Patti F. The combination of cyclophosphamide plus interferon beta as rescue therapy could be used to treat relapsing–remitting multiple sclerosis patients – twenty-four months follow-up. *J Neurol* 2005;**252**:1255–1261.

21. Zipoli V, Portaccio E, Hakiki B, Siracusa G, Sorbi S, Amato MP. Intravenous mitoxantrone and cyclophosphamide as second-line therapy in multiple sclerosis: An open-label comparative study of efficacy and safety. *J Neurol Sci* 2008;**266**:25–30.

22. Weiner HL, Mackin GA, Orav EJ, *et al.* Intermittent cyclophosphamide pulse therapy in progressive multiple sclerosis: Final report of the Northeast Cooperative Multiple Sclerosis Treatment Group. *Neurology* 1993;**43**:910–918.

therapy in the treatment of relapsing remitting multiple sclerosis. *Eur J Neurol* 2009;**16**:424–426.

23. Hohol MJ, Olek MJ, Orav EJ, *et al.* Treatment of progressive multiple sclerosis with pulse cyclophosphamide/methylprednisolone: Response to therapy is linked to the duration of progressive disease. *Mult Scler* 1999;5:403–409.

24. Makhani N, Gorman MP, Branson HM, Stazzone L, Banwell BL, Chitnis T. Cyclophosphamide therapy in pediatric multiple sclerosis. *Neurology* 2009;72:2076–82.

25. Goodkin DE, Rudick RA, VanderBrug MS, *et al.* Low-dose (7.5 mg) oral methotrexate reduces the rate of progression in chronic progressive multiple sclerosis. *Ann Neurol* 1995;37:30–40.

26. Goodkin DE, Rudick RA, VanderBrug MS, Daughtry MM, Van DC. Low-dose oral methotrexate in chronic progressive multiple sclerosis: Analyses of serial MRIs. *Neurology* 1996;47:1153–1157.

27. Vermersch P, Waucquier N, Michelin E, *et al.* Combination of IFN beta-1a (Avonex) and mycophenolate mofetil (Cellcept) in multiple sclerosis. *Eur J Neurol* 2007;14:85–89.

28. Frohman EM, Brannon K, Racke MK, Hawker K. Mycophenolate mofetil in multiple sclerosis. *Clin Neuropharmacol* 2004;27:80–83.

29. Hauser SL, Waubant E, Arnold DL, *et al.* B cell depletion with rituximab in relapsing–remitting multiple sclerosis. *N Engl J Med* 2008;358:676–688.

30. Carson KR, Evens AM, Richey EA, *et al.* Progressive multifocal leukoencephalopathy after rituximab therapy in HIV-negative patients: A report of 57 cases from the Research on Adverse Drug Events and Reports project. *Blood* 2009;113:4834–4840.

31. Karenfort M, Kieseier BC, Tibussek D, Assmann B, Schaper J, Mayatepek E. Rituximab as a highly effective treatment in a female adolescent with severe multiple sclerosis. *Dev Med Child Neurol* 2009;51:159–161.

32. Coles AJ, Compston DA, Selmaj KW, *et al.* Alemtuzumab vs. interferon beta-1a in early multiple sclerosis. *N Engl J Med* 2008;359:1786–1801.

33. Rose JW, Burns JB, Bjorklund J, Klein J, Watt HE, Carlson NG. Daclizumab phase II trial in relapsing and remitting multiple sclerosis: MRI and clinical results. *Neurology* 2007;69:785–789.

34. Rose JW, Watt HE, White AT, Carlson NG. Treatment of multiple sclerosis with an anti-interleukin-2 receptor monoclonal antibody. *Ann Neurol* 2004;56:864–867.

35. Bielekova B, Howard T, Packer AN, *et al.* Effect of anti-CD25 antibody daclizumab in the inhibition of inflammation and stabilization of disease progression in multiple sclerosis. *Arch Neurol* 2009;66:483–489.

36. Bielekova B, Richert N, Howard T, *et al.* Humanized anti-CD25 (daclizumab) inhibits disease activity in multiple sclerosis patients failing to respond to interferon beta. *Proc Natl Acad Sci USA* 2004;101:8705–8708.

37. Miller H, Newell DJ, Ridley A. Multiple sclerosis. Trials of maintenance treatment with prednisolone and soluble aspirin. *Lancet* 1961;1:127–129.

38. Zivadinov R, Rudick RA, De Masi R, *et al.* Effects of IV methylprednisolone on brain atrophy in relapsing–remitting MS. *Neurology* 2001;57:1239–1247.

39. Hesse D, Frederiksen JL, Koch-Henriksen N, *et al.* Methylprednisolone does not restore biological response in multiple sclerosis patients with neutralizing antibodies against interferon-beta. *Eur J Neurol* 2009;16:43–47.

40. Whitehead BF, Rees PG, Sorensen K, *et al.* Results of heart–lung transplantation in children with cystic fibrosis. *Eur J Cardiothorac Surg* 1995;9:1–6.

41. Zorzon M, Zivadinov R, Locatelli L, *et al.* Long-term effects of intravenous high dose methylprednisolone pulses on bone mineral density in patients with multiple sclerosis. *Eur J Neurol* 2005;12:550–556.

42. Gold R. Combination therapies in multiple sclerosis. *J Neurol* 2008;255(Suppl 1):51–60.

43. Ytterberg C, Johansson S, Andersson M, *et al.* Combination therapy with interferon-beta and glatiramer acetate in multiple sclerosis. *Acta Neurol Scand* 2007;116:96–99.

44. Pu"licken M, Bash CN, Costello K, *et al.* Optimization of the safety and efficacy of interferon beta 1b and azathioprine combination therapy in multiple sclerosis. *Mult Scler* 2005;11:169–174.

45. Lus G, Romano F, Scuotto A, Accardo C, Cotrufo R. Azathioprine and interferon beta(1a) in relapsing–remitting multiple sclerosis patients: Increasing efficacy of combined treatment. *Eur Neurol* 2004;51:15–20.

46. Confavreux C, Saddier P, Grimaud J, Moreau T, Adeleine P, Aimard G. Risk of cancer from azathioprine therapy in multiple sclerosis: A case-control study. *Neurology* 1996;46:1607–1612.

47. La ML, Mascoli N, Milanese C. Azathioprine. Safety profile in multiple sclerosis patients. *Neurol Sci* 2007;28:299–303.

48. Casetta I, Iuliano G, Filippini G. Azathioprine for multiple sclerosis. *J Neurol Neurosurg Psychiatry* 2009;80:131–132.

49. Jeffery DR, Chepuri N, Durden D, Burdette J. A pilot trial of combination therapy with mitoxantrone and interferon beta-1b using monthly gadolinium-enhanced magnetic resonance imaging. *Mult Scler* 2005;11:296–301.

50. O'Connor PW, Li D, Freedman MS, *et al.* A Phase II study of the safety and efficacy of teriflunomide in multiple sclerosis with relapses. *Neurology* 2006;**66**:894–900.

51. Cohen JA, Barkhof F, Comi G, *et al.* Oral fingolimod or intramuscular interferon for relapsing multiple sclerosis. *N Engl J Med* 2010;**362**:402–415.

52. Kappos L, Gold R, Miller DH, *et al.* Efficacy and safety of oral fumarate in patients with relapsing–remitting multiple sclerosis: A multicentre, randomised, double-blind, placebo-controlled phase IIb study. *Lancet* 2008;**372**:1463–1472.

53. Giovannoni G, Comi G, Cook S, *et al.* A placebo-controlled trial of oral cladribine for relapsing multiple sclerosis. *N Engl J Med* 2010;**362**:416–426.

54. Comi G, Pulizzi A, Rovaris M, *et al.* Effect of laquinimod on MRI-monitored disease activity in patients with relapsing–remitting multiple sclerosis: A multicentre, randomised, double-blind, placebo-controlled phase IIb study. *Lancet* 2008;**371**:2085–2092.

Symptomatic therapy in pediatric multiple sclerosis

Sunita Venkateswaran, Susan Bennett, and Jayne Ness

In children and adolescents, multiple sclerosis (MS) has an impact on the developing central nervous system and can result in transient or fixed deficits of gross motor and/or fine motor skills, sensory perceptual processing, bowel/bladder function, vision, balance, and coordination. The heterogeneous presentation and disease course of MS makes symptom prediction difficult. Large brain lesions may be present in non-eloquent regions and not produce symptoms. Conversely, small lesions in dense axonal tracts may produce multiple symptoms. We have the inability to predict, as of yet, which lesions will heal completely, and which will become permanent and produce residual symptoms. Heat-induced "pseudorelapses" may also occur and these must be clearly differentiated from a true clinical relapse, although to a patient the experience can be one and the same.

In addition to sensory and motor symptoms, pediatric MS patients may experience ongoing difficulties with fatigue and mental health issues, independent of relapses and lesion distribution, which significantly impact daily function and quality of life. Paroxysmal symptoms such as the sensation of tightness around the chest or intermittent muscle spasms can be very distressing.

Some deficits may be under-recognized due to the young age of the patient (i.e. visual or sensory symptoms in a pre-schooler or increased urinary frequency in the diaper-wearing toddler). Other deficits may not become apparent until new challenges arise as the child progresses in school (i.e. poor handwriting due to subtle weakness or visual motor deficit; poor physical endurance due to fatigue and/or heat sensitivity; difficulties completing tests and homework due to slower processing speed). Any of these symptoms can limit the child's participation in play and school and in an adolescent may have a profound impact on socialization and achieving independence during the formative years of development.

As in adult demyelinating disorders, the focus of medical treatment and rehabilitation is to promote neuroplasticity and cortical reorganization. When that is not possible, the focus is to manage new and residual symptoms and promote the highest level of functional recovery to normalize life between relapses. Objective age-appropriate measures of symptoms, mobility and activity are essential in optimizing medical and rehabilitation management.

As illustrated in Figure 12.1, there is considerable symptom overlap in pediatric demyelinating disorders. For ease of discussion, the evaluation and care of patients with symptoms resulting from the following pediatric demyelinating disease will be addressed as individual systems with discussion of anatomy and typical features, evaluation measures, and treatment options, including both non-pharmacologic and pharmacologic approaches.

1. Visual disturbances
2. Speech, language or swallowing problems
3. Motor function including spasticity, tremor, and gait
4. Autonomic symptoms including bowel and bladder difficulties
5. Sensory symptoms including pain and paroxysmal symptoms
6. Systemic issues including heat intolerance, fatigue, and mental health issues. Cognitive and psychosocial difficulties in pediatric demyelinating disorders are discussed separately in Chapters 13 and 14.

Demyelinating Disorders of the Central Nervous System in Childhood, ed. Dorothée Chabas and Emmanuelle L. Waubant. Published by Cambridge University Press. © Cambridge University Press 2011.

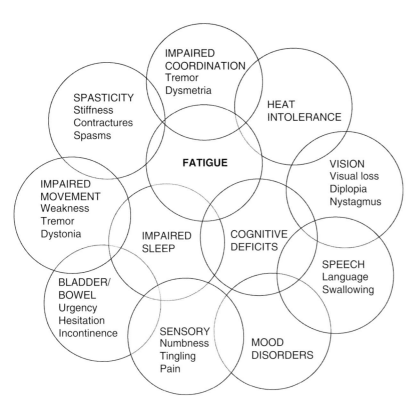

Figure 12.1 Intertwined symptoms in pediatric MS
Children and adolescents with MS may acquire fixed deficits following a relapse or develop symptoms independently of a relapse. Symptoms in one realm can exacerbate difficulties in other areas.

Evaluation and care of patients with visual abnormalities

Vision abnormalities are a common complaint in pediatric MS both as a presentation and as a relapse. Approximately 20% of children present with optic neuritis (ON) [1], and between 20 and 41% present with brainstem demyelination at their first demyelinating event [1–3]. It is likely that visual disturbances are underestimated in the pediatric MS population; in one series, pathological visual evoked potentials (VEPs) were present in one-third of 85 pediatric MS patients despite the absence of a clinical history of ON and the majority having normal visual acuity testing using standard vision charts [4].

Transient or fixed visual dysfunction in MS may result from demyelinating lesions at any point along the visual pathway from the optic nerve to the striate cortex. Common visual disorders in MS include decreased visual acuity and color perception due to ON, diplopia, nystagmus, oscillopsia and/or impaired visual tracking due to brainstem lesions, and visual field cuts resulting from lesions of the optic nerves, chiasm, optic radiations or striate cortex. In addition,

conditions such as anterior uveitis are much more common in MS patients. Cataracts and glaucoma must be screened for in children who have been on long-term steroids.

Optic neuritis

Although most children who have suffered from an episode of ON recover completely [5], common residual symptoms include decreased color vision, reduced contrast sensitivity and acuity, and increased sensitivity to light. Pain should not be present upon recovery, and for those children who are left with severe visual loss, alternative diagnoses must be considered (Leber's hereditary optic neuropathy, neuromyelitis optica). An in-depth discussion on ON is presented in Chapters 20 and 21 of this textbook.

Internuclear ophthalmoplegia (INO)

The most common eye movement abnormality in MS is an INO secondary to lesions in the medial longitudinal fasciculus (MLF). Examination of horizontal gaze in these patients reveals incomplete or slow adduction of the ipsilateral eye, and mononuclear nystagmus of the contralateral eye. This nystagmus is thought to be due to overcompensation, or increased signal to the contralateral eye, in attempts to adduct the weaker affected eye. More subtle INO can be brought out by asking the patient to make quick horizontal saccades or during optokinetic testing. Both unilateral and bilateral INO can occur in MS. Bilateral INO affecting both MLFs and with additional involvement of the midbrain oculomotor sub nuclei of the medial rectus can cause a phenomenon called wall-eyed bilateral INO (WEBINO) where both eyes are exotropic on primary gaze.

Patients with an INO may complain of oscillopsia or diplopia. More extensive lesions can also interrupt the vertical pursuit pathways or the vestibular pathways (via the superior vestibular nuclei), producing associated vertical gaze evoked and torsional nystagmus. Convergence can also be affected in patients with WEBINO.

The one-and-a-half syndrome, a combination of the absence of horizontal gaze in one eye and abnormal adduction of the other eye, is due to a lesion involving the parapontine reticular formation (PPRF) and the adjacent MLF ipsilateral to the eye with the complete gaze palsy. These children may also have associated facial nerve palsies due to the proximity of the lesion to the facial nerve nucleus.

Nystagmus

Neural integrators for vertical and horizontal gaze-holding are located in the midbrain (interstitial nucleus of Cajal) and medulla (medial vestibular nuclei and nucleus prepositus hypoglossi), respectively. These regions are also connected to cerebellar nuclei in the flocculus and paraflocculus to fine tune gaze. Damage to these areas causes failure of neural integration and gaze-evoked nystagmus.

Other types of nystagmus present in MS include pendular nystagmus, where there are bidirectional slow phases in any plane. This is also due to the failure of neural integration or lesions within Mollaret's triangle. This type of nystagmus can be especially disturbing [6], as it produces retinal slip, preventing stabilization of images and thereby affecting all activities from walking to reading.

Other visual abnormalities present in our patients include skew deviation, other cranial nerve palsies, and saccadic intrusions.

Evaluation of visual function

Evaluation of visual function includes basic components of the neurological examination (funduscopy, assessment of acuity, color vision, pupillary light reflex, visual fields). Although visual acuity is typically assessed using standard high contrast Snellen charts, low-contrast letter acuity (Sloan chart) has greater sensitivity in detecting visual dysfunction in adult MS patients and correlates with measures of disability, MRI lesion volume, and retinal nerve fiber thickness as measured by optical coherence tomography (OCT) [7]. However, low-contrast letter acuity has not been validated in the pediatric age group. Other measures of visual function including VEP and OCT are discussed in greater detail in the section on ON in children. Ishihara plates can be used as a screen for color vision dysfunction as plates become progressively more difficult to differentiate.

Neuro-ophthalmology colleagues can be of great assistance in evaluation of ocular alignment, motility, intrusions, pursuit, saccades, nystagmus, and vestibular function, as these evaluations are challenging without the appropriate equipment or expertise.

Management of visual dysfunction
Non-pharmacologic interventions for visual dysfunction

Prior unrecognized refractive error can contribute to the residual symptoms, so this should be initially corrected. Sunglasses or tinted corrective glasses can minimize photosensitivity, while prisms can help correct binocular vision which is critical for accurate depth perception.

Occupational therapy can help children to retrain the visual motor and visual perceptual system following a demyelinating event. Much of the theoretical framework for visual motor and visual perceptual training is based on the Hierarchy of Visual Skill Development Model developed by Warren [(8,9]. In this model, first, oculomotor skills and central and peripheral visual acuity are required to generate an image, followed by progression to visual scanning. This is followed by pattern recognition, visual memory and finally, visual cognition. This approach is used to identify and remediate visual dysfunction in adults with acquired brain injury. Many of the same principles can be applied to the child with demyelinating disease.

Table 12.1 Interventions for the visually impaired child

Provide good lighting in commonly used areas

Provide lighting that maximizes contrast and clarity

Provide contrast at desk or table, e.g. dark table or mat with white paper on top

Magnification of material to be read

Outline steps and pathways with contrast markings

Sunglasses outdoors and in settings with fluorescent lights

Assistive technology for visual functioning

Software which provides:

  Screen enlarger/magnifier

  Screen reader

  Scan and read

Work station placement to avoid glare

Non-glare screen on computer

Organize note-taking "buddy" at school

"Eyes Need Relaxing"

Instruct patients to close their eyes and cover with warm cloth or warmed hands to allow for muscle relaxation.

Repeat frequently throughout the course of the day

Using this framework of visual skill development, specific interventions have been designed to provide the visually impaired child with visual motor and perceptual challenges (Table 12.1).

Pharmacologic management of visual symptoms

Nystagmus and oscillopsia can be particularly disabling, resulting in persistent blurry vision, difficulties in visual tracking, and imbalance. Common medical approaches include use of baclofen or gabapentin, but improvement is often not sufficient enough to justify concurrent sedation. There are unfortunately no known pharmacological treatments for chronic gaze palsies or pursuit abnormalities [6]. Table 12.2 outlines medications available to treat eye movement abnormalities.

Evaluation and care of speech and swallowing difficulties

The majority of children with demyelinating disease do not experience symptoms related to communication or swallowing; however, a severely affected child with predominant brainstem attacks or a child with advanced MS may experience the following: delayed swallowing reflex; reduced pharyngeal peristalsis; reduced laryngeal function; reduced lingual function; reduced oral sensation.

The presence of any of these symptoms must be addressed by the speech language pathologist and the feeding and swallowing team, as there is the potential for choking and aspiration. In addition, children who have difficulty swallowing may be at risk for weight loss, malnutrition, and dehydration. Specific interventions to assist the child with swallowing problems are listed in Table 12.3.

Evaluation and management of motor, gait, and coordination difficulties
Spasticity and weakness

Spasticity is defined as "velocity dependent resistance" and affects >80% of adult MS patients [10]. Spasticity more commonly affects lower than upper extremities in MS [11], and has a definite impact on disability scores due to its effects on ambulaton. Lesions causing eventual spasticity can be widespread in both the brain and spinal cord and are the result of interruption of descending inhibitory pathways. Fixed contractures can be a result of spasticity, but can be prevented in milder cases if ongoing rehabilitation is maintained. Total elimination of spasticity is not always advantageous, as increased muscle tone in certain muscle groups may work to stabilize other weakened muscle groups by promoting postural support [12].

Spasticity is very intertwined with the other symptoms of MS as it can worsen fatigue, impact on coordination, and by affecting the speed of gait, make bowel and bladder abnormalities more difficult to handle.

Gait and coordination difficulties

Gait imbalance, whether due to transverse myelitis, multiple cortical lesions, cerebellar lesions, or encephalopathy, is a very common presentation, with up to 15% of children having ataxia at presentation [2]. This proportion is much higher (53%) in children under

Table 12.2 Pharmacological interventions for nystagmus and oscillopsia

Medication (Brandname)	Formulations	Starting pediatric dose and max. dose	Side effects	Comments
Gabapentin (Neurontin™) [68–71]	Tablet: 100, 300, 400, 600, 800 mg Liquid: 50 mg/ml	**Start:** 10–15 mg/kg div TID; or 300 mg od × 3 days **Goal:** titrate to 25–40 mg/kg/d div TID; or 300 mg od ×3 day, then 300 mg BID, then TID **Max:** 3600 mg per day div TID-QID	Dizziness, fatigue	Useful for pendular nystagmus
Memantine (Namenda™) [68–71] *NMDA receptor antagonist*	Tablet: 5, 10 mg Liquid: 2 mg/ml	No peds dosing **Start:** 5 mg od **Goal:** Increase in 1 week to 5 mg BID **Max:** 20 mg/day div BID	Lethargy, dizziness, confusion, headache, HTN	Useful for pendular nystagmus
4-aminopyridine Ampyra™ (dalfampridine) [72] *NMDA antagonist*	Tablet: 10 mg	**Adult dosing (no peds dosing):** **Start:** 10 mg qhs **Goal:** 20 mg/day div BID or 1 mg/kg/day **Max:** 30 mg/d div BID Increased seizure risk if >30 mg/day	Insomnia, headache, dizziness, peripheral and perioral paresthesias, palpitation, contraindicated if h/o seizures	FDA approval Jan 2010 for improved gait but also used in Europe for fatigue, spasticity
3,4-diaminopyridine [72]		**Start:** 5 mg/day **Goal:** Titrate to TID-QID dosing **Max:** 80 mg/day div QID	Parasthesias, abdominal pain	Avoid in patients with history of seizure
Carbemazepine (Tegretol™, Tegretol-XR™ Carbetrol™)	Tablet: 100, 200 mg Tablet extended release: 100, 200, 300, 400 mg Liquid: 20 mg/ml	**Start:** 10 mg/kg/day div BID-TID **Goal:** titrate to 15 mg/kg/day div BID-TID **Max:** 1600 mg/day div BID-QID; follow levels, side effects	Sedation, dizziness, ataxia, lymphopenia, decreased platelets	Useful for paraxosymal nystagmus Follow CBC, AST, ALT, and drug levels; 4–12 is typical range HLA-B*1502 (mainly Asian ancestry) have increased risk of Steven-Johnson Syndrome
Acetozolamide (Diamox™) *Carbonic anhydrase inhibitor*	Tablet: 125, 250, 500 mg extended release IV formulation	**Start:** 5–10 mg/kg/day div TID; or 125–250 mg od, titrate to TID-QID **Max:** 1000 mg/day div TID-QD	Fatigue, metallic taste, parasthesia, nausea/vomiting, diarrhea, polyuria	Useful for paraxosymal nystagmus

Table 12.3 Interventions for swallowing difficulties

Positioning of the head in 15 to 20 degrees of cervical flexion during swallowing
Maintain good posture and head position in wheelchair
Thickeners for liquids
Exercise for oral musculature
Adaptive feeding equipment

the age of 10 [2], and in children with acute mono-phasic transverse myelitis, where 90% are unable to walk at presentation, and only 36% are able to walk independently at follow-up [13]. The rate of tremor and other movement disorders have not been specifically studied in pediatric acquired demyelinating syndrome (ADS).

Evaluation of motor and coordination abnormalities

Measurement tools for motor development and activity performance in neurorehabilitation have been specifically developed for the pediatric population. However, the common standardized instruments used in pediatrics may not be sensitive enough to detect strength, coordination, and movement abnormalities unless there are significant impairments in mobility. Examples of standardized scales used in pediatric neurorehabilitation include: the Gross Motor Function Classification System (GMFCS) [14], Peabody Developmental Motor Scale, Pediatric Evaluation of Disability Inventory (PEDI), and Bruininks–Oseretsky Test of Motor Proficiency-2 (BOT-2). A comprehensive listing of pediatric standardized tests can be found at http://www.pediatricapta.org. In children with demyelinating disease, testing may need to be repeated if initial testing was performed at time of relapse or during recovery.

Adult studies traditionally use the Ashworth [15] and modified Ashworth Scales [16] to assess the degree of spasticity, although the Tardieu scale may be a more appropriate tool as it evaluates passive tone through both fast and slow velocities, abiding more closely to the definition of spasticity. It may also be more sensitive to changes post-treatment [17–19]. Examples of available and recommended standardized measures

that are applicable to our clinical population are described below.

BOT-2

The advantage of the BOT-2 is that it measures gross and fine motor skills of children aged 4–21, encompassing several functional areas in one test. There are eight subset scores that measure:

- fine motor precision – 7 items (e.g. cutting out a circle, connecting dots);
- fine motor integration – 8 items (e.g. copying a star, copying a square);
- manual dexterity – 5 items (e.g. transferring pennies, sorting cards, stringing blocks);
- bilateral coordination – 7 items (e.g. tapping foot and finger, jumping jacks);
- balance – 9 items (e.g. walking forward on a line, standing on one leg on a balance beam);
- running speed and agility – 5 items (e.g. shuttle run, one-legged side hop);
- upper-limb coordination – 7 items (e.g. throwing a ball at a target, catching a tossed ball); and
- strength – 5 items (e.g. standing long jump, sit-ups).

A short form of this battery of tests is available, but has decreased validity in children under the age of 6 [20].

Timed 25 foot walk [21–23]: the patient is allowed to walk with an assistive device or an orthotic. The patient starts in the standing posture at a taped line on the floor. When asked to begin, the patient walks 25 feet as quickly and safely as possible. The therapist records the time in seconds from first heel strike over the taped line to first heel strike over the second taped line positioned 25 feet away. Two trials are performed and the average time is recorded.

Timed up and go [24]: The patient is seated in a chair placed in the middle of the hallway. A large cone is placed 10 m from the patient. At the command to begin, the subject rises from the chair and walks as quickly and safely as possible to the large cone, walks around the cone, walks back to the chair and sits down. Time is measured in seconds and starts with the command to begin and ends when the patient has returned to a seated position in the chair.

Both of the above tests are limited by the age and height of the patient. Normative values in the pediatric population are not available.

Standardized test for upper extremity function/coordination

Nine-hole peg test (9HPT) [21–23]: This a timed, quantitative measure of upper extremity function where the patient must take nine pegs out of a container, place them in a block containing nine holes, remove the pegs, and return them to the container. Both the dominant and non-dominant hands are tested twice (two consecutive trials of the dominant hand, followed immediately by two consecutive trials of the non-dominant hand). It is important that the 9-HPT be administered on a solid table and that the 9-HPT apparatus is secured. This test is limited by coordination abilities that improve with age.

Management of motor and coordination difficulties

Spasticity

Non-pharmacologic treatment for spasticity

For pediatric practitioners accustomed to caring for children with cerebral palsy, physical and occupational therapy are obvious first-line interventions. However, rehabilitation centers accustomed to serving children with relatively static disorders such as cerebral palsy or intellectual disability may have difficulty addressing the fluctuating needs of children and adolescents with MS or other acquired demyelinating disorders. Obtaining appropriate accommodations may be even more challenging for patients with less obvious impairments due to fatigue, slowed processing speed, visual deficits, or disrupted bladder and bowel function. Depending on the severity of the spasticity, different degrees of intervention may be required. The goals of treating spasticity include: improving ambulation and general mobility, improving self-care, reducing pain and paroxysmal spasms, and preventing contractures [25]. Therapeutic exercise should always be a component of the treatment plan to address muscles weakness and for general cardiovascular training. The physical education program at school may need to be tailored to the child's level of physical ability and to prevent fatigue.

When weakness and spasticity predominate, prolonged stretching and prolonged cold application of spastic muscles can inhibit the excessive tone. Strengthening antagonist muscles also improves postural tone, by stimulating inhibition of spastic muscles at the spinal cord level. Spastic muscle groups should also be strengthened in their normal alignment and without generating synergistic activity. For example, biceps muscle contraction should be initiated in a gravity-neutral plane to avoid recruiting synergistic muscle of shoulder elevation. Whenever possible, strengthening activities should be performed in functional postures such as sitting, kneeling, or standing in order to reinforce truncal stability which is needed for performing all tasks. Persistent muscle weakness and spasticity may require an ankle foot orthotic, or static splint for the upper extremity.

There is increased interest in application of Constraint Induced Movement Therapy (CIMT) for MS patients [26]. Initially validated in hemiparetic adult stroke patients, CIMT entails restraining the non-involved arm or leg, in combination with intensive repetitive exercises of the paretic extremity. The goal is to approximate functional activities which become increasingly refined ("shaping"). Functional neuroimaging studies have demonstrated cortical reorganization with this type of therapeutic intervention. CIMT has been demonstrated to be effective in children with congenital hemiparesis [26].

Pharmacologic treatment of spasticity

There are limited randomized controlled trials comparing treatments for spasticity in children. For treatment of generalized spasticity, oral medications include baclofen, diazepam, tizanidine, and dantrolene. In a practice guideline for treatment of spasticity in the pediatric cerebral palsy population [19], only diazepam could be classified as "probably effective" in reducing spasticity based on Class I and Class II randomized, controlled trials [27,28]. Recommendations for other oral agents could not be determined due to insufficient data. Because of significant sedation plus risk of dependence, diazepam or its longer-acting counterpart clonazepam are not first-line treatments for spasticity in MS, although night-time dosing of a benzodiazepine may promote sleep initiation and reduce spasticity-induced jerks that can disrupt sleep.

Despite the paucity of randomized controlled trials demonstrating effectiveness, oral baclofen is typically the first-line treatment for spasticity in children. Starting doses of baclofen are typically 2.5–5 mg (1/4–1/2 of 10 mg tablet) given 2–3 times daily. A liquid formulation of baclofen at 5 mg/ml enables starting doses as low at 1 mg/ml. To limit sedation, baclofen should be slowly titrated to the minimal effective dose (maximal effective dose is typically 60 mg/day divided TID). Tizanidine is reported to be efficacious in children, but as sedation can be problematic, sublingual tizanidine may be a better option [29]. Dantrolene is also sedating and, additionally, is associated with increased irritability, weakness, seizure risk, and hepatotoxicity so is not used in pediatric disorders (i.e. cerebral palsy) or adult MS in North America.

In localized or segmental spasticity, injection of botulinum toxin (available as onabotulinumtoxinA, Botox; anabotulinumtoxinA, Dysport or botulinum toxin B, Myobloc or Neurobloc) provides 2–6 months of relaxation in the targeted muscles. In a 2008 evidence-based review of Botox treatment for spasticity for adults with MS and the 2010 spasticity practice parameter for children with cerebral palsy, Botox was given a level A recommendation for treatment of lower extremity spasticity, and a level B recommendation for its use in upper extremities [19,30]. No recommendation was made regarding other botulinum toxins or neurolytic agents such as phenol due to insufficient evidence. Repeated injections, given more frequently than 3-month intervals, may become less efficicacious over time due to the generation of botulinum antibodies. The larger muscle groups such as gastrocnemius are riskier targets due to the higher doses of botulinum toxin required and the potential for systemic distribution. Isolated reports of generalized weakness following local botulinum toxin injections prompted the FDA in 2009 to institute a black box warning for these agents.

In cases of medically intractable spasticity or intolerance to oral medications, a rare instance in pediatric MS, a baclofen pump placed in the lower abdomen with an intrathecal catheter (ITB) can deliver continuous baclofen. This has already proven to be efficacious in the adult MS population and in a significant number of children with cerebral palsy [31].

Dalfampridine, a slow-release formulation of 4-aminopyridine, has recently been approved by the FDA for specific use in adult MS gait disorders. Please refer to Table 12.4 for details on this medication.

Ataxia and tremor

Non-pharmacological intervention

Therapeutic intervention for ataxia and tremor is more challenging. Anecdotal evidence supports the use of compression sleeves on the extremities or weighting the distal extremities, trunk, or assistive device. A brace across a joint can also aid in minimizing random movement of the limb.

Balance requires ocular motor function, vestibular input, and somatosensory processing working in concert, and should be evaluated at each visit. Spontaneous nystagmus and diplopia not only impact the child's ability for reading, learning, and attention but also balance in any upright posture. Strategies for visual fixation and strengthening ocular muscles for visual tracking should be initiated by the occupational therapist or the physical therapist. Similarly, vestibular rehabilitation should be initiated with a child that is experiencing dizziness or imbalance related to a brainstem lesion. This is most often detected when testing the vestibular ocular reflex (VOR).

A new intervention in many physical therapy clinics is the Nintendo Wii™, a video game system which has games consisting of activities for fitness, balance, strengthening, yoga, and aerobics. In addition to the fitness programs there is software that simulates sports and recreational activity. The Wii™ is especially popular with children as it requires their active participation and provides immediate sensory feedback. It has been used successfully in children with cerebral palsy [32].

Pharmacological treatment of ataxia and tremor

The treatment of persistent tremor can be challenging, especially tremors of the trunk and neck. Table 12.4 lists potential medications used to treat tremor and their side effects. Treatment of intention (also called kinetic) tremors by beta-blockers such as propranolol or primidone, and benzodiazepines such as clonazepam, can sometimes be successful, but overall, cerebellar tremors are very disabling and difficult to treat. Non-pharmacological interventions, as mentioned above, may be more rewarding. Physiological tremors and medication-induced tremors, not due to MS itself, can be treated well by beta-blockers and decrease of medication dose, respectively.

Evaluation and care of bladder and bowel symptoms

Bladder and bowel incontinence is both a social inconvenience and embarrassment which greatly interferes with daily life. Once identified, the evaluation and management of these symptoms is important to prevent long-term complications.

Table 12.4 Medications for spasticity, tremor and mobility

Medication (Brandname)	Formulations	Starting pediatric dose and max. dose	Side effects	Comments
Spasticity				
Baclofen (Lioresal™) [19] *Binds GABA-B (inhibitory) receptor*	Tablets: 10, 20 mg Liquid: 5 mg/ml	**Start:** 1 mg–2.5 mg qhs, titrate to TID **Goal:** Minimum effective dose **Max:** 60–80 mg/day div TID-QID	Sedation, dizziness, weakness	Also used for periodic alternating nystagmus
Diazepam (Valium™) [19] *Binds benzo-diazepine receptor on GABA$_A$ channel, increases frequency of GABA$_A$ channel opening, enhances GABA binding*	Tablets: 2, 5,10 mg Liquid: 5 mg/ml.	**Start:** 0.5 mg **Goal:** 0.12–0.8 mg/kg/day PO div q6–8h **Max:** 30 mg/day div TID	Sedation, ataxia; short-term use recommended due to risk of physical dependence	Ketoconazole, omiprazole, fluvoxamimne, fluoxetine may prolong the effects of diazepam
Clonazepam (Klonopin™, Rivotril™, Clonopam™) [19] *Binds benzodiazepine receptor on GABA$_A$ channel, increases frequency of GABA$_A$ channel opening, enhances GABA binding*	Tablets: 0.5, 1, 2 mg ODT: 0.125, 0.25, 0.5, 1, 2 mg ODT: 0.125, 0.25, 0.5, 1, 2 mg Liquid: 0.1 mg/ml	**Start:** 0.125 mg qhs × 1 week then BID **Goal:** Min effective dose **Max:** 0.2 mg/kg per day or 10 mg/day	Sedation, ataxia; short-term use recommended due to risk of physical dependence	Taper off slowly over weeks to prevent withdrawal
Tizanidine (Zanaflex™) [19] *Alpha-2 agonist*	Capsule or tablet: 2, 4, 6 mg	**Start:** 0.05 mg/kg or 2 mg qhs × 1 week, then increase to BID **Goal:** 2–4 mg BID **Adults:** 12 mg TID (36 mg/day)	Sedation Hypotension Dizziness Hepatotoxicity (monitor transaminases)	Contraindicated with ciprofloxacin, fluvoxamine due to inhibition of hepatic metabolism of tizanidine
Dantrolene (Dantrium) [19] *Decrease Ca^{2+} release from sarcoplasmic reticulum*	Tablet: 25, 50, 100 mg tablet	**Start:** 0.5 mg/kg od × 7d, then 0.5 mg/kg TID **Goal:** 6–8 mg/kg/day div BID-QID **Max:** 12 mg/kg/day or 400 mg day	Sedation; anorexia, nausea/vomiting Hepatotoxicity, (monitor transaminases)	Discontinue if no improvement in 6 weeks
Mobility				
4-aminopyridine (Ampyra™) (dalfampridine) [49] *Blocks voltage gated K+ channel*	Tablet: 10 mg	**Adult dosing (no pediatric dosing reported):** **Start:** 10 mg qhs **Goal:** 20 mg/day div BID or 1 mg/kg/day **Max:** 30 mg/day div BID Increased seizure risk >30 mg/day	Insomnia, headache, dizziness, peripheral and perioral paresthesias, palpitation, contraindicated if h/o seizures	FDA approval Jan 2010 for improved gait but also used in Europe for fatigue, spasticity

Table 12.4 (cont.)

Medication (Brandname)	Formulations	Starting pediatric dose and max. dose	Side effects	Comments
Ataxia/tremor				
Primidone (Mysoline™) [73,74] *Mechanism of action unknown; active metabolite includes phenobarbitone*	Tablet: 50, 250 mg	**Start:** 10–20 mg/kg/day div BID-TID or 50–100 qhs **Titrate:** 50 BID × 1 week then TID or incr 25–50 mg qhs q week; goal 750 mg/day div qhs-TID **Max:** 2 g/day	Sedation, dizziness, diplopia	Avoid abrupt withdrawal
Propranolol (Inderal™, Inderal™ LA) [73,74] *Beta-blocker*	Tablet: 10, 20, 40, 60, 80 mg Extended release: 60, 80, 120, 160 mg Liquid: 4 or 8 mg/ml	**Start:** 1 mg/kg/day div BID-TID **Titrate:** 0.5–1 mg/day div BID-TID or 10–20 mg q 3–7 day **Max:** 4–8 mg/kg/day or 320 mg/day div BID-TID	Fatigue, dizziness, bradycardia, bronchospasm	Use with care in patients with asthma
Clonazepam (Klonopin™, Rivotril™, Clonopam™) [73,74] *Binds benzodiazepine receptor on GABA$_A$ channel, increases frequency of GABA$_A$ channel opening, enhances GABA binding*	Tablet: 0.5, 1, 2 mg ODT: 0.125, 0.25, 0.5, 1, 2 mg Liquid: 0.1 mg/ml	**Start:** 0.125 mg qhs × 1 week then BID **Goal:** Min effective dose **Max dose:** 0.2 mg/kg per day or 10 mg/day	Sedation, ataxia; short-term use recommended due to risk of physical dependence	Taper off slowly over weeks to prevent withdrawal
Leviteracetam (Keppra™) [75,76] *Unknown*	Tablet: 250, 500, 750 mg Extended release: 500XR, 750XR Liquid: 20 mg/ml	**Start:** 10–20 mg/kg/day div od-BID; titrate up q 3–7 days **Goal:** 20–40 mg/kg/day **Max:** 60–80 mg/kg/day or 3000 mg per day	Irritability, dizziness, ataxia	Does not interact with other medications Adjust for renal insufficiency

Bladder dysfunction

Both spinal cord pathology and brain pathology can lead to dysfunctional voiding and bowel habits. As a presentation of MS, it occurs approximatey one-fifth of the time [2,3], while in acute transverse myelitis, bladder function is compromised in approximately 85% of children at onset, and almost 70% at follow-up [13].

Bladder control occurs through a number of pathways under both autonomic (pelvic nerves for sensory input and motor parasympathetics; the hypogastric nerve for sympathetic input) and voluntary control (via the pudendal nerve, pons, and cerebral cortex). As the bladder fills, sensory neurons detect the amount of stretch in the detrusor muscle, initiating the micturation reflex. Via the pathways from the frontal lobes and the brainstem, the bladder then receives input from post-ganglionic parasympathetic neurons causing detrusor wall contraction. In order for the bladder to empty, there must be coordinated contraction of the bladder wall and relaxation of the external sphincter [33,34]. The higher cortical centers override autonomic bladder control.

In MS, there are three types of bladder dysfunction: detrusor sphincter dyssynergy (DSD), the

Table 12.5 Pharmacological management of the neurogenic bladder and bowel

Medication (Brandname)	Formulations	Starting pediatric dose and max. dose	Side effects	Comments
Neurogenic bladder				
Oxybutinin (Ditropan™, Oxybutyn™) (Gelnique™ – 10% topical) [77,78] *Anti-cholinenergic*	Tablet: 5 mg; Extended release (ETAB): 5, 10, 15 Liquid: 1 mg/ml 10% Topical: 1 g packets	**Start:** 5 mg od ETAB: 5 mg od **Titrate:** 5 mg BID-TID **Max:** 5 mg TID or ETAB: 30 mg od **Adult dosing for 10% topical (no pediatric dosing available):** apply 1 g pkg to abdomen, thighs, shoulder or upper arms qday; rotate sites	Dry mouth, dizziness, constipation; cognitive slowing Topical application: skin reaction, pruritis	Overactive or hyperreflexive bladder
Tolterodine (Detrol™, Detrol LA™) [77,78] *Anti-cholinergic*	Tablet: 1, 2 mg, Long-acting: 2, 4 mg long acting	**Adult dosing (no pediatric dosing available):** **Start:** 1–2 mg od **Max:** 4 mg od or 2 mg od if on CYP3A4 inhibitors		Contraindicated with potassium salts, avoid use with pramlintide, decrease dose with fluvoxamine, azole anti-fungal, erythromycins
Fesoterodine (Toviaz™) [77] *prodrug converted to 5-hydroxy-methyl tolterodine; Anti-cholinergic*	Tablet: 4, 8 mg ER	**Adult dosing (no prediatric dosing available):** **Start:** 4 mg od **Max:** 8 mg od or 4 mg od if on CYP3A4 inhibitors	Dry mouth, constipation, UTI, dry eyes, Serious reactions: heat stroke, angina, chest pain, QT prolong	Contraindicated with potassium salts, avoid use with pramlintide, decrease dose with fluvoxamine, azole anti-fungal, erythromycins
Solifenacin (Vesicare™) [77] *Selective M2, M3 muscarinic inhibitor*	Tablet: 5, 10 mg	**Adult dosing (no prediatric dosing available):** **Start:** 5 mg od **Max:** 10 mg od or 5 mg od if on CYP3A4 inhibitors	Dry mouth, constipation, UTI, dry eyes, Serious reactions: angioneurotic edema, QT prolong, hallucinations	Contraindicated with potassium salts, dronedarone, cisapride, pimozide pheonthiazine Avoid with multiple meds including haloperidol Decrease dose with fluxoxamine, azoles
Darifenacin (Enablex™) [77] *Selective M3 muscarinic inhibitor*	Tablet: 7.7 mg; 15 mg ER	**Adult dosing (no pediatric dosing available):** **Start:** 7.5 mg od **Goal:** increase to 15 mg od after 2 weeks **Max:** 15 mg od or 7.5 mg od if on CYP3A4 inhibitors	Dry mouth, constipation, UTI, abdominal pain, dizziness Urinary retention	Contraindicated with potassium salts, avoid use with pramlintide; decrease dose with azole anti-fungals, erythromycins, fluxoamine

Table 12.5 (cont.)

Medication (Brandname)	Formulations	Starting pediatric dose and max. dose	Side effects	Comments
Neurogenic bladder				
DDAVP (Desmopressin) [79]	Tablet: 0.1, 0.2 mg, Liquid: 4 µg/ml for IV or nasal	**Start:** 0.2 mg qhs **Goal:** 0.1–1.2 mg po BID-TID **Max:** 1.2 mg/day	Flushing, headache, rhinitis, nausea, abdominal pain	Hyponatremia which can cause seizures, thromobosis
Intravesicular injections			Performed by urologist	
Botox A [80]			Sedation required for procedure	
Oxybutinin [81]			Lower incidence of systemic side effects	
Atropine [82]			Repeat injections required after 3–36 months	
Neurogenic bowel				
Docusate sodium (Colace™)	Tablet: 1, 2, 4, 8 mg	**Start:** 5 mg/kg/day od		constipation
Polyethylene glycol (PEG 3350; MiraLax™)	Powder: 17 g per capful; mix in 4–8 oz liquid	Mild–moderate constipation: 0.8–1 g/kg/day; max 17 g (1 capful) per day Severe constipation or impaction: 25 ml/kg/h **Max:** 2 l/h for 2	Caution with renal disease	Severe constipation with impaction
PEG-electrolyte liquid (PegLyte™, GoLytely™)	Powder, mixed in liquid	**Start and max:** 17 g od	Caution with renal disease	Maintenance for moderate constipation
Loperamide	Tablet: 2 mg	**Start:** 0.08–0.24 mg/kg/day **Max:** 2 mg/dose		Incontinence

flaccid bladder, and the spastic bladder, each warranting a different type of treatment. The spastic bladder is the most common form of neurogenic bladder in MS and is due to loss of voluntary control of the external sphincter leading to frequency, urgency, and incontinence. DSD results from lesions anywhere from the cortex to the lower spinal cord, but is usually due to cervical cord lesions [35]. Incoordination between the external sphincter and the bladder wall causes both incontinence, urgency, delayed emptying, and retention. Detrusor hyporeflexia or the flaccid bladder has been associated with pontine lesions [35]. Urinary retention can result in urinary tract infections and rarely renal scarring due to urinary reflux.

Evaluation and management of the neurogenic bladder

The physical exam of a child with a neurogenic bladder should include a perineal and rectal tone examination. The patient should also be evaluated with a voiding cystourethrogram to determine bladder capacity and residual bladder volumes. Residual volumes of over 50 cc in a young child or 100 cc in an adolescent or teenager is abnormal.

Strategies to prevent urinary incontinence for the spastic bladder and DSD include minimizing caffeinated fluids, restricting fluids, and voiding prior to bedtime. Pharmacological treatments to decrease urgency and frequency include anti-cholinergic medications such as oxybutinin which increase bladder capacity. Botulinum toxin injections of 300 units is a safe alternative therapy and can be repeated at 6–9-month intervals. Desmopressin (DDAVP^{TM}) is useful for nocturnal enuresis, but there is a risk of hyponatremia. For severe incontinence due to a paralytic pelvic floor, surgical options are available and include sex-specific sling procedures [36].

If the issue is urinary retention, it is extremely important to allow complete bladder emptying at regular intervals by attempting timed voidings, by bladder massage (Credé maneuver) or pelvic floor exercises. Some patients may actually be able to initiate the micturition reflex by stimulation of the perineal area. For more severe cases, clean intermittent catheterization (CIC) with the largest possible catheter may be necessary. CIC can also be used in combination with oxybutinin in children with DSD to allow for bladder filling and controlled voiding. When a child presents with urinary frequency or urgency, investigations for a urinary tract infection and diabetes should be part of the work-up.

Bowel dysfunction

Bowel dysfunction in MS is another area which is not well understood. Bowel continence requires intact sympathetic and parasympathetic innervation to the colon and the anal sphincter, as well as descending voluntary control from the medial frontal lobes. Sensory feedback signaling colonic distension coordinated with relaxation of both the internal and external sphincters is necessary for proper voiding to take place. Lesions in the spinal cord may initially cause flaccid paralysis of the anal sphincter resulting in incontinence, while lesions in the frontal lobes may cause incontinence or constipation due to lack of voluntary control. Constipation appears to be more common than incontinence in MS patients.

Evaluation and care of the neurogenic bowel

Both diarrhea and constipation are diagnosed by volume, consistency, and frequency of stools. Constipation is defined as difficulty with defecation for at least two weeks, with less than three bowel movements a week.

Constipation can be managed by a combination of diet modification, increased liquids, and increased physical activity [37]. It is important to rule out other common causes of constipation such as thyroid disease, and secondary constipation due to other medications such as tricyclic antidepressants.

Bulking agents such as psyllium to increase fiber intake can help but too much fiber intake can cause discomfort from bloating. Stool softeners such as docusate sodium (Colace^{TM}) can be given for short courses at a dose of 5 mg/kg/day with the usual dose of 100–200 mg/day. Pro-kinetic agents and stimulants are not recommended in children. For severe or chronic constipation, polyethylene glycol is an effective treatment, with good safety records in the pediatric population. It can be given to an adolescent as a liquid formulation at 2 l/h (max. 4 l) until fecal impaction is cleared. This can also be used on a daily basis mixed in a beverage for ongoing management at a dose of approximately 1 g/kg/day to a maximum of 17 g/day.

Bowel incontinence is the most difficult to manage and understandably causes the most discomfort and embarrassment. It can be aggravated by mobility issues and cause secondary self-esteem issues. Sometimes incontinence can occur with severe constipation and is termed overflow incontinence, and this can resolve if the constipation is treated. Fecal incontinence should be differentiated by history from chronic diarrhea which may have infectious, malabsorptive, or inflammatory etiologies. If other causes are suspected, or if growth is affected, a consultation with gastroenterology is essential. Other causes such as trauma should also be ruled out. Fortunately, this is a rare complication of MS, especially in the pediatric population. Pharmacological treatment with anti-motility drugs such as loperamide is still the mainstay of treatment.

Sensory symptoms – pain and paroxysmal symptoms

Pain is a common symptom in MS with estimates ranging from 29% to 86% in adult studies [38,39]. There are no estimates of pain in the pediatric MS population. The underlying pathophysiology of central neuropathic pain is not well described but may result from ephaptic discharges originating from demyelinated axons and spreading to normal neurons.

Studying pain is difficult in the MS population as there are a myriad of reasons for a patient to have pain and the type, severity, and duration of pain can vary based on the etiology. For this reason, there has been an attempt to describe and categorize the types of pain syndromes and associated etiologies [40]. Differentiating neuropathic pain caused by demyelination and axonal damage to somatosensory pathways (Lhermitte's sign, dysesthesias), from non-neuropathic pain due to disruption of motor neurons (tonic spasms) can have important treatment implications. Localized non-neuropathic pain may also be secondary to medication injection and contractures.

Management of specific pain syndromes

Treating pain syndromes is not a simple task. Although pain can be due to MS itself, other causes of pain should be ruled out. As acute or chronic pain can compound other comorbidities such as depression and sleep disorders, symptoms should be managed as promptly as other physical symptoms.

Injection-induced pain can be managed by non-steroidal anti-inflammatories, or acetaminophen prior to injection. Injection sites should be alternated and after the injection, gentle pressure and a cool or warm pack can help alleviate pain. For flu-like episodes associated with the pain, a small dose of oral steroids pre- and post-injection during the first few weeks of treatment may diminish symptoms.

Episodic pain such as Lhermitte's phenomenon, likely due to cervical spinothalamic tract lesions, are difficult to predict, and are usually infrequent and last for a limited number of weeks. Tonic spasms, on the other hand, can occur several times per day lasting for several months. These may be due to lesions of the pyramidal or extrapyramidal tracts, or commonly due to a lesion in the contralateral posterior limb of the internal capsule or cerebral peduncle [41]. Anti-epileptic drugs may be beneficial for tonic spasms. Trigeminal neuralgia is not reported to be a frequent occurrence in pediatric MS patients, but in adult patients is much more common than in the general population [40]. It is due to a lesion in the trigeminal root entry zone into the brainstem. If it does occur in a pediatric patient, first-line medications include carbamazepine or oxcarbazepine.

Central dysesthetic pain is probably the most difficult to treat. This type of pain is usually present in more advanced MS. It commonly affects both legs, and is often described as constant throbbing and burning that is worse at night and with activity. It is always associated with sensory loss and does not follow a dermatomal distribution. Lesions in the spinal cord and thalamus

are usually present [42]. Many of the medications listed in Table 12.6 can be tried, but there are no trials demonstrating the efficacy of one over the other.

Systemic symptoms – heat intolerance, fatigue, and mental health issues

The chronic and relapsing–remitting unpredictable nature of MS makes it a very difficult disease to manage. Unfortunately, without clinical or laboratory-based biomarkers, each child must be prepared for an unknown disease course. Children and adolescents can have serious anxieties about the physical implications, medication administration, and investigations. These factors make dealing with MS a difficult process that requires social and psychological supports initiated at the time of diagnosis.

Heat intolerance

Transient deterioration of function in both physical and cognitive domains can occur when a patient with MS experiences increased body temperature through physical activity, fever, or the external environment [43,44]. This is called Uthoff's phenomenon and if prolonged, may appear to be a clinical relapse. During recovery from a relapse, the conduction in demyelinated axons is altered due to redistribution of sodium channels. Even small increases in core body temperature can induce conduction block or delay in demyelinated axons [45]. Complicating matters, plaques in thermoregulating centres, such as the intermediolateral tract in the spinal cord, can add to temperature instability by disrupting autonomic and endocrine mechanisms involved in maintaining normal core body temperatures.

It is necessary to differentiate "pseudorelapses" from true clinical relapses in order to avoid unnecessary acute treatment. The child, family and school teachers should be educated that heat may exacerbate previous signs and symptoms, and that the child may take a break from activity if he feels that symptoms are being triggered. Pushing a child to complete an activity can be dangerous, especially if gait becomes impaired and results in an injury.

Management strategies

Non-pharmacological preventative measures should be taken to reduce the chance of heat-induced symptoms. Pre-cooling may be an option for a child who knows

Table 12.6 Pharmacological management of pain and paroxysmal symptoms

Medication (Brandname)	Formulations	Starting pediatric dose and max. dose	Side effects	Comments
Neuropathic pain				
Amitriptyline (Elavil) [83] *Inhibits norepinephrine and serotonin reuptake*	Tablet: 10, 25, 50, 75, 100, 150 mg Liquid: 10 mg/ml	**Start:** 1–3 mg/kg/day div TID; 10 mg qhs; **Titrate:** 0.5 mg/kg or 5–10 mg q week-month (may need 3–4 weeks before assessing if dose effective) **Max:** 5 mg/kg/day; 200 mg/day	Sedation, dry mouth, constipation, arrhythmia	Baseline and periodic EKG due to risk of arrhythmia Taper off slowly
Nortriptyline (Pamelor™) [83] *Inhibits norepinephrine and serotonin reuptake*	Tablet: 10, 25, 50, 75 mg; Liquid: 2 mg/ml	**Start:** 5–10 mg qhs **Titrate:** 5–10 mg q week-month (may need 3–4 weeks before assessing if effective) **Max dose:** 150 mg/day	Sedation, dry mouth, constipation, arrhythmias	Baseline and periodic EKG due to risk of arrhythmia Taper off slowly
Gabapentin (Neurontin™) *Binds voltage-gated Ca2+ channel, blocks Ca2+ flux*	Tablet: 100, 300, 400, 600, 800 mg; Liquid: 50 mg/ml	**Start:** 10–15 mg/kg div TID; start 300 mg od ×3 day, then BID, then TID **Goal:** 25–40 mg/kg div TID; or 300–1200 mg TID **Max:** 3600 mg per day	Sedation, dizziness, nystagmus	Leukopenia; Adjust for decreased renal function
Pregabalin (Lyrica™) [83,84] *Binds Ca2+ channel, blocks neurotransmitter release*	Tablet: 25, 50, 75, 100, 150, 200, 225, 300	**Adult dosing (no pediatric dosing guidelines) Start:** 25–50 mg BID-TID **Goal:** 50–100 mg BID-TID **Max:** 300 mg/day	Dizziness, sedation, peripheral edema, weight gain, blurred vision	Rarely, thrombocytopenia, angioedema, rhabdomyolysis
Carbemazepine (Tegretol™, Tegretol-XR™ Carbetrol™) *Blockade Na+ channels*	Tablet: 100, 200 Extended release: 100, 200, 300, 400 Liquid: 20 mg/ml	**Start:** 10 mg/kg/day div BID-TID **Goal:** 15 mg/kg/day div BID-TID **Max:** 1600 mg/day div BID-QID	Sedation, dizziness, ataxia Lymphopenia, decreased plts	Follow CBC, AST, ALT Follow CBZ levels; 4–12 is typical range HLA-B*1502 (mainly Asian ancestry) have increased risk of Steven-Johnson
Topiramate (Topamax™) *Blocks Na+, Ca2+, AMPA/KA channels; enhances GABA, K+ currents*	Sprinkle: 15, 25 mg Tablet: 25, 50, 100, 150, 200 Liquid not available	**Start:** 1 mg/kg/day div BID; titrate in 1 mg/kg/day **Goal:** 5–10 mg/kg/day **Max:** 400 mg BID or unacceptable side effects	Cognitive slowing, oligohydrosis, weight loss, risk of renal stones	Encourage adequate hydration

Table 12.6 (*cont.*)

Medication (Brandname)	Formulations	Starting pediatric dose and max. dose	Side effects	Comments
Neuropathic pain				
Leviteracetam (Keppra™) [85] *Unknown*	Tablet: 250, 500, 750 mg Extended release: 500XR, 750XR Liquid: 20 mg/ml	**Start:** 10–20 mg/kg/day div od-BID; titrate up q 3–7 days **Goal:** 20–40 mg/kg/day **Max:** 60–80 mg/kg/day or 3000 mg per day	Irritability, dizziness, ataxia	Does not interact with other medications Adjust for renal insufficiency
Paroxysmal Symptoms				
Carbamazepine (Tegretol, Tegretol-XR™ Carbetrol™) [86,87] *Sodium channel blocker*	Tablet: 100, 200 Extended release: 100, 200, 300, 400 Liquid: 20 mg/ml	**Start:** 5–10 mg/kg/day div BID-TID **Goal:** 15 mg/kg/day div BID-TID **Max:** 1600 mg/day div BID-QID	Sedation, dizziness, ataxia Lymphopenia, decreased plts, hyponatremia	Follow CBC, AST, ALT Follow CBZ levels; 4–12 is typical range HLA-B*1502 (mainly Asian ancestry) have increased risk of Steven-Johnson
Oxcarbazepine (Trileptal™) [87,88] *Blockade of Na+ and L-type Ca2+ channels*	Tablet: 150, 300, 600 mg Liquid: 60 mg/ml	**Start:** 10 mg/kg/day div BID **Goal:** 20–40 mg/kg/day div BID **Max:** 60 mg/kg/day or 2400 mg/day div BID	Sedation, dizziness, hyponatremia, leukopenia, thrombocytopenia (lower risk than carbemazepine)	May need to monitor Na
Gabapentin (Neurontin™) [86,87,89] *Binds voltage-gated Ca2+ channel, blocks Ca2+ flux*	Tablet: 100, 300, 400, 600, 800 mg Liquid: 50 mg/ml	**Start:** 10–15 mg/kg div TID; start 300 mg od ×3 days, then BID, then TID **Goal:** 25–40 mg/kg div TID; or 300–1200 mg TID **Max:** 3600 mg per day	Sedation, dizziness, nystagmus	Leukopenia; adjust for decreased renal function
Pregabalin (Lyrica™) [83,84] *Binds Ca2+ channel, blocks neurotransmitter release*	Tablet: 25, 50, 75, 100, 150, 200, 225, 300	**Adult dosing (no pediatric dosing guidelines):** **Start:** 25–50 mg BID-TID **Goal:** 50–100 mg BID-TID **Max:** 300 mg/day	Dizziness, sedation, peripheral edema, weight gain, blurred vision	Thrombocytopenia, angioedema, rhabdomyolysis
Acetozolamide (Diamox™) [41,90] *Carbonic anhydrase inhibitor*	Tablet: 125, 250, 500 extended release IV formulation	**Start:** 5–10 mg/kg/day div TID; or 125–250 mg od, titrate to TID-QID **Max:** 1000 mg/day div TID-QD	Fatigue, metallic taste, paresthesia, nausea/vomiting, diarrhea, polyruia	

that they want to participate in a strenuous activity and this may allow the child several hours of protection from heat-induced symptoms [46]. Cooling garments, such as a cooling sleeve, may also allow extended periods of exercise without symptom exacerbation, but may have the disadvantage of being a heavy weight during the activity [47]. If a child begins experiencing heat-invoked symptoms, they should be excused from the activity, and go to a cooler environment to help reverse the symptoms.

Dalfampridine (extended release 4-aminopyridine), a potassium channel blocker, was approved in 2010 by the FDA for amelioration of MS symptoms. Its mechanism of action is thought to be increased action potential duration and amplitude (reviewed in [48]), thereby increasing transmitter release and conduction velocity. In a randomized controlled trial of adult MS patients, speed of ambulation improved marginally in the treatment group throughout the treatment period [49]. Serious side effects include decreased seizure threshold (serum concentration-dependent), while milder side effects include anxiety, dizziness, and interestingly gait instability [48].

Fatigue

Fatigue is poorly understood but the most common symptom experienced by MS patients and is adversely correlated with quality of life [50,51]. In a child, this lack of energy and profound tiredness can interfere with schooling and socialization, and impacts extracurricular activities [52].

Over 40% of children with MS experience fatigue [52–54], and EDSS scores significantly relate to fatigue and quality of life measures [54]. Fatigue, just like other neurological symptoms, can fluctuate, be triggered by heat and excessive activity, and may be present without other obvious neurological impairments.

Evaluation of fatigue

Minimizing fatigue in the pediatric MS population requires a multifaceted approach of eliminating unnecessary energy demands, improving sleep hygiene and optimizing symptomatic medication and disease-modifying treatment (DMT) regimens. Also, screening for other conditions such as depression and hypothyroidism and encouraging regular exercise is necessary.

It is important not to solely rely on parent accounts of their child's level of energy, as parents of children

with MS tend to over-report fatigue in their children [54]. This study also noted that parental reports of fatigue correlated better with neurological impairment, meaning that parents may be misinterpreting their child's neurological impairment as fatigue.

The PedsSQ Multidimensional Fatigue Scale has been validated and used in other pediatric chronic diseases such as cancer, inflammatory bowel disease, and rheumatological diseases [55]. Both night-time sleep habits and daytime sleep patterns should be evaluated. If fatigue is interfering with schoolwork, extracurricular activities, or socialization, strategies should be in place to optimize energy levels by both behavioral and pharmacological means.

Management of fatigue

Despite fatigue being one of the most prevalent symptoms in MS, there are few treatments for fatigue and even fewer controlled trials of pharmacologic or non-pharmacologic interventions for fatigue. This is likely due to poor understanding of the pathophysiology of fatigue in MS. The first step to managing fatigue should be lifestyle modification. Suggestions for minimizing energy expenditure on a day-to-day basis are outlined in Table 12.7. One useful self-reporting fatigue scale is the Fatigue Severity Scale [56], which is designed to help distinguish the symptoms of fatigue from those of depression.

Table 12.8 lists medications for alleviating fatigue which may be appropriate in the pediatric population. Amantadine was initially marketed as an anti-influenza A agent, but was identified anecdoctally as being useful for ameliorating fatigue in MS and other disorders. The most recent Cochrane Database Review of amantadine for fatigue in MS revealed that there are inadequate studies demonstrating efficacy and tolerability [57]. There is one randomized crossover trial of carnitine and amantidine which also did not clearly show efficacy [58]. Modafinil, a mainstay of narcolepsy therapy, has been shown to reduce daytime sleepiness due to MS in some studies [59] but not in others [60].

Fatigue related to DMT

Flu-like symptoms and fatigue are common with all three available forms of IFNB therapy. Interestingly, a recent small study has shown that the level of fatigue does not differ between children on DMTs and those who are not [54]. Fatigue following interferon beta

(IFNB) injections can be minimized if injections are given in the evening and weekly IM IFNB-1a can be administered on an evening convenient for the patient to recover from post-injection symptoms.

Table 12.7 Non-pharmacological strategies to manage fatigue

Providing 2 sets of books so that the student can keep one set of books at school, and another set at home in order to avoid carrying heavy bags between home/school

Rolling bookbag to carry books and other school items

Limiting homework assignments: assign enough problems to demonstrate mastery of a subject but avoid unnecessary repetition

Encourage daily exercise

Limit overheating by unlimited access to water, including keeping a water bottle at the desk

Unrestricted restroom access

Identifying a "buddy" in each class who can help with scribing notes in class

Strengthen organizational skills so less energy is expended on trying to "catch up"

o Keeping lists

o Daily assignment book reviewed by teachers (or classroom buddy) before going home and review by family before returning to school

Maintain regular schedule at home for homework and sleep

Fatigue related to symptomatic therapy

Tricyclic antidepressants, often used more for neuropathic pain or headache prophylaxis than for depression, have sedating effects that contribute to fatigue. Bedtime dosing can help ameliorate tricyclic-induced sedation and may also improve sleep in some patients. Similarly, anti-convulsants used for treatment of associated MS symptoms can also contribute to sedation. Anti-convulsants with prominent sedation include carbemazepine and leviteracetam (used for neuropathic pain, ephaptic symptoms, mood disorders), topiramate (headache prophylaxis), and valproic acid (headache prophylaxis, mood disorders). Use of an extended release formulation at bedtime may reduce sedation (available for carbemazepine as Tegretol XR, for valproic acid as Depakote ER, and for levitiracetam as Keppra XR).

Sedation is also the main side effect of anti-spasticity agents, including baclofen, tizanidine, and diazepam. Strategies for reducing sedation related to anti-spasticity agents include using the smallest effective dose, giving bigger doses at night-time if necessary or limiting the use of more sedating agents such as tizanidine to bedtime only.

Depression

Depression is a common comorbidity in adults with MS, estimated to affect 50–70% of adults at some point in their disease course. Preliminary data from pediatric MS cohorts suggest that the rate of depression is similar, if not higher [61], using a structured psychiatric

Table 12.8 Pharmacological management of depression

Medication (Brandname)	Formulations	Starting pediatric dose and max. dose	Side effects	Comments
Fluoxetine (Prozac™) *Selective serotonoin reuptake inhibitor*	Tablet: 10, 20, 40 mg Liquid: 4 mg/ml	**Start:** 5–10 mg od **Goal:** 10–40 mg/day **Max:** 60 mg/day (30 mg in smaller pts)	Nausea, headache, insomnia, anxiety, anorexia	FDA indication for depression in pts ≥8 years; Black box warning re: risk of increased suicidality during 1st month of treatment
Escitalopram (Lexapro™) *Selective serotonoin reuptake inhibitor*	Tablet: 5, 10, 20 mg Liquid: 5 mg/5 ml	**Start:** 10 mg po od **Titrate:** May increase to 20 mg od after 3 weeks **Max:** 20 mg/od	Nausea, headache, insomnia, diarrhea, sedation	FDA indication for depression ≥12 years Black box warning re: risk of increased suicidality during 1st month of treatment

evaluation. Anxiety, although studied to a lesser extent, is reported in up to a third of adult MS cohorts but has not been evaluated specifically in pediatric MS.

Adolescents are less likely to seek help for mood disorders, and this is especially true for African-Americans and Asians. This is very important, as recent studies of pediatric MS have demonstrated rising incidence rates and perhaps a more severe phenotype in non-Caucasian populations [62,63], and they are more likely to internalize their symptoms [64]. Therefore, self-reporting scales may underestimate the true incidence of depression in these children [52].

Evaluation of depression

Screening for mood disorders should occur at every visit. Adolescents and teenagers should have the opportunity to be interviewed separately so that a confidential, honest discussion can take place. If suspected, the Children's Depression Inventory [65] is a validated self-reporting scale that can be an adjunct to the clinical history.

Ideally, a social worker, psychologist and/or psychiatrist should be available to deal promptly with crisis issues that may reveal themselves during an otherwise regular follow-up appointment. Once again, a team approach, with multiple specialties meeting with the patient during one period of time, would help an otherwise stressful situation.

Management

Selective serotonin reuptake inhibitors (SSRIs) are considered first-line for depression in both adult and pediatric populations, but there have been concerns of increased suicide in adolescents treated with SSRIs, especially during the first few weeks of treatment before the antidepressant takes effect. Fluoxetine is FDA-approved for depression in children ≥8 years and Escitalopram is FDA-approved for depression in children ≥12 years of age. Based on findings from 23 published and post-marketing studies that showed increased suicidal ideation after initiation of SSRI antidepressants, in 2004, the FDA issued a black box warning for increased suicide risk in adolescents treated with SSRIs. Further study has revealed that the benefits of treating depression in children clearly outweighs the risks [66]. Table 12.8 lists the types of SSRIs that may be used with caution in children and adolescents.

The FDA recommends close monitoring by family members after initiation of antidepressant therapy plus weekly clinic visits for the first month on SSRI therapy, then every two weeks for the second month and every three months thereafter. In practice, this recommended schedule of frequent follow-up visits has been difficult to maintain. Therefore, the American Psychiatric Association suggests that follow-up following institution of SSRI therapy in children and adolescents be individually tailored, with family instructed to monitor the patient closely in the first month after SSRI. Once treatment has begun, it should not be abruptly stopped as this can lead to withdrawal symptoms. Cognitive behavioral therapy combined with SSRIs has been shown to be effective in treating depression in adolescents [67].

Conclusion

Clinicians should be cognizant of the variety of symptoms that may surface in a child with MS. Many of these symptoms may be physical, but others may not be as apparent, such as fatigue, depression, and episodic pain. Individualized multidisciplinary care is needed to optimize recovery and function for these children.

Long-term management is most important in pediatric-onset MS, and although a child may appear to be asymptomatic, periodic thorough evaluations may reveal difficulties in daily living. Children and families should be connected to appropriate resources in order to optimize their quality of life.

References

1. Mikaeloff Y, Suissa S, Vallee L, *et al*. First episode of acute CNS inflammatory demyelination in childhood: Prognostic factors for multiple sclerosis and disability. *J Pediatr* 2004;**144**:246–252.

2. Banwell B, Ghezzi A, Bar-Or A, Mikaeloff Y, Tardieu M. Multiple sclerosis in children: Clinical diagnosis, therapeutic strategies, and future directions. *Lancet Neurol* 2007;**6**:887–902.

3. Yeh EA, Chitnis T, Krupp L, *et al*. Pediatric multiple sclerosis. *Nat Rev Neurol* 2009;**5**:621–631.

4. Pohl D, Rostasy K, Treiber-Held S, Brockmann K, Gartner J, Hanefeld F. Pediatric multiple sclerosis: Detection of clinically silent lesions by multimodal evoked potentials. *J Pediatr* 2006;**149**:125–127.

5. Wilejto M, Shroff M, Buncic JR, Kennedy J, Goia C, Banwell B. The clinical features, MRI findings, and outcome of optic neuritis in children. *Neurology* 2006;**67**:258–262.

6. Frohman EM, Frohman TC, Zee DS, McColl R, Galetta S. The neuro-ophthalmology of multiple sclerosis. *Lancet Neurol* 2005;**4**:111–121.

7. Balcer LJ, Frohman EM. Evaluating loss of visual function in multiple sclerosis as measured by low-contrast letter acuity. *Neurology* 2010;**74**(Suppl 3): S16–23.

8. Warren M. A hierarchical model for evaluation and treatment of visual perceptual dysfunction in adult acquired brain injury, Part 2. *Am J Occup Ther* 1993;**47**:55–66.

9. Warren M. A hierarchical model for evaluation and treatment of visual perceptual dysfunction in adult acquired brain injury, Part 1. *Am J Occup Ther* 1993;**47**:42–54.

10. Rizzo MA, Hadjimichael OC, Preiningerova J, Vollmer TL. Prevalence and treatment of spasticity reported by multiple sclerosis patients. *Mult Scler* 2004;**10**:589–595.

11. Barnes MP, Kent RM, Semlyen JK, McMullen KM. Spasticity in multiple sclerosis. *Neurorehabil Neural Repair* 2003;**17**:66–70.

12. Milla PJ, Jackson AD. A controlled trial of baclofen in children with cerebral palsy. *J Int Med Res* 1977;**5**: 398–404.

13. Pidcock F, Krishnan C, Crawford T, Salorio C, Trovato M, Kerr D. Acute transverse myelitis in childhood: Center-based analysis of 47 cases. *Neurology* 2007;**68**:1447–1449.

14. Palisano R, Rosenbaum P, Walter S, Russell D, Wood E, Galuppi B. Development and reliability of a system to classify gross motor function in children with cerebral palsy. *Dev Med Child Neurol* 1997;**39**:214–223.

15. Ashworth B. Preliminary trial of carisoprodol in multiple sclerosis. *Practitioner* 1964;**192**:540–542.

16. Bohannon RW, Smith MB. Interrater reliability of a modified Ashworth scale of muscle spasticity. *Phys Ther* 1987;**67**:206–207.

17. Gracies JM, Burke K, Clegg NJ, et al. Reliability of the Tardieu Scale for assessing spasticity in children with cerebral palsy. *Arch Phys Med Rehabil* 2010;**91**: 421–428.

18. Haugh AB, Pandyan AD, Johnson GR. A systematic review of the Tardieu Scale for the measurement of spasticity. *Disabil Rehabil* 2006;**28**:899–907.

19. Quality Standards Subcommittee of the American Academy of Neurology and the Practice Committee of the Child Neurology Society, Delgado MR, Hirtz D, et al. Practice parameter: Pharmacologic treatment of spasticity in children and adolescents with cerebral palsy (an evidence-based review): Report of the Quality Standards Subcommittee of the American Academy of Neurology and the Practice Committee of the Child Neurology Society. *Neurology* 2010;**74**:336–343.

20. Venetsanou F, Kambas A, Aggeloussis N, Serbezis V, Taxildaris K. Use of the Bruininks–Oseretsky test of motor proficiency for identifying children with motor impairment. *Dev Med Child Neurol* 2007;**49**:846–848.

21. Cutter GR, Baier ML, Rudick RA, et al. Development of a multiple sclerosis functional composite as a clinical trial outcome measure. *Brain* 1999;**122** (Pt 5): 871–882.

22. Fischer JS, Rudick RA, Cutter GR, Reingold SC. The Multiple Sclerosis Functional Composite Measure (MSFC): An integrated approach to MS clinical outcome assessment. National MS Society Clinical Outcomes Assessment Task Force. *Mult Scler* 1999; **5**:244–250.

23. Rudick R, Antel J, Confavreux C, et al. Recommendations from the National Multiple Sclerosis Society Clinical Outcomes Assessment Task Force. *Ann Neurol* 1997;**42**:379–382.

24. Wall JC, Bell C, Campbell S, Davis J. The Timed Get-up-and-Go test revisited: Measurement of the component tasks. *J Rehabil Res Dev* 2000;**37**:109–113.

25. Ward AB. Long-term modification of spasticity. *J Rehabil Med* 2003;**41**(Suppl):60–65.

26. Mark VW, Taub E, Bashir K, et al. Constraint-Induced Movement therapy can improve hemiparetic progressive multiple sclerosis. Preliminary findings. *Mult Scler* 2008;**14**:992–994.

27. Engle HA. The effect of diazepam (Valium) in children with cerebral palsy: A double-blind study. *Dev Med Child Neurol* 1966;**8**:661–667.

28. Mathew A, Mathew MC, Thomas M, Antonisamy B. The efficacy of diazepam in enhancing motor function in children with spastic cerebral palsy. *J Trop Pediatr* 2005;**51**:109–113.

29. Vakhapova V, Auriel E, Karni A. Nightly sublingual tizanidine HCl in multiple sclerosis: Clinical efficacy and safety. *Clin Neuropharmacol* 2010;**33**:151–154.

30. Simpson DM, Gracies JM, Graham HK, et al. Assessment: Botulinum neurotoxin for the treatment of spasticity (an evidence-based review): Report of the Therapeutics and Technology Assessment Subcommittee of the American Academy of Neurology. *Neurology* 2008;**70**:1691–1698.

31. Gooch JL, Oberg WA, Grams B, Ward LA, Walker ML. Care provider assessment of intrathecal baclofen in children. *Dev Med Child Neurol* 2004;**46**:548–552.

32. Deutsch JE, Borbely M, Filler J, Huhn K, Guarrera-Bowlby P. Use of a low-cost, commercially available gaming console (Wii) for rehabilitation of an adolescent with cerebral palsy. *Phys Ther* 2008;**88**:1196–1207.

33. Blumenfeld H. *Neuroanatomy Through Clinical Cases, Second Edition.* Sunderland, MA: Sinauer Associates, Inc.; 2010.

34. Brazis PW, Masdeu JC, Biller J. *Localization in Clinical Neurology*, 5th ed. Philadelphia, PA: Lippincott Williams & Wilkins; 2006.

35. Araki I, Matsui M, Ozawa K, Takeda M, Kuno S. Relationship of bladder dysfunction to lesion site in multiple sclerosis *J Urol* 2003;**169**:1384–1387.

36. Chrzan R, Dik P, Klijn AJ, de Jong TP. Sling suspension of the bladder neck for pediatric urinary incontinence. *J Pediatr Urol* 2009;**5**:82–86.

37. Buie T, Fuchs GJ 3rd, Furuta GT, *et al.* Recommendations for evaluation and treatment of common gastrointestinal problems in children with ASDs. *Pediatrics* 2010;**125**(Suppl 1):S19–29.

38. Stenager E, Knudsen L, Jensen K. Acute and chronic pain syndromes in multiple sclerosis. A 5-year follow-up study. *Ital J Neurol Sci* 1995;**16**:629–632.

39. Clifford DB, Trotter JL. Pain in multiple sclerosis. *Arch Neurol* 1984;**41**:1270–1272.

40. O'Connor AB, Schwid SR, Herrmann DN, Markman JD, Dworkin RH. Pain associated with multiple sclerosis: Systematic review and proposed classification. *Pain* 2008;**137**:96–111.

41. Waubant E, Alize P, Tourbah A, Agid Y. Paroxysmal dystonia (tonic spasm) in multiple sclerosis. *Neurology* 2001;**57**:2320–2321.

42. Osterberg A, Boivie J, Thuomas KA. Central pain in multiple sclerosis – Prevalence and clinical characteristics. *Eur J Pain* 2005;**9**:531–542.

43. Petajan JH, Gappmaier E, White AT, Spencer MK, Mino L, Hicks RW. Impact of aerobic training on fitness and quality of life in multiple sclerosis. *Ann Neurol* 1996;**39**:432–441.

44. Dutta R, McDonough J, Yin X, *et al.* Mitochondrial dysfunction as a cause of axonal degeneration in multiple sclerosis patients. *Ann Neurol* 2006;**59**:478–489.

45. Rasminsky M. The effects of temperature on conduction in demyelinated single nerve fibers. *Arch Neurol* 1973;**28**:287–292.

46. White AT, Wilson TE, Davis SL, Petajan JH. Effect of precooling on physical performance in multiple sclerosis. *Mult Scler* 2000;**6**:176–180.

47. Grahn DA, Murray JV, Heller HC. Cooling via one hand improves physical performance in heat-sensitive individuals with multiple sclerosis: A preliminary study. *BMC Neurol* 2008;**8**:14.

48. Bever CT Jr. 10 Questions about 4-aminopyridine and the treatment of multiple sclerosis. *Neurologist* 2009;**15**:161–162.

49. Goodman AD, Brown TR, Krupp LB, *et al.* Sustained-release oral fampridine in multiple sclerosis: A randomised, double-blind, controlled trial. *Lancet* 2009;**373**:732–738.

50. Freal JE, Kraft GH, Coryell JK. Symptomatic fatigue in multiple sclerosis. *Arch Phys Med Rehabil* 1984;**65**:135–138.

51. Krupp LB, Alvarez LA, LaRocca NG, Scheinberg LC. Fatigue in multiple sclerosis. *Arch Neurol* 1988;**45**:435–437.

52. Amato MP, Zipoli V, Portaccio E. Cognitive changes in multiple sclerosis. *Exp Rev Neurother* 2008;**8**:1585–1596.

53. Weisbrot DM, Ettinger AB, Gadow KD, *et al.* Psychiatric comorbidity in pediatric patients with demyelinating disorders. *J Child Neurol* 2010;**25**:192–202.

54. MacAllister WS, Christodoulou C, Troxell R, *et al.* Fatigue and quality of life in pediatric multiple sclerosis. *Mult Scler* 2009;**15**:1502–1508.

55. Varni JW, Burwinkle TM, Szer IS. The PedsQL Multidimensional Fatigue Scale in pediatric rheumatology: Reliability and validity. *J Rheumatol* 2004;**31**:2494–2500.

56. Krupp LB, LaRocca NG, Muir-Nash J, Steinberg AD. The fatigue severity scale. Application to patients with multiple sclerosis and systemic lupus erythematosus. *Arch Neurol* 1989;**46**:1121–1123.

57. Pucci E, Branas P, D'Amico R, Giuliani G, Solari A, Taus C. Amantadine for fatigue in multiple sclerosis. *Cochrane Database Syst Rev* 2007;1:CD002818.

58. Tomassini V, Pozzilli C, Onesti E, *et al.* Comparison of the effects of acetyl L-carnitine and amantadine for the treatment of fatigue in multiple sclerosis: Results of a pilot, randomised, double-blind, crossover trial. *J Neurol Sci* 2004;**218**:103–108.

59. Rammohan KW, Rosenberg JH, Lynn DJ, Blumenfeld AM, Pollak CP, Nagaraja HN. Efficacy and safety of modafinil (Provigil) for the treatment of fatigue in multiple sclerosis: A two centre phase 2 study. *J Neurol Neurosurg Psychiatry* 2002;**72**:179–183.

60. Stankoff B, Waubant E, Confavreux C, *et al.* Modafinil for fatigue in MS: A randomized placebo-controlled double-blind study. *Neurology* 2005;**64**:1139–1143.

61. MacAllister WS, Belman AL, Milazzo M, *et al.* Cognitive functioning in children and adolescents with multiple sclerosis. *Neurology* 2005;**64**:1422–1425.

62. Banwell B, Kennedy J, Sadovnick D, *et al.* Incidence of acquired demyelination of the CNS in Canadian children. *Neurology* 2009;**72**:232–239.

63. Boster AL, Endress CF, Hreha SA, Caon C, Perumal JS, Khan OA. Pediatric-onset multiple sclerosis in African-American black and European-origin white patients. *Pediatr Neurol* 2009;**40**:31–33.

64. Anderson ER, Mayes LC. Race/ethnicity and internalizing disorders in youth: A review. *Clin Psychol Rev* 2010;**30**:338–348.

65. Kovacs M. The Children's Depression, Inventory (CDI). *Psychopharmacol Bull* 1985;**21**:995–998.

66. Bridge JA, Iyengar S, Salary CB, *et al.* Clinical response and risk for reported suicidal ideation and suicide attempts in pediatric antidepressant treatment: A meta-analysis of randomized controlled trials. *JAMA* 2007;**297**:1683–1696.

67. March J, Silva S, Petrycki S, *et al.* Fluoxetine, cognitive-behavioral therapy, and their combination for adolescents with depression: Treatment for Adolescents With Depression Study (TADS) randomized controlled trial. *JAMA* 2004;**292**:807–820.

68. Thurtell MJ, Joshi AC, Leone AC, *et al.* Crossover trial of gabapentin and memantine as treatment for acquired nystagmus. *Ann Neurol* 2010;**67**:676–680.

69. Starck M, Albrecht H, Pollmann W, Dieterich M, Straube A. Acquired pendular nystagmus in multiple sclerosis: An examiner-blind cross-over treatment study of memantine and gabapentin. *J Neurol* 2010;**257**:322–327.

70. Starck M, Albrecht H, Pollmann W, Straube A, Dieterich M. Drug therapy for acquired pendular nystagmus in multiple sclerosis. *J Neurol* 1997;**244**:9–16.

71. Bandini F, Castello E, Mazzella L, Mancardi GL, Solaro C. Gabapentin but not vigabatrin is effective in the treatment of acquired nystagmus in multiple sclerosis: How valid is the GABAergic hypothesis? *J Neurol Neurosurg Psychiatry* 2001;**71**:107–110.

72. Strupp M, Kalla R, Glasauer S, *et al.* Aminopyridines for the treatment of cerebellar and ocular motor disorders. *Prog Brain Res* 2008;**171**:535–541.

73. Koch M, Mostert J, Heersema D, De Keyser J. Tremor in multiple sclerosis. *J Neurol* 2007;**254**:133–145.

74. Mills RJ, Yap L, Young CA. Treatment for ataxia in multiple sclerosis. *Cochrane Database Syst Rev* 2007; 1:CD005029.

75. Solaro C, Mancardi G. Symptomatic therapies in multiple sclerosis. Introduction. *Neurol Sci* 2008;**29** (Suppl 4):S347.

76. Striano P, Coppola A, Vacca G, *et al.* Levetiracetam for cerebellar tremor in multiple sclerosis: An open-label pilot tolerability and efficacy study. *J Neurol* 2006;**253**:762–766.

77. Fowler CJ. The effectiveness of bladder rehabilitation in multiple sclerosis. *J Neurol NeurosurgPsychiatry* 2010;**81**:944.

78. Nicholas RS, Friede T, Hollis S, Young CA. Anticholinergics for urinary symptoms in multiple sclerosis. *Cochrane Database Syst Rev* 2009; 1: CD004193.

79. Fowler CJ, Panicker JN, Drake M, *et al.* A UK consensus on the management of the bladder in multiple sclerosis. *Postgrad Med J* 2009;**85**:552–559.

80. Sahai A, Dowson C, Khan MS, Dasgupta P, GKT Botulinum Study Group. Repeated injections of botulinum toxin-A for idiopathic detrusor overactivity. *Urology* 2010;**75**:552–558.

81. Guerra LA, Moher D, Sampson M, Barrowman N, Pike J, Leonard M. Intravesical oxybutynin for children with poorly compliant neurogenic bladder: A systematic review. *J Urol* 2008;**180**:1091–1097.

82. Fader M, Glickman S, Haggar V, Barton R, Brooks R, Malone-Lee J. Intravesical atropine compared to oral oxybutynin for neurogenic detrusor overactivity: A double-blind, randomized crossover trial. *J Urol* 2007;**177**:208–13; discussion 213.

83. Pollmann W, Feneberg W. Current management of pain associated with multiple sclerosis. *CNS Drugs* 2008;**22**:291–324.

84. Solaro C, Boehmker M, Tanganelli P. Pregabalin for treating paroxysmal painful symptoms in multiple sclerosis: A pilot study. *J Neurol* 2009; **256**:1773–1774.

85. Rossi S, Mataluni G, Codeca C, *et al.* Effects of levetiracetam on chronic pain in multiple sclerosis: Results of a pilot, randomized, placebo-controlled study. *Eur J Neurol* 2009;**16**:360–366.

86. Schapiro RT. Management of spasticity, pain, and paroxysmal phenomena in multiple sclerosis. *Curr Neurol Neurosci Rep* 2001;**1**:299–302.

87. Leandri M. Therapy of trigeminal neuralgia secondary to multiple sclerosis. *Exp Rev Neurother* 2003; **3**:661–671.

88. Solaro C, Tanganelli P, Messmer Uccelli M. Pharmacological treatment of pain in multiple sclerosis. *Exp Rev Neurother* 2007;**7**:1165–1174.

89. Yetimalar Y, Gurgor N, Basoglu M. Clinical efficacy of gabapentin for paroxysmal symptoms in multiple sclerosis. *Acta Neurol Scand* 2004;**109**: 430–431.

90. Voiculescu V, Pruskauer-Apostol B, Alecu C. Treatment with acetazolamide of brain-stem and spinal paroxysmal disturbances in multiple sclerosis. *J Neurol Neurosurg Psychiatry* 1975; **38**:191–193.

Chapter 3

Cognitive dysfunction in pediatric-onset multiple sclerosis

Laura J. Julian, Maria Trojano, Maria Pia Amato, and Lauren B. Krupp

Although multiple sclerosis (MS) is more frequently diagnosed in adulthood, an estimated 2–5% of persons with MS have a pediatric-onset MS (POMS) [1,2]. The disease results in motor, cognitive, and neuropsychiatric symptoms. Historically, cognitive impairment in MS patients has been considered a less important disease-related consequence as compared to physical disability. However, in recent years both clinicians and researchers have become increasingly aware of the prevalence of MS-related cognitive impairment and its impact on patients' everyday functioning. Cognitive problems in MS occur in 40–65% of adult patients with MS [3,4]. The profile of cognitive impairment shows prominent involvement of episodic memory, complex attention, executive functions, speed of information processing, and visuospatial abilities; whereas semantic memory, attentive span, language functions, and overall intelligence appear to be relatively preserved [4]. Relationships between cognitive impairment and clinical variables in terms of disease duration and disability level typically measured by the Expanded Disability Status Scale (EDSS) [5] are usually mild to moderate. Additionally, cognitive impairment can be detected in patients in the earliest stages of the disease with low levels of physical disability [4]. There is great inter-patient variability and overall, the extent of cognitive impairment appears to progress over time [4].

Cognitive dysfunction in POMS has been less well studied, but children may be especially prone to cognitive impairment given that the neuropathologic processes of MS, including inflammation, blood–brain barrier breakdown, and demyelination, co-occur with the developmental process of myelination in the developing central nervous system (CNS), thereby potentially damaging critical structural regions involved in cognition and cognitive development [6]. In particular, experimental and functional imaging studies suggest the involvement of myelin in cognition, learning, memory, and the development of a range of skills [6]. Indeed, myelination of appropriate brain regions coincides with the development of specific cognitive functions, such as reading, development of vocabulary and the development of a range of executive functions. Moreover, myelination correlates with normal cognitive development and intelligence, and has been associated with normal variations in reading skills and working memory [6]. It is also understood that MS is a condition not restricted to white matter and both cortical and deep gray matter structures are also vulnerable to MS-related disease processes [7,8], which may also confer effects on cognition and learning. In this population, disease-related mechanisms are occurring during key formative years for cognitive development and have the propensity to significantly interfere with present and future academic achievements as well as with psychosocial development and function [9] (see Chapter 14).

This chapter covers the nature and course of POMS-related cognitive impairment, its clinical correlates, assessment considerations, impact on functional activities, and future directions directed towards improving our detection of cognitive impairment, the potential for treatments, and management of POMS-related cognitive impairment in clinical practice.

Prevalence, pattern, and clinical correlates of cognitive impairment in POMS

Very little published material is available on neuropsychological aspects of childhood and juvenile MS

Demyelinating Disorders of the Central Nervous System in Childhood, ed. Dorothée Chabas and Emmanuelle L. Waubant.
Published by Cambridge University Press. © Cambridge University Press 2011.

and therefore broad generalizations and accurate prevalence rates of cognitive dysfunction are unknown. The majority of studies evaluating cognitive impairment in POMS have been based on single case reports or small clinical series [10–14]. Many of these studies are limited by small sample sizes, lack of adequate control groups, and variability of measurement techniques. However, given the increased attention paid to MS in childhood coupled with increasing awareness of the importance of considering cognitive function, we anticipate that very informative larger-scale studies will be available in the near future. Below we review four recent studies suggesting that, similar to adults with MS, cognitive function contributes significantly to the overall burden of disease in children and adolescents.

First, Banwell and co-workers [13] examined a series of 10 cases in Canada classified as "recent onset" (i.e. presented with the first MS attack within 12 months of testing, $n = 3$), and "remote onset" (i.e. mean time since the first attack 5.1 years, $n = 7$) group. In this study a comprehensive neuropsychological test battery including measures of general intelligence, verbal and visual memory, attention, receptive and expressive language, and executive functioning was utilized and available published normative data were used to classify patient performance. Compared to normative data, all patients demonstrated impairment on at least one test, with some children showing deficits on most or all areas. Impairment was most pronounced in patients belonging to the "remote onset" group, suggesting that longer disease duration and/or younger age at disease onset may be important risk factors for cognitive impairment. Importantly, disease severity as measured by the EDSS was low (range 1.0–3.0) in this sample, confirming that, as in adult-onset cases, cognitive deficits can occur independently of the physical manifestations of the disease.

Second, in the United States, McAllister and colleagues [14] examined 37 cases using a standardized neuropsychological battery designed to assess attention, language, memory, visuospatial, and motor functions. In this study, 35% of the patients showed significant cognitive impairment, defined by impaired cognitive performance on at least two cognitive tasks as compared with normative data. A total of 59% had an impaired performance on at least one measure. The most frequently impaired domain in this study was complex attention, affecting 30% of cases. Unlike

studies in adult MS, language, measured by the Boston Naming Test [15], and receptive language, measured by the Listening to Paragraphs subtest of the Clinical Evaluation of Language Fundamentals – III [16], was impaired in a significant proportion of this cohort, affecting 19% and 14%, respectively. Other domains including visual memory and verbal fluency were either intact or impaired in a small proportion of the sample. In this study, there were clear relationships between cognitive performance and clinical variables. In particular, poor cognitive performance was associated with higher EDSS, total number of relapses, and disease duration. In multivariate analyses, EDSS and the number of MS relapses emerged as the strongest predictors of cognitive function, even after controlling for dominant hand dexterity.

Two studies have been published to date from an Italian pediatric research group, constituting the only studies including a control group rather than normative data. The first study is based on an Italian cohort of 63 children and adolescents with MS, compared with 57 demographically matched healthy controls [17]. All the patients had a relapsing–remitting disease course and a mean EDSS score of 1.5. The neuropsychological test battery assessed intelligence (IQ) through the Weschsler Intelligence Scale for children (WISC-R) [18], verbal and visuospatial memory, sustained attention, abstract reasoning, expressive and receptive language. In this study, the MS group appeared to have reduced verbal and performance IQ scores when compared to matched controls, with 28% of the patients with reduced scores on the WISC-R and 8% having Full Scale IQ scores below 70, reaching the range of intellectual disability according to the *Diagnostic and Statistical Manual of Mental Disorders*, Fourth Edition (DSM-IV) [19]. Significant cognitive impairment was present in 31% of this cohort, defined as the failure of at least three tests, using as performance at or below the fifth percentile of control performance. Additionally, 53% exhibited minor degrees of cognitive dysfunction as defined by impairment on at least two measures. Analysis of domains suggested that 27% of the sample was impaired on at least one of three cognitive domains. Similar to previous studies, the nature of the cognitive dysfunction was within verbal functioning (39–53% of the cases), visuospatial memory (18–56%), complex attention (28–50%), and aspects of executive functions (41%). Moreover, semantic and phonemic verbal fluencies were reduced in

22 and 17% of the cases, respectively, whereas verbal comprehension performance was compromised in 28–39% of the patients. In this study, the only significant predictor of cognitive impairment was an IQ score less than 90. In a further analysis, considering as the dependent variable an IQ score less than 70, the only significant predictor was a younger age at disease onset.

A more recent study from the Italian group found that overall, cognitive impairment was identified in 41% of children and adolescents with MS, using a threshold of at least 4 measures impaired [20]. The mean number of impaired tests in MS patients was 4.4 tests compared to 1 test in the healthy control group. Using a comprehensive battery of tests, MS patients were found to perform significantly worse than controls on a range of domains including overall verbal and nonverbal abilities, episodic memory, executive functioning, attention, and language.

Finally, a prevalence between 10 and 24% of learning and memory deficits has been reported after only one year from the disease onset [21]. Moreover, separate examination of acute disseminated encephalomyelitis (ADEM) and MS patients suggested incremental impact of recurrent demyelinating disease on cognitive functions [22].

On the whole, we estimate that at least one-third of children and adolescents with MS can exhibit significant cognitive dysfunction. Available evidence suggests that the profile of cognitive dysfunction in POMS shares common features with the known profile in adult-onset MS, including involvement of memory functions, complex attention and processing speed, and aspects of executive functions. While studies are limited, it is important to know that the breadth of the deficits in POMS may be broader and may encompass other cognitive domains including language functions and overall intelligence. We hypothesize that given the fact that this condition may occur during a critical phase for the development of linguistic faculties, language functions may be particularly vulnerable in this age range. Another peculiar aspect of cognitive functioning in this age range is the findings to date of affected intelligence or overall ability level in children with MS, particularly in the patients with younger age at the disease onset. Importantly, specific aspects of the assessment of intelligence or ability in children heavily demand specific cognitive processes known to be compromised in MS, including speeded processing. However,

this cannot account for all of the decreased ability observed in these cohorts. Perhaps there exists some relationship among diffuse neuropathological damage in the CNS, and the global impact on the development of intellectual faculties and, consequently, on intelligence and/or overall ability levels.

As in adult-onset cases, the relationship with the main clinical features in terms of disease duration, disability scores, and relapse frequency appears unclear. So far, increasing disability levels and disease duration appear to be associated with cognitive impairment. Yet, cognitive dysfunction is still observed in disability-free subjects. Longitudinal studies starting from the early disease stages may possibly clarify the time dependent nature of these relationships.

Based on the available evidence on the frequency and functional impact of cognitive problems, neuropsychological assessment should be included in the routine clinical evaluation of children and adolescents with MS to monitor symptoms over time in order to assist in educational planning and inform decisions regarding MS therapy.

The longitudinal course of cognitive functioning in POMS

Longitudinal studies of adults with MS have generally shown some degree of cognitive loss over time. In a 3-year study of 42 adults with MS, there was evidence of cognitive decline in both patients that were initially cognitively intact at baseline, and evidence that there may be more pronounced cognitive loss in patients who initially presented with some cognitive impairments [23]. A 10-year longitudinal study on a cohort of 50 MS patients in the incipient phase of the disease similarly documented a decline of cognitive capacities over time. Multiple regression analysis indicated that a secondary progressive course, higher EDSS scores and increasing age were independently associated with a worse longitudinal cognitive outcome [24].

To date, there is a dearth of longitudinal studies of cognitive function in children and adolescents. In the study reviewed above by McAllister *et al.* [25], 12 MS children and adolescents underwent two neuropsychological assessments, separated by a mean inter-assessment duration of 8 months. At baseline, all but two participants demonstrated impairment on at least one neuropsychological task (defined as 1.5 SD below normative data). At follow-up evaluation, the frequency at which patients performed in the impaired range increased on several tasks, with the Trail Making Test part B, assessing complex attention and aspects of executive functioning, showing the largest increase in impairment frequency. A statistically significant association with baseline EDSS score and an increase in number of impaired measures was observed. Additionally, number of interim relapses neared significance with longitudinal cognitive outcomes [25]. Using a longer inter-assessment duration, the above-mentioned Italian cohort was also re-assessed after approximately 2 years [26]. Preliminary results pointed to a deteriorating cognitive performance in the majority (i.e. 70%) of a cohort that was predominantly treated with disease-modifying therapies (DMTs) and had a relatively stable MRI course. A reduced IQ and a younger age at the disease onset appeared to be major predictors of poorer cognitive outcomes [26].

To summarize the literature with respect to the prognosis of cognitive functioning in POMS, we find that in the very few studies conducted, a reasonable proportion of these patients decline over time (up to 70% as in the Italian study). With two longitudinal studies conducted to date, definitive conclusions cannot be made. Systematic larger-scale longitudinal studies will be critical to determine the overall course of cognitive functioning as well as the relationships with the trajectory of expected cognitive developments.

Neuropsychological assessment techniques to detect cognitive impairment in POMS

Although we believe a routine cognitive evaluation would be beneficial for most patients with known or suspected POMS, this option is not always available for a variety of reasons (i.e. access to neuropsychological services, costs of comprehensive neuropsychological evaluations, and time). However, given the estimated prevalence of cognitive impairment in this population, systematic approaches to identifying patients with cognitive dysfunction are warranted.

A screening evaluation, the Brief Neuropsychological Battery for Children (BNBC), has been evaluated and proposed by Portaccio and colleagues [20] and is presented in Table 13.1. This battery, comprised of measures of verbal knowledge, information processing speed, executive functioning, and verbal memory,

Table 13.1 Existing neuropsychological batteries in use for children/adolescents with pediatric onset multiple sclerosis

Brief Neuropsychological Battery for Children (BNBC)	NMSS Pediatric Centers of Excellence Neuropsychological Battery
WISC-R Vocabulary [49]	WASI Vocabulary [50]
Symbol Digit Modalities Test [38]	WASI Similarities
Trail Making Test – A [51]	WASI Block Design
Trail Making Test – B	WASI Matrix Reasoning
SRT-Consistent Long Term Retrieval [52]	CVLT- Children/CVLT-II [53,54]
SRT-Long Term Storage	WISC-IV Coding/WAIS-III Digit Symbol Test [55, 56]
	WISC-IV/ WAIS-III Digit Span Test
	Contingency Naming Test [57]
	D-KEFS Trail Making Test [58]
	D-KEFS Verbal Fluency
	Continuous Performance Test II [59]
	Grooved Pegboard [60]
	Beery VMI [61]
	Expressive One Word Picture Vocabulary Test [62]
	WIAT-II Pseudoword Decoding Test [63]

Abbreviations: NMSS, National Multiple Sclerosis Society; WISC-R, Wechsler Intelligence Scale for Children Revised; WASI, Wechsler Abbreviated Scale of Intelligence; CVLT, California Verbal learning Test; WISC-IV, Wechsler Intelligence Scale for Children – II; D-KEFS, Delis–Kaplan Executive Function System; VMI, Beery–Buktenica Developmental Test of Visual-Motor Integration; WIAT, Wechsler Individual Achievement Test.

was tested against a larger neuropsychological battery. Using a fairly liberal cut-off of one or more tests impaired on this battery (defined as performance below the 5th percentile compared to healthy controls), sensitivity and specificity of this battery reached 96 and 81%, respectively, suggesting reasonable detection of cognitive impairment in this cohort.

In the USA, the Pediatric MS Centers of Excellence (sponsored by the National MS Society) include a neuropsychological assessment core. The neuropsychological battery utilized in this network is also presented in Table 13.1. This battery requires approximately 2.5–3 h of testing, and incorporates a number of measures considered to be sensitive to the kinds of impairment commonly seen in MS, including an estimate of overall ability, measures of verbal learning and memory, attention and working memory, visual–spatial functioning, processing speed, and a number of aspects of executive functioning. As of the writing of this chapter, this battery is currently in use in six Pediatric MS Centers across the United States. Data investigating the utility of this battery for detecting cognitive impairment in MS have not been published.

Considerations for testing and interpretation

Psychological distress

It is well-known that psychological distress, including depression and anxiety, is quite common in adults with MS and is an important factor influencing neuropsychological performance. The burden of depression and anxiety on cognitive function has not been systematically evaluated in POMS. Although published studies evaluating psychological characteristics in children and adolescents find rates of psychological distress ranging from very rare to over half of patients, there is increasing evidence to suggest a similar burden of psychological distress in children and adolescents with POMS as compared to adults [9,14,17]. Depression is known to negatively impact cognition in MS [27–29]. Furthermore, although studied to a lesser extent, anxiety appears to exert similar effects [30].

Studies to explore the impact of psychological distress on cognitive function in children and adolescents with MS are warranted. In adults, the relationships among depression and cognitive impairment are likely complex and interactive. Cognitive functioning may be a functional result of depressive symptomatology (e.g. lack of concentration, attentional problems, etc.); however, both depression and cognitive function may originate from damage to similar neuropathological pathways. Lesion–depression relationships have been identified in MS [31,32], and the presence of cognitive impairment has been shown to

identify MS patients who have responded poorly to conventional antidepressant therapies [33].

Pain

Again, while pain is not well understood in POMS, it is another frequent symptom of MS with a well-established negative impact on cognitive functioning. Persons with MS can experience pain due to spasticity, paroxysmal symptoms, headache, and neuropathic pain. Pain produces both direct and indirect effects on cognitive functioning through decreased attention, processing speed, and difficulties with encoding. Pain medications including narcotic pain medications and anti-epileptic medicines can also produce changes in cognitive functioning, particularly difficulties with attention and processing speed.

Fatigue

Although this has not been studied in depth, reports suggest that over half of children and adolescents report fatigue of at least mild severity (one-third report severe fatigue) [34]. Fatigue is the most common clinical symptom of adults with MS and can negatively impact cognition related to physical fatigue and cognitive fatigue. Cognitive fatigue is defined as a decline in cognitive performance over a brief period of time, such as a neuropsychological testing session or part of a school day. Although the patient is not participating in any physically fatiguing activities, this decline is often still observed. Krupp and colleagues oberved that patients with MS demonstrate clear declines in performance on measures of verbal memory and executive functioning over a 4-h session. In contrast, medically healthy controls demonstrate improvement in memory and executive functioning over the same period of time, an observation likely due to practice effects [35]. As such, it is particularly important for MS patients to adequately pace themselves to keep fatigue to a minimum. There are obvious implications for neuropsychological testing, and, as such, patients should be prepared as much as possible for testing sessions, and testing over multiple sessions may be necessary.

Other physical symptoms

The neuropsychological assessment of an MS patient can be complicated by other specific impairments commonly occurring as part of the disease processes.

MS frequently is accompanied by specific symptoms of the visual and motor system which can impact a child's ability to complete neuropsychological testing or can influence the resulting test interpretation.

Studies indicate that up to half of children and adolescents present with optic neuritis (ON) [36], which can impact overall visual acuity and color vision. It is important to note that even mild changes in visual acuity negatively impact neuropsychological test results [37], thereby prompting caution in test interpretation. Testing approaches to accommodate visual symptoms include initial screening for visual acuity, the use of measures with large stimuli or increased font size on questionnaires, and the use of measures without visual acuity demands as necessary. In general, it should be standard practice to consider visual acuity to ensure a valid neuropsychological testing approach.

Cerebellar, brainstem, and/or spinal involvement can impact functioning of upper extremities which would influence gross and fine motor functioning, including the ability to write. Often, patients can write, but speed and coordination are impacted. In these cases, the use of motor control tasks may be helpful to aid the separation of hand-motor function from other cognitive functions in test performance. In those patients with more severely compromised fine motor speed and manipulation, the use of measures that rely less on fine motor speed and coordination may be particularly useful. An example of this from the adult MS literature is through the use of the Oral Version of the Symbol Digit Modalities Test [38], which has emerged as one of the most sensitive screening tests available to detect cognitive dysfunction [38,39]. Although this measure was not originally validated for children and adolescents, a recent Italian study using this measure found that it successfully discriminated children and adolescents with MS from healthy controls [20]. Although the use of measures that avoid hand-motor coordination and speed demands may be useful for some patients, we must also remain mindful of other aspects of motor functioning that can influence performance on cognitive tests. For example, recent studies have evaluated the deleterious impact of dysarthria and oral-motor speed on neuropsychological test performance [40,41].

Finally, treatment effects must be considered for the timing of a neuropsychological assessment. For example, although relatively uncommon, adverse behavioral effects have been observed during methylprednisolone treatment after acute relapse [42]. Therefore, it may be advisable to conduct behavioral/neuropsychological assessments distal to the acute relapse and related treatment (e.g. 30 days).

In sum, there are a number of physical and psychological features related to MS that can influence the feasibility of a standard neuropsychological evaluation. Fortunately, in the neuropsychology community, clinicians and researchers have long been struggling with these issues, and, as a result, there are a number of assessment approaches available for use depending on the clinical needs of each patient. Additionally, any number of these other physical and psychological features can influence interpretation of test results. Therefore, neuropsychologists must use appropriate caution in considering the multifaceted manifestations that may account for test performance.

Impact of cognitive function on functional activities

The onset of POMS can occur during very important developmental stages critical for social, academic, and daily functioning. It is not uncommon that children with POMS require academic support or experience reductions in their involvement in social and other activities. Given the nature of the cogntive dysfunction observed in POMS, extrapolation of these findings would predict a considerable functional impact. Although the functional impact of cognitive impairment in children with MS is not clearly documented in studies conducted so far, one might postulate that these impairments would translate to an increased need for school-based interventions and accommodations. We briefly review those neuropsychological studies to date that highlight the impact of neuropsychological impairment on everyday functioning in children and adolescents with POMS.

Amato and colleagues suggested that beyond the impact of physical disability, cognitive problems were reported to negatively affect school, social, and everyday activities of daily living in approximately one-third of their Italian cohort [17]. In this study, parent interviews were conducted for a subset of children included in their cohort. Parents of 41 children reported that 22% of their children required additional school supports related to cognitive difficulties, and 12% missed school related to cognitive difficulties. Furthermore, of the 34% with decreased participation in hobbies and sports, 64% of these children had evidence of cognitive impairment. Although the specific impact of cognitive impairment on functional outcomes was not assessed, MacAllister suggested that 35% of their cohort required school related assistance or a modification of their academic curriculum [14].

Well-designed studies targeted towards understanding the relative contribution of cognition, in addition to other physical impairments, are needed. Additionally, lengthier follow-up studies will be required to more definitively address the long-term prognosis for these children and adolescents as they age into adulthood with respect to their occupational and social functioning related to cognitive decline. Certainly, cognitive decline, increased disability, and a progressive course have all been found to influence social and work-related function in adults with early-onset MS [24]. These findings underline the need for multidisciplinary care, with particular attention being paid to social and academic development, as well as the emotional well-being of this vulnerable patient population.

Neuropsychology and future directions in POMS

Cognitive dysfunction clearly represents a major problem in children with MS. These children are at risk for poor academic performance and this could adversely affect their future ability to achieve their academic potential, go on to gainful employment, and be fully independent.

Future research should include further characterization of the nature of cognitive dysfunction, identification of risk factors, analysis of the relation between neuroradiologic correlates, and of cognitive impairment to other disease factors, and further elucidation of the contribution of concurrent symptoms and diagnoses of affective disorders. Additional research should also focus on treatment.

Future research directions:

- further delineating the cognitive domains most vulnerable to disruption;
- identifying risk factors for cognitive impairment;
- describing functional outcomes associated with cognitive impairment;
- determination of the rate of cognitive decline;
- characterizing the effects of pediatric cognitive functioning as children transition into adulthood;
- delineating neuroimaging and other clinical correlates;

- assessing the therapeutic benefits of disease-modifying agents;
- testing non-pharmacologic, rehabilitative interventions;
- clinical trials with well-tolerated, safe, and effective therapeutic agents.

A major unknown, and one of great concern, is the rate of cognitive decline. It appears that cognitive decline in pediatric MS may occur at a faster rate than in adults. The changes over a short period of time such as over two years can be dramatic [25,43]. Exploration of these changes should include assessment of the relative rates of decline according to each cognitive domain as well as overall cognitive performance. Finally, although this is poorly understood, a relative stasis of cognitive abilities may occur that is unique to children and adolescents (i.e. they remain stable while their peers continue to follow a normal developmental trajectory). If the deterioration of cognitive ability is in fact as severe as the data suggest, there will be additional hurdles for these individuals as they transition to early adulthood. Whether the rate of decline will attenuate once adulthood is reached is unknown.

Cross-sectional and longitudinal studies of the association between neuroimaging and cognitive dysfunction should further elucidate the pathologic processes underlying cognitive impairment. Presumably global atrophy and underlying gray and white matter atrophy contribute to cognitive dysfunction. Thalamic atrophy identified in pediatric MS [44] needs to be assessed with respect to its contribution to cognitive deficits. The cognitive consequences of other neuroimaging abnormalities such as lesion burden and loss of neuronal integrity need to be addressed in future research.

Critical to the care of children and adolescents with MS is identification of effective interventions. Identifying the problem can lead to simple adjustments in the academic setting including providing additional time for tests, allowing the use of computers if handwriting is adversely affected, providing access to accommodations, special services, and other educational interventions. However, we need more direct therapies to enhance cognitive functioning in these children.

Pharmacologic intervention is another approach which should be studied in pediatric MS. There is some suggestion in adult MS that early intervention with DMT can be relatively beneficial for cognitive functioning. Whether such benefits are also applicable to pediatric MS deserves further study. Direct therapy for cognitive dysfunction has received relatively limited research in adult MS. At the moment, some data indicate that donepezil can improve memory performance in adult MS [45]. If positive treatment effects and an encouraging safety profile with donepezil can be further demonstrated in adult MS then such treatment might be considered for study in children with the disease.

The developing brain should have greater plasticity and, as such, could be expected to derive particular benefit from compensatory mechanisms. In adult-onset cases, functional MRI studies have documented cortical reorganization that occurs from the early stages of the disease [46]. In patients with normal performance on a cognitive task, several studies have reported more widespread activation of a greater number of cerebral areas during the task [46]. This is generally interpreted as a compensatory mechanism due to brain plasticity that allows the subject to perform in the normal range despite brain damage. On the other hand, the lack of diffused activation observed in patients with an impaired task performance is interpreted as due to increasing brain pathology that exceeds compensatory abilities [46]. On the whole, these findings point to the need of early therapeutic interventions. The search for effective therapeutic strategies is clearly a priority for future research in the area.

Learning such compensatory strategies could greatly benefit navigating daily life and improving school performance. Cognitive rehabilitation has been incompletely studied in adult MS although there are some studies to suggest benefit in the areas of verbal learning and memory [47,48]. Cognitive rehabilitation studies for children with MS are sorely needed. Children could represent a special population in which such interventions might best succeed.

Conclusion

It is well known that, overall, cognitive impairment is both a common and debilitating symptom in MS. Given the estimated frequency and functional impact of cognitive problems in children and adolescents with MS, there is little reason to suspect that those with POMS are less affected. In fact, there may be some evidence to suggest that, at least initially, children and adolescents with MS may be more affected

than their adult counterparts. It is well-understood that cognitive impairment is an important clinical outcome of MS and a syndrome that results from disease-related neuropathological changes, but may also be a product of concomitant conditions including depression, fatigue, and pain. Determining the means to systematically evaluate cognition in POMS to identify patients at risk for cognitive impairment is critical in order to target and potentially prevent a significant source of disability. Taken together, there are many challenges and multiple directions for future research regarding cognitive functioning in pediatric MS. The consequences of cognitive impairment are severe; further understanding and treatment are critical.

References

1. Duquette P, Murray TJ, Pleines J, *et al.* Multiple sclerosis in childhood: Clinical profile in 125 patients. *J Pediatr* 1987;**111**:359–363.

2. Ghezzi A, Deplano V, Faroni J, *et al.* Multiple sclerosis in childhood: Clinical features of 149 cases. *Mult Scler* 1997;**3**:43–46.

3. Rao SM, Leo GJ, Ellington L, Nauertz T, Bernardin L, Unverzagt F. Cognitive dysfunction in multiple sclerosis. II. Impact on employment and social functioning. *Neurology* 1991;**41**:692–696.

4. Amato MP, Zipoli V, Portaccio E. Cognitive changes in multiple sclerosis. *Expert Rev Neurother* 2008;**8**:1585–1596.

5. Kurtzke JF. Rating neurologic impairment in multiple sclerosis: An expanded disability status scale (EDSS). *Neurology* 1983;**33**:1444–1452.

6. Fields RD. White matter in learning, cognition and psychiatric disorders. *Trends Neurosci* 2008;**31**:361–370.

7. Filippi M, Rocca MA. MR imaging of gray matter involvement in multiple sclerosis: Implications for understanding disease pathophysiology and monitoring treatment efficacy. *Am J Neuroradiol* 2009. A1944.

8. Elizabeth F, Jar-Chi L, Kunio N, Richard AR. Gray matter atrophy in multiple sclerosis: A longitudinal study. *Ann Neurol* 2008;**64**:255–265.

9. MacAllister WS, Boyd JR, Holland NJ, Milazzo MC, Krupp LB. The psychosocial consequences of pediatric multiple sclerosis. *Neurology* 2007;**68**(Suppl 2):S66–69.

10. Bye AM, Kendall B, Wilson J. Multiple sclerosis in childhood: A new look. *Dev Med Child Neurol* 1985;**27**:215–222.

11. Amato MP, Ponziani G, Pracucci G, Bracco L, Siracusa G, Amaducci L. Cognitive impairment in early-onset

multiple sclerosis. Pattern, predictors, and impact on everyday life in a 4-year follow-up. *Arch Neurol* 1995;**52**:168–172.

12. Dale RC, de Sousa C, Chong WK, Cox TC, Harding B, Neville BG. Acute disseminated encephalomyelitis, multiphasic disseminated encephalomyelitis and multiple sclerosis in children. *Brain* 2000;**123**:2407–2422.

13. Banwell BL, Anderson PE. The cognitive burden of multiple sclerosis in children. *Neurology* 2005;**64**: 891–894.

14. MacAllister WS, Belman AL, Milazzo M, *et al.* Cognitive functioning in children and adolescents with multiple sclerosis. *Neurology* 2005;**64**:1422–1425.

15. Kaplan EF, Goodglass H, Weintraub S. *The Boston Naming Test (2nd edn)*. Philadelphia, PA: Lea & Febiger; 1983.

16. Semel E, Wiig EH, Secord WA. *Clinical Evaluation of Language Fundamentals – 3*. San Antonio, TX: Psychological Corporation a Pearson Brand; 1995.

17. Amato MP, Goretti B, Ghezzi A, *et al.* Cognitive and psychosocial features of childhood and juvenile MS. *Neurology* 2008;**70**:1891–1897.

18. Wechsler D. *Wechsler Intelligence Scale for Children – Revised*. New York, NY: The Psychological Corporation; 1974.

19. American Psychiatric Association. *Diagnostic and Statistical Manual of Mental Disorders (4th edn)*. Washington, DC: American Psychiatric Association; 1994.

20. Portaccio E, Goretti B, Lori S, *et al.* The brief neuropsychological battery for children: A screening tool for cognitive impairment in childhood and juvenile multiple sclerosis. *Mult Scler* 2009;**15**:620–626.

21. Julian L, Im-Wang S, Chabas D. Learning and memory in pediatric multiple sclerosis. *Paper presented at: ACTRIMS/ECTRIMS meeting*, 2008; Montreal, Canada.

22. Parrish J, Yeh E, Jackson L, Weinstoch-Guttman B, Benedict R. Neurocognitive status in patients with demyelinating desease and healthy controls assessed with the pediatric MS Centres of Excellence Consensus Neuropsychological Battery. *Paper presented at Neurology*, 2009.

23. Kujala P, Portin R, Ruutiainen J. The progress of cognitive decline in multiple sclerosis. A controlled 3-year follow-up. *Brain* 1997;**120**:289–297.

24. Amato MP, Ponziani G, Siracusa G, Sorbi S. Cognitive dysfunction in early-onset multiple sclerosis: A reappraisal after 10 years. *Arch Neurol* 2001;**58**:1602–1606.

25. MacAllister WS, Christodoulou C, Milazzo M, Krupp LB. Longitudinal neuropsychological assessment in pediatric multiple sclerosis. *Dev Neuropsychol* 2007;**32**:625–644.

26. Amato M, Goretti B, Ghezzi A, *et al.* Cognitive and psychosocial features of childhood and juvenile multiple sclerosis. A reappraisal after two years. *Paper presented at: American Academy of Neurology meeting*, 2009; Seattle.

27. Arnett PA, Higgenson CI, Randolph JJ. Depression in multiple sclerosis: Relationship to planning ability. *J Int Neuropsychol Soc* 2001;**7**:665–674.

28. Arnett PA, Higginson CI, Voss WD, Bender WI, Wurst JM, Tippin JM. Depression in multiple sclerosis: Relationship to working memory capacity. *Neuropsychology* 1999;**13**:546–556.

29. Arnett PA, Higginson CI, Voss WD, *et al.* Depressed mood in multiple sclerosis: Relationship to capacity-demanding memory and attentional functioning. *Neuropsychology* 1999;**13**:434–446.

30. Julian LJ, Arnett PA. Relationships among anxiety, depression, and executive functioning in multiple sclerosis. *Clin Neuropsychol* 2009;**23**:1–11.

31. Zorzon M, de Masi R, Nasuelli D, *et al.* Depression and anxiety in multiple sclerosis. A clinical and MRI study in 95 subjects. *J Neurol* 2001;**248**:416–421.

32. Zorzon M, Zivadinov R, Nasuelli D, *et al.* Depressive symptoms and MRI changes in multiple sclerosis. *Eur J Neurol* 2002;**9**:491–496.

33. Julian LJ, Mohr DC. Cognitive predictors of response to treatment for depression in multiple sclerosis. *J Neuropsychiatry Clin Neurosci* 2006;**18**:356–363.

34. MacAllister WS, Christodoulou C, Troxell R, *et al.* Fatigue and quality of life in pediatric multiple sclerosis. *Mult Scler* 2009;**15**:1502–1508.

35. Krupp LB, Elkins LE. Fatigue and declines in cognitive functioning in multiple sclerosis. *Neurology* 2000;**55**:934–939.

36. Ness JM, Chabas D, Sadovnick AD, Pohl D, Banwell B, Weinstock-Guttman B. Clinical features of children and adolescents with multiple sclerosis. *Neurology* 2007;**68**(Suppl 2):S37–45.

37. Bruce JM, Bruce AS, Arnett PA. Mild visual acuity disturbances are associated with performance on tests of complex visual attention in MS. *J Int Neuropsychol Soc* 2007;**13**:544–548.

38. Smith A. *Symbol Digit Modalities Test (SDMT). Manual (Revised)*. Los Angeles, CA: Western Psychological Services; 1982.

39. Parmenter BA, Zivadinov R, Kerenyi L, *et al.* Validity of the Wisconsin Card Sorting and Delis–Kaplan Executive Function System (DKEFS) Sorting Tests in multiple sclerosis. *J Clin Exp Neuropsychol* 2007;**29**:215–223.

40. Smith MM, Arnett PA. Dysarthria predicts poorer performance on cognitive tasks requiring a speeded oral response in an MS population. *J Clin Exp Neuropsychol* 2007;**29**:804–812.

41. Arnett PA, Smith MM, Barwick FH, Benedict RH, Ahlstrom BP. Oralmotor slowing in multiple sclerosis: Relationship to neuropsychological tasks requiring an oral response. *J Int Neuropsychol Soc* 2008;**14**:454–462.

42. Lyons PR, Newman PK, Saunders M. Methylprednisolone therapy in multiple sclerosis: A profile of adverse effects. *J Neurol Neurosurg Psychiatry* 1988;**51**:285–287.

43. Amato M, Goretti B, Ghezzi A, *et al.* Cognitive and psychosocial features of childhood and juvenile multiple sclerosis: A reappraisal after 2 years. *Neurology* 2009;**72**(Suppl 3):A97.

44. Mesaros SM, Rocca MAM, Absinta MM, *et al.* Evidence of thalamic gray matter loss in pediatric multiple sclerosis SYMBOL. *Neurology* 2008; **70**(13, Part 2 of 2):1107–1112.

45. Krupp LB, Christodoulou C, Melville P, Scherl WF, MacAllister WS, Elkins LE. Donepezil improved memory in multiple sclerosis in a randomized clinical trial. *Neurology* 2004;**63**:1579–1585.

46. Chiaravalloti ND, DeLuca J. Cognitive impairment in multiple sclerosis. *Lancet Neurol* 2008;7:1139–1151.

47. O'Brien AR, Chiaravalloti N, Goverover Y, Deluca J. Evidenced-based cognitive rehabilitation for persons with multiple sclerosis: A review of the literature. *Arch Phys Med Rehabil* 2008;**89**:761–769.

48. Goverover Y, Hillary FG, Chiaravalloti N, Arango-Lasprilla JC, DeLuca J. A functional application of the spacing effect to improve learning and memory in persons with multiple sclerosis. *J Clin Exp Neuropsychol* 2009;**31**:513–522.

49. Wechsler D. *Wechsler Intelligence Scale for Children – Revised.* New York, NY: Psychological Corporation; 1974.

50. Corporation TP. *The Wechsler Abbreviated Scale of Intelligence.* San Antonio, TX: Harcourt Assessment; 1999.

51. *Army Individual Test Battery: Manual of Directions and Scoring.* Washington, DC: War Department, Adjutant General's Office; 1944.

52. Buschke F, Fuld PA. Evaluating storage, retention and retrieval in disordered memory and learning. *Neurology* 1974;**24**:1019–1025.

53. Delis D, Kramer J, Kaplan E, Ober B. *California Verbal Learning Test Manual: Second Edition, Adult Version.* San Antonio, TX: Psychological Corporation; 2000.

54. Delis JH, Kramer JH, Kaplan E, Ober B. *California Verbal Learning Test – Children's Version.* San Antonio, TX: The Psychological Corporation; 1994.

55. Wechsler D. *Wechsler Adult Intelligence Scale – III.* New York, NY: The Psychological Corporation; 1991.

56. Wechsler D. *WISC-IV Administrative and Scoring Manual.* San Antonio, TX: The Psychological Corporation; 2003.

57. Taylor HG, Albo VC, Phebus CK, Sachs BR, Bierl PG. Postirradiation treatment outcomes for children with acute lymphocytic leukemia: Clarification of risks. *J Pediatr Psychol* 1987;**12**:395–411.

58. Delis DC, Kaplan E, Kramer JH, Ober BA. *Delis–Kaplan Executive Function Scale (D-KEFS).* San Antonio, TX: The Psychological Corporation; 2001.

59. Conners CK. *Connor's Continuous Performance Test II. Technical Guide and Software Manual.* North Tonawada, NT: Multi-Health Systems; 2000.

60. Matthews CG, Klove H. *Instruction Manual for the Adult Neuropsychological Test Battery.* Madison, WI: University of Wisconsin Medical School; 1964.

61. Beery KE, Beery NA. *The Beery–Buktenica Developmental Test of Visual–Motor Integration – 5th edn.* Minneapolis, MN: NCS Pearson, Inc.; 2006.

62. Expressive One-Word Picture Vocabulary Test. [computer program]. *Version.* Novato, CA: Academic Therapy Publications; 1979.

63. *Wechsler Individual Achievement Test: Second Edition.* San Antonio, TX: Harcourt Assessment, Inc.; 2005.

Living with pediatric multiple sclerosis: patient well-being

Sunny Im-Wang, Maria Milazzo, and Ellen M. Mowry

The stress of having a chronic illness has countless effects on both a child or adolescent and his/her family, especially when there is uncertainty surrounding the prognosis of the illness, as is true of multiple sclerosis (MS) [1]. In general, lack of information and inadequate support hinder parents' efforts to cope with their child's disease [2,3].

The diagnosis of a chronic illness such as MS is confusing at any age but may be particularly challenging to older children, as the natural developmental instinct for children as they grow is to gain independence. These children are placed in a developmental bind where the dependence on others that is introduced by the illness conflicts with this natural drive for independence. Older children facing chronic illness are more likely to experience increased anxiety when their illness and its related issues, such as treatment, conflict with body image issues and desire for independence [4,5]. Since older children and adolescents are normally focused on the physical changes occurring in their bodies, fears or distortions related to chronic illness will intensify these concerns. In MS, for example, children may fear that their injection area will show and limit their ability to wear certain clothes.

While the relationship between chronic illness and psychological adjustment is complicated and indirect, children with such illnesses are at risk for mental health and adjustment problems [6]. Depression and anxiety are more likely in children with chronic illness; these symptoms may be a primary feature or secondarily connected to the illness. For instance, the intrusiveness of treatment involved with the illness and required medical regimen correlates with the level of mental health problems.

There are daily stresses that all children and adolescents face, including peer problems, academic failure,

and exposure to inter-parental conflict, which are expected and considered to be normal [4,5]. Children and adolescents worry about their relationships with their friends at school and their level of academic success or failure. In addition, they are affected by their parents' relationship when conflict exists between the two. These stressors are thought to be experiences that will serve as groundwork for children to learn from for later use in their social and intellectual worlds. However, for children and adolescents who are chronically ill, these normal developmental stressors are compounded as a result of their illness, potentially affecting social and emotional functioning.

In this chapter, we discuss the concepts introduced above as they pertain to children and adolescents with MS and discuss how health care can ameliorate these stressors. We will discuss how children with MS and their parents rate the impact of the disease on their overall daily functioning, or health-related quality of life. We will then focus on the influence of MS on school and psychosocial aspects of life in children and adolescents, offering practical information about how to most effectively address potential problems.

Health-related quality of life in multiple sclerosis

MS has substantial impacts on the lives of those diagnosed with the disorder. Both attacks and progressive symptoms associated with MS can contribute to the net burden of disease. There are many tools that are used in clinical trials to quantify this burden. The Expanded Disability Status Scale (EDSS) is one such tool, providing a nonlinear score based predominantly on the neurologic examination [7]. Despite its widespread use as an endpoint in clinical trials, the EDSS has been

Demyelinating Disorders of the Central Nervous System in Childhood, ed. Dorothée Chabas and Emmanuelle L. Waubant. Published by Cambridge University Press. © Cambridge University Press 2011.

criticized due to limitations in its psychometric properties [8] and because it does not equally account for the various functional systems (e.g. vision, cognitive changes) or other aspects of health (e.g. mood, sleep) that may be affected by MS.

In parallel, there has been an increasing interest in patient-reported outcomes in recent years. Health-related quality of life represents one type of patient-reported outcome and is thought to capture the impact of an illness on the patient's own experience of physical and psychosocial well-being. In adults with MS, measures of health-related quality of life are considered more comprehensive in capturing the disease burden than are conventional disability scales, such as the EDSS [9,10]. The Food and Drug Administration now mandates that health-related quality of life measures are incorporated into MS clinical trials [11].

Health-related quality of life in adult-onset MS

Adults with MS tend to report reductions in health-related quality of life even when compared with those with other chronic diseases [12]. Patients who have recently been diagnosed and have little objective disability still report poorer health-related quality of life scores than healthy controls [10,13–15], and improvement of health-related quality of life following a relapse lags behind disability improvement [16].

The assessment of health-related quality of life has been incorporated into several trials of disease-modifying therapies (DMTs) [17–24]. Interferon therapy had no impact on health-related quality of life in three studies [18,20,24], while in two others, patients on treatment had improved quality of life, primarily in measures of physical function [22,23]. More recently, natalizumab has been shown to have a positive effect on health-related quality of life [17]. There are no studies specifically assessing the impact of glatiramer acetate (Copaxone) on health-related quality of life.

Some aspects of health-related quality of life are associated with brain atrophy on magnetic resonance imaging [25]. This finding is important since atrophy, thought to be caused by neuro-axonal loss, is predictive of the long-term development of disability in patients with MS [26–29]. Two small reports demonstrated that some aspects of health-related quality of life are weakly associated with subsequent decline in

physical function, even after accounting for baseline disability [30,31]. These studies collectively suggest that health-related quality of life may be a marker of disease burden in adult-onset MS, raising the question of whether such patient-reported outcomes may help distinguish patients most at risk for a worse subsequent disease course.

The impact of pediatric MS on health-related quality of life

Since MS has the potential to disrupt a child's developmental trajectory, it is plausible that the disease may cause substantial burden in affected children. There are a few reports of patient-reported outcomes in pediatric MS. One group reported that almost half of the 37 children assessed experienced fatigue [32]. A single study of only nine children with MS examined self-perception, which was fairly normal except in the domain of social acceptance [33].

Three studies have addressed health-related quality of life in pediatric MS [34–36]. The first compared quality of life scores from a group of children with MS or monophasic demyelinating events to scores from healthy children; the former group reported worse quality of life [34]. A second study assessed quality of life using the Pediatric Quality of Life Inventory (PedsQL), a validated, widely used instrument that measures global self- and parent/proxy-reported health-related quality of life in children [37]. The PedsQL assesses both physical and psychosocial aspects of quality of life; the latter score is formed by taking into account emotional, social, and school-related functioning. In the study, physical and social functioning were inversely correlated with physical disability (higher EDSS score) per the children and their parents; parents' assessment of school functioning was also inversely correlated with physical disability [35]. In a third study, health-related quality of life in 50 children with MS or clinically isolated syndrome was compared to that of their siblings and to that of children with chronic neuromuscular conditions, again using the PedsQL [36]. Self-reported scores for children with MS were meaningfully lower than scores for their siblings (Table 14.1). The difference was more pronounced for psychosocial than for physical aspects of functioning; school functioning was particularly impaired in children with MS. Compared to children with neuromuscular disorders, those with MS/clinically isolated syndrome reported better physical and social functioning but more difficulties

Table 14.1 Health-related quality of life scores in pediatric multiple sclerosis

Mean scores (± SD)	MS/CIS	Neuromuscular controls	Sibling controls	p value*	p value§
Child self-report	n=41	n=38	n=12		
Total	71±17	65±17	87±10	0.11	0.004
Physical	73±23	56±24	91±10	0.002	0.010
Psychosocial	70±17	70±17	84±11	0.90	0.008
Emotional	65±24	74±19	78±21	0.055	0.079
Social	85±15	68±20	93±8	<0.0001	0.088
School ζ	60±23	70±22	82±16	0.049	0.003
Parent proxy-report	n=45	n=51	n=10		
Total	69±20	53±17	90±13	<0.0001	0.004
Physical	68±25	46±24	93±10	<0.0001	0.003
Psychosocial	70±20	57±18	89±15	0.001	0.007
Emotional	64±26	60±21	88±19	0.38	0.010
Social	82±20	53±24	93±10	<0.0001	0.096
School ζ	64±21	56±21	85±20	0.086	0.008

Note:
ζ not available for some subjects as not all children attend school. MS/CIS versus *neuromuscular controls; § sibling controls

with school and emotional functioning. The results were similar for parent proxy reports (Table 14.1). For children with MS or clinically isolated syndrome, greater physical disability (as assessed by the EDSS) and, to some extent, non-white race were associated with worse health-related quality of life. Their parents reported worse scores for girls and tended to report worse scores if their child was non-white or had a longer disease duration.

These results suggest that children with MS experience substantial deficits in health-related quality of life, particularly as compared to healthy children. Further studies in larger cohorts with concurrent controls are needed to further explore the magnitudes of the differences in overall and individual aspects of functioning. Since there are no MS-specific quality of life instruments for children, the full impact of the disease on daily functioning may not be captured by this measure. For example, in adults with the disease, a global quality of life measure akin in scope to the PedsQL 4.0, the SF-36, was found to be a poor measure of the impact of the subtle visual dysfunction known to affect patients with MS [38]. The underlying contributors to reduced

health-related quality of life in children must also be explored. Finally, the impact of MS on the functioning of the family deserves considerable attention.

Pediatric multiple sclerosis and school

Like work for adults, school is a large part of a child's life. School and social adjustment in children with chronic illness can be impacted by parental perceptions of their child's vulnerability [39]. Parents of pediatric MS patients are naturally faced with numerous questions about school issues, including academic and emotional issues. The task of gathering the appropriate information to help their child cope as well as to advocate for him/her in school can be a daunting experience for parents of children with MS. Research suggests that interventions aimed at enhancing child adjustment to chronic illness are best if parents are included into the intervention [39].

For children and adolescents, their school-related concerns are frequently related to psychosocial aspects, such as how their friends will view them and how they want to be perceived, and are driven by not wanting to feel different. Therefore, even if there is a need for accommodation in the classroom and/or school facility and a specific plan has been established, children and adolescents often do not like to use those resources and/or may under-report active symptoms in order to avoid embarrassment about being different.

The impact of cognitive functioning on school

MS can affect a child's cognitive functioning, including reasoning, processing, attention span, information processing and retrieval, and other thinking abilities [40]. Cognitive dysfunction can, in turn, impact the learning and memory and, consequently, the academic performance of children with MS. In addition, since acute attacks or residual symptoms can cause numbness or weakness, this can also affect writing and handwriting [41].

The impact of MS on children's cognitive abilities and their functioning in school is particularly strong for younger children who experience disease activity prior to completing their core educational building blocks [33,42]. A child whose learning process is disrupted prior to acquiring skills such as mathematics or advanced sentence structure will likely develop substantially different deficits compared with an adult who has already mastered these subjects [42]. It is imperative that every effort is made to recognize and address these problems before they have a significant impact on a child's school experience [32]. Therefore, it is essential that parents of children with MS are aware of possible changes in order to aid with necessary intervention and/or accommodation at school.

Social–emotional functioning in school

The impact of MS on the social and emotional functioning of children and adolescents depends on their developmental stages. Developmental issues can complicate a child or adolescent's view of him or herself and how he or she approaches the MS treatment plan. Children with MS are faced with being responsible for their own health management. This new responsibility of self-care may be compounded by the stress of injection treatments, which can further increase stress levels and influence routines at school. In addition, medical appointments and symptoms can influence school attendance, which can affect emotional well-being [43–46].

Changes in their social and emotion functioning due to illness-related factors such as increased amounts of absences and possible psychosocial dynamic changes in friends may, in turn, affect the school lives of children and adolescents. Emotional stress can decrease levels of attention and concentration, which can influence academic performance. Therefore, close monitoring of school performance should be done to assess for changes in grades or classes. When such changes are noted, an underlying social or emotional stressor, in addition to neurological or cognitive impairment, should be considered as a potential contributor.

Socialization as a part of school life may suffer either due to active symptoms, such as fatigue or pain, or due to lack of interest in socialization because of embarrassment, self-esteem issues, and/or depression [41]. The impact of MS symptoms, whether primary, secondary, or tertiary, on the pediatric population depends on where they are in their developmental trajectory.

Peer relationships are an important component of child and adolescent development. Children worry about what their peers would think if something related to their chronic disease occurs. Academically, there are homework assignments and fast-paced lessons in the classroom. If a child is absent for a period of time due to a chronic illness, schoolwork easily accumulates, making it difficult for him/her to catch up. Compounded by potential cognitive changes, having to catch up with learning new materials in class can further stress any youth. When chronic illness is diagnosed in a family, it adds extreme financial and emotional strain on the parents. This can further stress the child beyond normal expected levels [5].

Accommodation/intervention

Available accommodations and/or interventions vary by location. For example, in the United States, all students are entitled to free public education, and if there are factors that hinder their learning, such as a medical condition, these students are entitled to an Individualized Educational Plan (IEP) and/or Section 504 Plan, if they meet criteria or eligibility. These types of formal accommodations and/or interventions require a physician's letter describing the disease. An example used by some Pediatric MS Centers is shown in Figure 14.1.

Since MS is unpredictable by nature and characterized by varying degrees of active clinical symptoms, it is highly recommended that the future potential

Date: _____

RE: _____, _____
     (Last name, First name)   (Date of Birth)

Dear School Staff:

Our patient above has been diagnosed with:

- ☐ Multiple Sclerosis
- ☐ Devic's Disease
- ☐ Other demyelinating disease (including Clinically Isolated Syndrome and Acute Disseminated Encephalomyelitis)

This is a neurologic medical condition that may have an effect on this student's cognitive/academic performance and other functioning at school. Potential symptoms may include, but are not limited to: fatigue, muscle weakness, numbness, tingling, urinary urgency or frequency, urinary or bowel "accidents," imbalance, poor coordination, blurry or double vision, loss of vision (temporary), difficulty thinking or concentrating, slurred speech, headache, and pain.

Since change in cognitive functioning is one of the symptoms of this disease, the learning process may be affected. In addition, due to unpredictability of this disease, ongoing monitoring of this student's cognitive functioning at school is highly recommended.

Sincerely,

{Also provide consent signature from the patient's legal guardian}

Figure 14.1 A sample letter to school indicating impact of medical diagnosis on functioning at school.

need for accommodation and intervention is discussed, even when significant and/or serious clinical symptoms are not currently present. This will ensure that the process of receiving accommodations is smoother should a need arise. Some of general recommendations that have been made to schools can be found in Figure 14.2.

Psychosocial aspects of pediatric multiple sclerosis

The psychosocial impact of pediatric MS

Psychosocial issues have been described in the adult MS population but are poorly understood in pediatric MS. An examination of the literature on other chronic pediatric medical conditions identifies areas of concern and needs further investigation. Growing up with a chronic illness can be a challenge, placing a child or teen at increased psychosocial risk of psychological dysfunction in general. However, the pediatric MS group is unique in that the process of demyelination occurs in a developing brain, the disease is relatively rare with few similarly affected peers or role models, and there is a general lack of familiarity with the condition in the medical or lay community.

For the school-aged child, in whom a healthy identity is dependent on developing a stage of accomplishment, time away from school or modified activities in school (for example, an adaptive gym class) can lead to a sense of inferiority, helplessness, and apathy. The child may be angry about the illness and the unfairness that others are not similarly affected. Chronic illness in the adolescent interferes with the normal developmental processes of gaining autonomy, establishing a sense of identity, forming mature peer relationships, developing abstract reasoning, and planning for the future [47]. The manner in which the illness is managed by the adolescent, family (including establishing a balance between higher than normal levels of parental supervision and teen independence), peers, and health care providers will influence the normal progress of developmental tasks.

Teens with chronic illness are at risk for development of mental health and adjustment problems [48,49]. They are more likely to internalize their feelings and exhibit disorders such as anxiety, depression, excessive fear, rather than externalizing symptoms such as aggression [49,50]. The studies in the pediatric MS population are few, small and have had mixed results. In one early study, children with MS did not see themselves as being different from their peers in

Dear School Staff:

Pediatric Multiple Sclerosis (MS) is a neurologic medical condition that may have an effect on this student's cognitive/academic performance and other functioning at school. Potential symptoms may include, but are not limited to: fatigue, muscle weakness, numbness, tingling, urinary urgency or frequency, urinary or bowel "accidents," imbalance, poor coordination, blurry or double vision, loss of vision (temporary), difficulty thinking or concentrating, slurred speech, headache, and pain.

Since change in cognitive functioning is one of the symptoms of this disease, the learning process may be affected. In addition, due to unpredictability of this disease, ongoing monitoring of this student's cognitive functioning at school is highly recommended.

Following are some general accommodations that are based on the most **common** symptoms of Multiple Sclerosis; therefore, each student's needs should be determined based on his/her individual needs.

A Brief List Of Recommended General Accommodations For <u>Common</u>[i] MS Primary/Secondary Symptoms:

1. Speed of information processing difficulties
   a. Provide extra time for completion of assignments and examinations/quizzes
   b. Allow student to tape record assignments/homework - assists in recall and processing deficits
   c. Notes given prior to class
2. Information retrieval difficulties—students with MS commonly present difficulties with retrieving information on demand
   a. Whenever possible, provide multiple choice type exams
   b. Allow open book exams
   c. Provide cues to help retrieve information. For example, categorizing
   d. Allow visual cues. For example, if the student needs to use a formula to solve a math problem, have formulas available on index cards to be used during quizzes and in class assignments
3. Fatigue
   a. Allow student to have an extra set of books at home – assists in reducing fatigue
   b. Reduced homework assignments
   c. Allow for short breaks between assignments
   d. Closer proximity between classrooms
   e. Give frequent short quizzes, not long exams
4. Physical weakness/bladder difficulties
   a. Sit student near door to allow easy exit
   b. Allow student to leave classroom early to get to next classroom
   c. Sit student near window/AC unit for cooling during hot days to prevent increased fatigue
   d. Allow student to have water at his/her desk
   e. Allow student to have time out of seat to stretch to avoid spasms in legs, arms, etc…
   f. Allow frequent use of bathroom pass for any bowel/bladder urgencies or difficulties (Laminated hall pass)
   g. Extra clothing kept in RN office (bowel/bladder)
5. Motor difficulties
   a. Assistive technology, i.e. computer – for student's who have difficult with handwriting, etc…
   b. Provide peer note taker
   c. Do not grade on handwriting
   d. May need PT/OT services
6. Visual difficulties
   a. Seat student near the teacher or blackboard
   b. Notes enlarged for students with visual problems
   c. Read test item to student
7. Attention/Concentration difficulties (a) due to cognitive change (neurological in nature) or (b) secondary to being diagnosed with a chronic illness (emotional functioning)
   a. Promote organizational skills by providing course outline for the week, month, semester allowing student to plan
   b. Standing near the student when giving directions or presenting lessons
   c. Cue students to stay on task (nonverbal signal)
   d. Simplify complex directions—make sure directions/instructions are understood
   e. If difficulty is due to emotional functioning, in addition to teaching skills to improve attention and concentration, individual counseling may be needed since the student's emotional functioning is getting in the way of learning

If you would like further information and/or consultation, please contact[ii]:

_____ , _____
Name   Title
Sincerely,

_____

[i] These symptoms are common, however not all students will experience these symptoms. Some may experience less and some may experience more symptoms that would need additional support/accommodations.

[ii] Consultation on a specific student must have prior written consent from the student's legal guardian.

Figure 14.2 A sample general accommodation recommendation letter to school: for diagnosis of pediatric MS.

areas of scholastic and athletic competence, physical appearance, behavioral conduct, romantic appeal, or global self-worth. The children scored above the norm in the area of social acceptance [33]. In another study, the frequency of behavioral concerns including anxiety, depression, and adjustment disorder was almost as high as 50% [32]. A third study reported depression in fewer than 10% of the subjects, although the sensitivity of the instrument was low [40].

Family coping is a strong predictor of the child's psychosocial adjustment [51–53]. The time period around the diagnosis is a time of crisis. In pediatric MS, parents feel isolated and find a limited support network when facing a rare diagnosis. Positive adjustment to chronic illness has been found to be related to a sense of family cohesion, dual parental involvement, reasonable but not rigid compliance with the treatment plan, and a supportive marital relationship that is sensitive to the ongoing needs of the siblings [54]. Additional intervention or external support from the health care team is necessary when such conditions are absent.

Signs of psychosocial distress

Signs of psychosocial distress in children and teens include unexplained medical complaints, poor compliance with treatment plans, school refusal, and risk-taking behaviors [55]. A multidisciplinary team, experienced in working with children living with chronic illness, is necessary in order to recognize these indicators of distress.

Unexplained medical complaints

In one study, the Pediatric Symptom Checklist was used to screen school-aged children for psychosocial dysfunction. Chronically ill children with internalizing symptoms had a higher use of health care than either the healthy control group or other chronically ill children without these symptoms [56]. Unexplained medical symptoms, not attributable to a medical cause, can be distressing to the child, family, and health care providers. School performance and other social interactions will likely be affected. Repeat visits may be made to the physician and hospital for evaluation and treatment. For example, in pediatric MS, complaints of headache and fatigue may be related to the disease process itself, but can be an indication of underlying psychological distress. Evaluation of elusive symptoms includes a medical assessment as well as assessment of family adaptation to illness and psychosocial functioning. Treatment of the child within the family unit may be indicated.

Treatment adherence

Poor compliance may vary in degree and has the potential to result in a poor outcome. Medical compliance is based on the assumption that the child and family acknowledge the diagnosis and accept the treatment plan developed by the health care team. Causes for non-compliance include poor family functioning, a lack of disease-specific education, and lack of resources. Treatment compliance will change with the maturation of the child. For the younger child, the responsibility falls to the parent. Later, the burden of responsibility shifts toward the adolescent. Those with greater parental involvement have higher rates of compliance [57]. For the adolescent, medical compliance requires a recognition and acceptance of the illness. Nonetheless, complying with medication is a constant reminder that they are different from their peers. Non-compliance may be due to psychosocial dysfunction, due to a sense of loss of control, anger at the diagnosis, and concerns about one's future. Further, complying with treatment may produce untoward adverse effects. For the teen with an acute MS relapse, the short-term weight gain and acne associated with steroid treatment may be too distressing to agree to treatment. Injectable disease-modifying medications can cause difficulty with compliance for many children and teens.

Family-centered interventions in promoting compliance include an open discussion of treatment options such as frequency, side-effect profiles, and monitoring schedules, as well as family lifestyle. Promoting the teen's autonomy and including parental preference will maximize satisfaction with the treatment plan. It is important to anticipate that compliance in adolescence may be inadequate and assessment of compliance must be included in follow-up visits. Treatment choices may change over time with maturation and change in lifestyle. A careful psychosocial assessment of non-compliance is a critical feature in patient management.

School avoidance

School is a place where children and teens carry out their developmental work including interacting with peers and developing an independent identity [56].

Missed days of school may be caused by or a cause of psychosocial dysfunction. Anxiety or depressive disorders, social or school problems, anxious parents, or a combination of these factors, may be a cause of school absences. Absences often increase around the time of diagnosis. Even during periods of relative disease inactivity, children may be absent from school for medical visits, tests or treatments, or due to symptoms such as fatigue.

Most children want to attend school to see friends and be immersed in their usual routine. School re-entry programs can facilitate the transition back to the classroom for children with chronic illness. They prepare the student, family, educators, and peers for the return to the classroom [58]. Specific details for a transition back to school are discussed earlier in this chapter.

Risk-taking behaviors

Engaging in high-risk behaviors involving sex and substance use is a sign of psychosocial distress [55]. Fortunately, teens with chronic illness report fewer risk-taking behaviors [59] and similar or lower rates of substance use [60]. Decreased rates of risk-taking may be related to delayed physical and psychosocial maturation. Additionally, increased interaction with, and in some cases, over-protection by parents, teachers, health care providers, and other adults may minimize the possibility of risk-taking behaviors [61]. It is important to include time during office visits for discussion without the parent so that the teen can speak freely about sensitive issues.

Improving psychosocial function in pediatric MS

Working with the family

Parents of children with MS need and want information regarding the illness, the diagnostic process, treatment options, and future expectations. They often have some experience with adults with MS, but need information about the disease in children. Medical care for these children is often fragmented, as there may be a number of providers involved in care. Information may not always move smoothly and in a timely fashion, and conflicting information may be given. Primary care providers may ask the families to check in with the specialist before routine immunizations and the neurologists may refer routine pediatric issues to the pediatrician. An emergency room visit may lead to interactions with physicians unfamiliar with the underlying diagnosis. Consistent with the recommendations of the American Academy of Pediatrics "Medical Home" [62], a physician coordinator of the care is essential. Since multiple specialists can be involved the physician coordinating the care can provide a unified plan for the family. Children with MS often need a multidisciplinary team with each member providing their own perspective specific to their role, e.g. a physical therapist addressing motor needs while a social worker will be concerned with psychosocial and educational needs. The lead person on the team liaisons with the family to assure a seamless bidirectional transfer of information.

Including the child/teen

The age, developmental level, and emotional maturity of the youngster at the onset of symptoms will influence the extent of their involvement in the assessment, discussion of diagnosis, and treatment plan. The parent's knowledge of the child's coping style and readiness for information is vital in developing a plan for discussion of the diagnosis with the child [63]. Including the child in open communication about treatment options results in improved adherence [64–66]. In reviews of pediatric oncology studies, disclosure of the diagnosis to the child results in an improved relationship between child and parents, improved self-esteem, and better long-term emotional health.

Although teens with chronic illness do have lower rates of substance use, the most common substance of abuse is alcohol [67]. Teens with MS may be more at risk for the side effects of alcohol, such as interactions with medications and worsening of disease-related symptoms such as ataxia and dysarthria.

Disclosure

When and how to disclose the diagnosis of pediatric MS to others may be a difficult decision. The lack of awareness and education about pediatric MS can lead to a response such as "You can't have MS . . . you are not old enough," when a teen does disclose to a teacher or other respected adult. The need to first defend the diagnosis, and then ask for support can be difficult, and may result in the lack of disclosure. It is important to work with the family to identify a strategy for sharing the diagnosis with others. Close family members and friends may be told early on, working out from the

Table 14.2 Resource list

Resource	Provides
"Directions" Manual Massachusetts Department of Public Health http://www.mass.gov/dph/fch/directions	A resource for families to organize health records and locate resources for their child's health care
Family Village http://www.familyvillage.wisc.edu/	Website listing resources for families of children with disabilities
Individuals with Disabilities http://idea.ed.gov/	Resource for families and educators regarding special education law
Children and Teens with MS: A Network for Families 1–866–543–7967	Psychological and educational services for children, teens, and families Includes:
	• Kids Get MS Too: A Guide for Parents Whose Child or Teen has MS
	• Managing School-Related Issues: A Handbook for Parents
	• Handbook for School Personnel regarding Pediatric MS
	• Mighty Special Kids: An activity book for kids 5–12
	• DVD for Children and Teens with MS and their Families
	• MS World: chat rooms for teens, college students, and parents
MS Association of America http://www.msaa.com	MS Resource for clinicians and families
MS Society of Canada http://www.mssociety.ca	MS resource for clinicians and families - Canada
National MS Society http://www.nmss.org	MS resource for clinicians and families - USA
National Center for Medical Home Initiatives http://www.medicalhomeinfo.org	Resource for clinicians who wish to implement the medical home
Teen Adventure Camp Program http://www.pediatricmscenter.org	Camp program for teens with MS
Wrights Law http://wrightslaw.com	Resource for families and educators regarding education law and advocacy

inner circle over time, as child and family gain resilience and adjust to living with MS.

Educators are in a unique place to help children and should be included early in the disclosure process. This will ensure that the school staff can best understand the ongoing need for accommodations, and planning for the future. It might be beneficial to meet with a selected member of the school staff to start the dialogue. Supporting documentation from the medical team will be useful in explaining the unique needs of a child with MS in the school setting.

Building support

Reaching out to support groups may be helpful for the child and family. Since pediatric MS is rare, the likelihood of knowing another family in a similar situation is low. The parents of a child with MS often describe feelings of isolation and loneliness and want social contact with other families [68–70]. Introducing the parent of a newly diagnosed child to another who has a shared experience, either in person, by phone, or electronically can be beneficial in developing a sense of support and community. The experienced parent can share information and strategies that they have developed to cope with living with pediatric MS. Available resources for the affected children and teens include internet chat rooms, telephone support groups, and camp programs. See Table 14.2 for a brief list. Programs such as camps and retreats can build a sense of community for affected youth. One teen attending a

Table 14.3 Suggested means of empowering patients and their caregivers

Individual/arena associated with child with MS	Area of concerns	Suggestions
Self/patient	- Feels lack of control over their lives - Medication adherence - Desire to "fit in" with peers	- Involve child in the discussion and choice of treatments - Ensure discussions occur at the patient's level of understanding - Promote self-advocacy
Family/parent	- Anxiety due to lack of knowledge about their child's disease	- Empower parents with knowledge - Encourage transitional plan; planning ahead - Encourage involvement with support groups
School	- Poor understanding of pediatric MS and its potential impact on school performance and life	- Educate school staff about symptoms and nature of MS - A letter explaining patient's active symptoms and/or nature of MS may be warranted
Medical team	- Few studies about outcomes in pediatric MS - Multiple facets of illness to address with patients and families	- Involve multidisciplinary team (child neurologist, social worker, nurse, psychologist, occupational therapist, and physical therapist)

camp program said, "At home I am sick, here I am well." Another stated, "I am not alone, I do not have to explain how I feel, the rest of you just know."

Accessing care

Caring for children with MS is a family-centered process. When working with children with a chronic illness, the multidisciplinary team approach is best suited to meet changing needs over time. Team members will vary, but can include parents/guardians, siblings, and perhaps other identified family members such as a grandparent or close family friend. The health care team could include some or all of the following members: child neurologist, adult neurologist or MS specialist, pediatrician or primary care provider, nurse, psychologist, neuropsychologist, occupational therapist, physical therapist, social worker, and school liaison. It is essential that members of this multidisciplinary team communicate with one another and coordinate their care for the patient and family. Developing a strong collaborative relationship with the family, including an understanding of the family's belief system, goals for the future, past experience with the health care system, skills, and resources will allow for the most positive relationship.

Transitioning to adult care

As the teen matures chronologically, cognitively, and emotionally, plans for transitioning care from a child- to an adult-centered model need to be developed. Transition is an ongoing process with the goal to provide high-quality, uninterrupted health care that is patient-centered, and developmentally appropriate. Promoting skills in communication, decision making, and self-advocacy will enhance a sense of control in health care and maximize life-long function and potential as affected children make the transition to adulthood [71].

Improving the well-being of children with multiple sclerosis

Multiple sclerosis affects all aspects of the life of the child or adolescent and his or her family. As such, individuals involved in each aspect of an individual's life can contribute to his or her living well with MS. In Table 14.3, suggestions regarding ways in which health care providers can ensure that individuals involved in a child's life, development, and health care may contribute to his or her well-being are presented.

While medical professionals and school officials can contribute to the success of a child with MS, the

153

parental influence is more pervasive. Studies have shown that in chronic pediatric illnesses, educating and empowering parents and providing resources and support for them increases the likelihood that children will be able to adjust to and cope with their illnesses [46,53]. This can be accomplished by providing easily understood resources and knowledge about their child's illness and accompanying responsibilities, and also encouraging parents to seek support for their own emotional well-being. It is also important to highlight and plan on upcoming transitions, emphasizing on the importance of planning ahead, which will decrease anxiety from uncertainty of what is to come and will become a positive factor in helping parents and their child feel more in control and empowered. To help families adjust and manage the disease, a family systems approach is useful in providing directions for assessment and intervention. While few family interventions, particularly behavioral family interventions, have been rigorously evaluated, multisystemic models show promise for improving children's health outcomes and family adaptation to chronic illnesses.

While the well-being of children and adolescents with chronic disease in general has been studied at length, pediatric MS has only gained attention in recent years. Further studies of the specific impact of MS on children and their families, as well as of approaches to minimize any associated negative consequences, are needed.

References

1. Murray TJ. The psychosocial aspects of multiple sclerosis. *Neurol Clin* 1995;**13**:1997–223.

2. Barlow J, Harrison K, Shaw K. The experience of parenting in the context of juvenile chronic arthritis. *Clin Child Psychol Psychiatry* 1998;**3**:445–463.

3. Barlow JH, Ellard DR. Psycho-educational interventions for children with chronic disease, parents and siblings: An overview of the research evidence base. *Child Care Hlth Dev* 2004;**30**: 637–645.

4. Reiter-Purtill J, Noll RB. Peer relationships of children with chronic illness. In *The Handbook of Pediatric Psychology*, 3rd edn, ed. MC Robert. New York, NY: Guilford Press; 2003:176–197.

5. Repetti RL, McGrath EP, Ishikawa SS. Daily stress and coping in childhood and adolescence. In *Handbook of Pediatric and Adolescent Health Psychology*, ed. AJ Goreczny, M Hersen. Needham Heights, MA: Allyn & Bacon; 1999:343–357.

6. Robert MC. *Handbook of Pediatric Psychology*, 2nd edn. New York, NY: Guilford Press; 1995:127.

7. Kurtzke J. Rating neurologic impairment in multiple sclerosis: An expanded disability status scale (EDSS). *Neurology* 1983;**33**:1444.

8. Hobart J, Freeman J, Thompson A. Kurtzke scales revisited: The application of psychometric methods to clinical intuition. *Brain* 2000;**123**:1027–1040.

9. Nortvedt MW, Riise T, Myhr KM, Nyland HI. Quality of life in multiple sclerosis: Measuring the disease effects more broadly. *Neurology* 1999;**53**: 1098–1103.

10. Amato MP, Ponziani G, Rossi F, Liedl CL, Stefanile C, Rossi L. Quality of life in multiple sclerosis: The impact of depression, fatigue, and disability. *Mult Scler* 2001;**7**:340–344.

11. Miller DM, Kinkel RP. Health-related quality of life assessment in multiple sclerosis. *Rev Neurol Dis* 2008;**5**:56–64.

12. Rudick RA, Miller D, Clough JD, Gragg LA, Farmer RG. Quality of life in multiple sclerosis. Comparison with inflammatory bowel disease and rheumatoid arthritis. *Arch Neurol* 1992;**49**:1237–1242.

13. Mitchell AJ, Benito-Leon J, Morales Gonzalez JM, Rivera-Navarro J. Quality of life and its assessment in multiple sclerosis: Integrating physical and psychological components of wellbeing. *Lancet Neurol* 2005;**4**:556–566.

14. Janssens ACJW, van Doorn PA, de Boer JB, van der Meche FGA, Passchier J, Hintzen RQ. Impact of recently diagnosed multiple sclerosis on quality of life, anxiety, depression, and distress of partners. *Acta Neurol Scand* 2003;**108**:389–395.

15. Canadian Burden of Disease Study Group. Burden of illness of multiple sclerosis part II: Quality of life. *Can J Neurol Sci* 1998;**25**:31–38.

16. Bethoux F, Miller DM, Kinkel RP. Recovery following acute exacerbations of multiple sclerosis: From impairment to quality of life. *Mult Scler* 2001;**7**: 137–142.

17. Rudick RA, Miller D, Hass S, *et al.* Health-related quality of life in mulitple sclerosis: Effects of natalizumab. *Ann Neurol* 2007;**62**:335–346.

18. Zivadinov R, Zorzon M, Tommasi MA, *et al.* A longitudinal study of quality of life and side effects in patients with multiple sclerosis treated with interferon beta-1a. *J Neurol Sci* 2003;**216**:113–118.

19. Cohen JA, Cutter GR, Fischer JS, *et al.* Benefit of interferon beta-1a on MSFC progression in secondary progressive MS. *Neurology* 2002;**59**:679–687.

20. Vermersch P, deSeze J, Delisse B, Lemaire S, Stojkovic T. Quality of life in multiple sclerosis:

Influence of interferon beta-1a (Avonex) treatment. *Mult Scler* 2002;**8**:377–381.

21. Freeman JA, Thompson AJ, Fitzpatrick R, *et al.* Interferon-beta 1b in the treatment of secondary progressive MS: Impact on quality of life. *Neurology* 2001;**57**:1870–1875.

22. Arnoldus JH, Killestein J, Pfennings LE, *et al.* Quality of life during the first six months of interferon-beta treatment in patients with MS. *Mult Scler* 2000;**6**: 338–342.

23. Rice GP, Oger J, Duquette P, *et al.* Treatment with interferon beta-1b improves quality of life in multiple sclerosis. *Can J Neurol Sci* 1999;**26**:276–282.

24. Schwartz CE, Coulthard-Morris L, Cole B, Vollmer T. The quality-of-life effects of interferon beta-1b in multiple sclerosis: An extended Q-TWIST analysis. *Arch Neurol* 1997;**54**:1475–1480.

25. Mowry EM, Beheshtian A, Waubant E, *et al.* Quality of life in multiple sclerosis is associated with lesion burden and brain volume measures. *Neurology* 2009;**72**:1760–1765.

26. Losseff NA, Wang L, Lai HM, *et al.* Progressive cerebral atrophy in multiple sclerosis: A serial MRI study. *Brain* 1996;**119**:2009–2019.

27. Fisher E, Lee JC, Nakamura K, Rudick RA. Gray matter atrophy in multiple sclerosis: A longitudinal study. *Ann Neurol* 2008;**64**:255–265.

28. Fisniku LK, Chard DT, Jackson JS, *et al.* Gray matter atrophy is related to long-term disability in multiple sclerosis. *Ann Neurol* 2008;**64**:247–254.

29. Fisher E, Rudick RA, Cutter G, *et al.* Relationship between brain atrophy and disability: An 8-year follow-up study of multiple sclerosis patients. *Mult Scler* 2000;**6**:373–377.

30. Visschedijk MA, Uitdehaag BM, Klein M, *et al.* Value of health-related quality of life to predict disability course in multiple sclerosis. *Neurology* 2004;**63**: 2046–2050.

31. Nortvedt MW, Riise T, Myhr KM, Nyland HI. Quality of life as predictor for change in disability in MS. *Neurology* 2000;**55**:51–54.

32. MacAllister WS, Belman AL, Milazzo M, *et al.* Cognitive functioning in children and adolescents with multiple sclerosis. *Neurology* 2005;**64**: 1422–1425.

33. Kalb RC, DiLorenzo TA, LaRocca NG, *et al.* The impact of early-onset multiple sclerosis on cognitive and psychosocial indices. *Int J MS Care* 1999;**1**:1–6.

34. Ketelslegers IA, Neuteboom RF, Boon M, Catsman-Berrevoets CE, Hintzen RQ. Fatigue and depression in pediatric multiple sclerosis and monophasic variants. *Mult Scler* 2008;**14**:S143.

35. MacAllister WS, Christodoulou C, Troxell R, *et al.* Fatigue and quality of life in pediatric multiple sclerosis. *Mult Scler* 2009;**15**:1502–1508.

36. Mowry EM, Julian L, Chabas D, *et al.* Health-related quality of life is reduced in children with multiple sclerosis. *Mult Scler* 2008;**14**:S147.

37. Varni JW, Seid M, Kurtin PS. PedsQL 4.0: Reliability and validity of the pediatric quality of life inventory version 4.0 generic core scales in healthy patient populations. *Med Care* 2001;**39**:800–812.

38. Mowry EM, Loguidice MJ, Daniels AB, *et al.* Vision-related quality of life in multiple sclerosis: Correlation with new measures of low- and high-contrast letter acuty. *J Neurol Neurosurg Psych* 2009;**80**:767–772.

39. Anthony KK, Gil KM, Schanberg LE. Brief report: Parental perceptions of child vulnerability in children with chronic illness. *J Pediatr Psychol* 2003;**28**:185–190.

40. Amato MP, Goretti B, Ghezzi A, *et al.* Cognitive and psychosocial features of childhood and juvenile MS. *Neurology* 2008;**70**:1891–1897.

41. National Multiple Sclerosis Society. *Kids Get MS Too: A Guide for Parents Whose Child or Teen has MS.* Denver, CO: National Multiple Sclerosis Society, 2003.

42. Banwell BL. Multiple sclerosis in children. *Mult Scler Q Rep* 2004;**23**:1–13.

43. Madan-Swain A, Katz ER, LaGory J. School and social reintegration after a serious illness or injury. In *The Handbook of Pediatric Psychology in School Settings*, ed. RT Brown. Mahwah, NJ: Lawrence Erlbaum Associates; 2004:637–655.

44. Madan-Swain A, Frederick LD, Wallander JL. Returning to school after a serious illness or injury. In: *Cognitive Aspects of Chronic Illness in Children*, ed. RT Brown. New York, NY: Guilford Press; 1999:312–332.

45. Worchel-Prevatt FF, Heffer RW, Prevatt BC, *et al.* A school reentry program for chronically ill children. *J School Psychol* 1998;**36**:261–279.

46. Garwick A, Millar H. *Promoting Resilience in Youth with Chronic Conditions & Their Families.* Maternal & Child Health Bureau. Health Resources & Services Administration. U.S. Public Health Service. 1995.

47. Garrison WT, McQuiston S. *Chronic Illness during Childhood and Adolescence: Psychological Aspects.* Newbury Park, CA, Sage Publications, 1989.

48. Armstrong GD, Wirt RD, Nesbit ME, *et al.* Multidimensional assessment of psychological problems in children with cancer. *Res Nurs Health* 1982;**15**:205–211.

49. Cadman D, Boyle M, Szatmari P, *et al.* Chronic illness, disability, and mental and social well-being findings of the Ontario Child Health Study. *Pediatrics* 1987;**79**: 805–813.

50. Lavigne J, Faier-Routman J. Psychological adjustment to pediatric physical disorders: A meta-analytic review. *J Pediatr Psychol* 1992;**17**:133–158.

51. Hamlett KW, Pelligrini DS, Katz KS. Childhood chronic illness as a family stressor. *J Pediatr Psychol* 1992;**17**:33–47.

52. Brown RT, Kaslow NJ, Hazzard AP, *et al.* Psychiatric and family functioning in children with leukemia and their parents. *J Am Acad Child Adolesc Psychiatry* 1992;**31**:495–502.

53. Wallender JL, Thompson RJ Jr. Psychological adjustment of children with chronic physical conditions. In: *Handbook of Pediatric Psychology*, 2nd edn, ed. MC Roberts. New York, NY: Guildford Press; 1995:121–141.

54. Wallender J, Varni J, Babani L, *et al.* Children with chronic physical disorders: Maternal reports of their psychological adjustment. *J Pediatr Psychol* 1988;**13**:197–213.

55. Geist R, Grdisa V, Otley A. Psychosocial issues in the child with chronic conditions. *Best Pract Res Gastroenterol* 2003;**17**:141–152.

56. Jellinek MS, Murphy M, Little M, *et al.* Use of the pediatric symptom checklist to screen for psychosocial problems in pediatric primary care. *Arch Pediatr Adolesc Med* 1999;**153**:254–260.

57. Anderson B, Ho J, Brackett J, *et al.* Parent involvement in diabetes management tasks: Relationships to blood glucose monitoring adherence and metabolic control in young adolescents with insulin-dependent diabetes mellitus. *J Pediatr* 1997;**130**:257–265.

58. Sexson SB, Madan-Swain A. School reentry for the child with chronic illness. *J Learn Disabil* 1993;**26**:115–137.

59. Britto MT, Garrett JM, Dugliss MA, *et al.* Risky behavior in teens with cystic fibrosis or sickle cell disease: A multicenter study. *Pediatrics* 1998;**101**:250–256.

60. Cromer BA, Enrile B, McCoy K, *et al.* Knowledge, attitudes and behavior related to sexuality in adolescents with chronic disability. *Dev Med Child Neurol* 1990;**32**:602–610.

61. Stevens SE, Steele CA, Jutai JW, *et al.* Adolescents with physical disabilities: Some psychosocial aspects of health. *J Adolesc Hlth* 1996;**19**:157–164.

62. Starfield B, Shi L. The medical home, access to care, and insurance: A review of evidence. *Pediatrics* 2004;**113**:1493–1498.

63. Gupta VB, Willert J, Pian M, *et al.* When disclosing a serious diagnosis to a minor conflicts with family values. *J Dev Behav Pediatr* 2008;**29**:231–233.

64. Schor EL. Report of the task force on the family. *Pediatrics* 2003;**111**:1541–1571.

65. Lewis CC, Pantell RH, Sharp L. Increasing patient knowledge, satisfaction, and involvement: Randomized trial of a communication intervention. *Pediatrics* 1991;**88**:351–358.

66. McCabe MA. Involving children and adolescents in medical decision-making: Developmental and clinical considerations. *J Pediatr Psychol* 1996;**21**:505–516.

67. Valencia LS, Cromer BA. Sexual activity and other high risk behaviors in adolescents with chronic illness: A review. *J Pediatr Adolesc Gynecol* 2000;**13**:53–64.

68. MacAllister WS, Boyd JR, Holland NJ. The psychosocial consequences of pediatric multiple sclerosis. *Neurology* 2007;**68**:S66–69.

69. Montgomery V, Oliver R, Reisner A, *et al.* The effect of severe traumatic brain injury on the family. *J Trauma Inj Infect Crit Care* 2002;**56**:1121–1124.

70. Walker DK, Epstein SG, Taylor AB, *et al.* Perceived needs of families of children who have chronic health conditions. *Child Health Care* 1989;**18**:196–201.

71. McDonagh JE, Kelly DA. Transitioning care of the pediatric recipient to adult caregivers. *Pediatr Clin N Am* 2003;**50**:1561–1583.

15

Pediatric MS: biological presentation and research update

Tanuja Chitnis and Amit Bar-Or

Multiple sclerosis (MS) is a chronic immune-mediated disease resulting in inflammation, demyelination and neurodegeneration. Pediatric MS is an increasingly recognized disorder, identified in 3–5% of adults with MS [1–4]. Acute demyelinating syndromes including clinical presentations of acute disseminated encephalomyelitis (ADEM) and the clinically isolated syndromes (CIS) of optic neuritis (ON) and transverse myelitis also occur in children at a frequency of approximately 0.7/100 000 [5], and in some cases result in the subsequent diagnosis of MS.

Currently, the understanding of the pathogenic mechanisms that lead to the development and progression of MS in children and adolescents is limited; however, several initiatives are being developed to explore these questions. Addressing these questions is critical for the following reasons.

First, MS in children and adolescents is rare, suggesting that specific factors unique to the pediatric immune and central nervous system (CNS) may either prevent or fail to facilitate this immune-mediated process, or enhance repair. Thus, understanding the mechanisms that cause a sub-group of children to develop MS may identify potentially critical disease mechanisms important for disease initiation and propagation. Identifying these factors is most important in children who have experienced an ADS, and thus are at increased risk for developing MS.

Second, it is unknown whether the pathogenesis of pediatric-onset MS differs from adult-onset MS. Key differences in the pediatric immune system and CNS may result in differential disease course and response to therapy. This is particularly important, as "adult" MS therapies are being applied to children, and understanding the commonalities and differences in

pathobiology would allow for informed treatment and management of this disorder in children.

Third, compared to adult-onset MS, children with MS are relatively environmentally naïve, have had limited time for expansion of their immune cell repertoire, and may have a heightened genetic load leading to susceptibility for recurrent demyelination at such a young age. Hence, studies of the pathogenesis of childhood-onset MS may provide unique insights into the earliest events and triggers of MS in general.

Fourth, a better understanding of the pathobiology of the various forms of pediatric demyelinating disorders including ADEM [6], transverse myelitis and neuromyelitis optica would help to optimize treatment and management.

Lastly, the identification of biomarkers that may be used to predict disease onset, and to monitor disease course, severity and response to treatment in this population would be invaluable in aiding the management of these patients.

Here, we will summarize the current knowledge regarding the pathology, immune mechanisms and disease biomarkers of pediatric MS and acute demyelinating syndromes as well as future directions for research.

Pathology

There are limited data regarding underlying disease mechanisms of pediatric MS, and studies of disease pathology in early onset MS are particularly lacking. In adult-onset MS, the hallmark of MS pathology has historically been the perivascular inflammatory lesion, associated with demyelination and axonal injury [7]. The concept of disease heterogeneity was introduced

Demyelinating Disorders of the Central Nervous System in Childhood, ed. Dorothée Chabas and Emmanuelle L. Waubant.
Published by Cambridge University Press. © Cambridge University Press 2011.

several years ago based on MS autopsy and biopsy studies [8], where four distinct pathological sub-types of perivascular demyelinating lesions were described. Two patterns (I and II) showed close similarities to T-cell/macrophage-mediated or T-cell/macrophage plus antibody-mediated autoimmune encephalomyelitis, respectively. Patterns III and IV demonstrated oligodendrocyte apoptosis or oligodendrocyte death, respectively, in addition to a lesser macrophage and T-cell inflammation. It is presently unknown whether the pathology of pediatric MS exhibits pathologic heterogeneity, or whether it represents a distinct more homogeneous pathologic entity.

Additional features of adult-onset MS pathology include demyelination within the cortex, which can manifest both as typical perivascular demyelinating lesions, as well as in a sub-pial distribution, which is not perivascular in nature and invokes another, as yet unknown, mechanism of injury. These latter lesions involving cortical demyelination appear particularly common in pathology studies of secondary progressive multiple sclerosis (SPMS) and primary progressive multiple sclerosis (PPMS) brains [9]. To what extent they occur in early stages of adult-onset MS, and whether they are relevant to pediatric-onset MS, is unknown.

Another pathologic finding highlighted recently in studies of adult MS pathology relates to collections of immune cells identified within the pia-arachnoid, some of which appear to recapitulate features of lymph node tissue including characteristics of germinal centers (GC). These structures, referred to as "ectopic" or "tertiary" lymphatics, appear to be more common in later stages of the disease and may represent a more general phenomenon of chronic inflammation within the target organ of autoimmune diseases, as has been described for rheumatoid arthritis (RA), type 1 diabetes (T1D) and Sjögren's [10,11]. The relevance of such "tertiary" lymphatic tissue to pediatric-onset MS is unknown. Complicating the study of the evolution of pathological features of sub-pial demyelination and meningeal "follicle-like" structures has been the inability to readily visualize these structures using MRI.

There is ample imaging evidence in adults with MS suggesting the presence of rather diffuse tissue pathology, extending beyond the focal perivascular lesions in the white matter, as demonstrated by studies using diffusion tensor imaging (DTI) [12]. Studies contrasting adult-onset ADEM and MS found higher mean diffusivity in the normal-appearing white matter (NAWM) of MS patients, presumably reflecting widespread tissue destruction seen in MS, which was not present in adult ADEM, suggesting key differences in disease pathogenesis [13].

There are few reports of pathological changes in cases of pediatric MS and ADEM. The majority are in cases of tumefactive demyelination, which may represent a bias in the tendency to biopsy these particular cases [14–18]. Those cases with detailed pathology report a dense accumulation of lymphocytes and macrophages in a prominent perivascular distribution, with rare B cells. Demyelination is present in a predominantly perivascular pattern, while axonal damage is typically absent [14]. No systematic studies have been carried out specifically evaluating the pathology of pediatric MS.

ADEM [6], an acute inflammatory demyelinating syndrome involving encephalopathy and sometimes fever and meningismus, is considerably more common in children than in adults. Most children with ADEM are younger and have a monophasic event, and typically do not require chronic treatment; however, the acute event itself can be fulminant and severe in terms of neurological disability [19]. Distinguishing the pathology and pathophysiology of ADEM from MS is thus important, although this has been complicated by recent observations that a substantial minority (16–20%) of children with confirmed MS, had a presenting episode indistinguishable from ADEM [20]. The pathology of ADEM appears to be somewhat distinct from pediatric MS; however, it is unclear whether this is due to differences in disease pathogenesis, or differences in average age of patients at onset. An unbiased study from the Mayo Clinic examined pathological specimens from children and adults with demyelinating disease [21]. They found that a history of "encephalopathy" was associated with a perivascular type of inflammatory infiltrate with limited demyelination restricted primarily to the margin of the blood vessel. In contrast, specimens from patients with MS demonstrated demyelination, well beyond the perivascular space, involving large areas of white matter. We have observed similar findings in our own review of specimens (Chitnis, unpublished results) (Figures 15.1 and 15.2). Larger, comprehensive studies are required to define the pathological features of sub-types of demyelinating diseases in children.

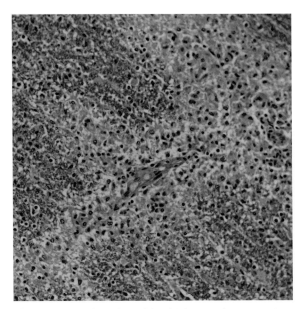

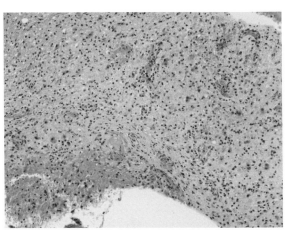

Figure 15.2 Luxol Fast Blue and Cresyl Violet stained biopsy section from the subcortical white matter of a 17-year-old girl with a diagnosis of pediatric multiple sclerosis (10×). Note the diffuse pattern of myelin loss and nodular inflammatory cell infiltration. Acknowledgments: Department of Pathology, Children's Hospital, Boston. (See plate section for color version).

Figure 15.1 Luxol Fast Blue and Cresyl Violet stained autopsy section from the subcortical white matter of a 17-year-old boy with a diagnosis of ADEM (10×). Note the perivascular pattern of myelin loss and inflammatory cell infiltration. Acknowledgments: Department of Pathology, Children's Hospital, Boston. (See plate section for color version).

CSF profiles

Cerebrospinal fluid (CSF) profiles including cellular profiles, oligoclonal bands and IgG Index have been used to characterize MS and differentiate it from other diseases. Oligoclonal bands are typically found in over 85% of established adult MS cases; however, they are a non-specific finding, and may be seen in other infectious or inflammatory conditions. Elevated IgG Index (usually over 0.7) may be observed in up to 80% of established adult MS cases. One of the challenges in studying oligoclonal banding patterns in the CSF of MS patients is the wide variety of techniques used to elucidate this measure, which includes gel electrophoresis, and the preferred technique of isoelectric focusing. Studies using the latter measure have a higher sensitivity than gel electrophoresis. In adults, an elevated IgG index or the presence of CSF-restricted IgG oligoclonal bands (OCB) are biological hallmarks of MS and thus are included in the diagnostic criteria [22,23]. When present at the time of an initial demyelinating event, these biological findings increase the likelihood of a second attack [24].

The CSF profile of patients with established pediatric MS appears to largely be affected by the age of the patient, but may also be affected by disease duration. The percentage of pediatric MS patients with OCB (8–92%), an elevated IgG index (64–75%), or pleocytosis (33–73%) varies widely between studies [25–30]. These inconsistencies between studies may be related to timing of lumbar puncture with respect to disease onset, the various age ranges studied, and different techniques used for CSF analysis. In addition, there are limited longitudinal data regarding the CSF profile in children and adolescents with MS. However, a recent larger study ($n = 107$), inclusive of a significant number of prepubescent children, found that younger children with established MS were more likely to be oligoclonal band negative, and had a higher percentage of neutrophils in their CSF profile compared with adolescents [31]. This study also found that the IgG index was elevated in almost 70% of adolescents with MS (>11 years), but in just over 25% of the younger children (<11 years). Besides age at onset, the authors found an independent and cumulative influence of disease duration on CSF findings. Thus, it is possible that an age-related immaturity of the immune system explains these differences, or that the innate immunity, potentially related to a more recent exposure to an environmental potential triggering factor (e.g. first viral exposure), is activated before the adaptive antigen-specific immunity in MS in general. Finally, this study included longitudinal data suggesting that the initial CSF cellular profile tends to become more typical of adult MS as the

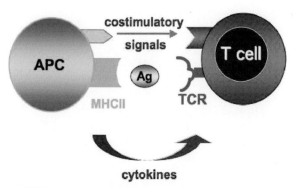

Figure 15.3 T-cell activation by antigen (Ag) and costimulatory molecules. In the peripheral immune system, T cells recognize antigen (Ag) presented to their T-cell receptor (TCR), by MHC class II on antigen-presenting cells (APC). The interaction of costimulatory molecules such as B7 and CD28 on APCs and T cells facilitates T-cell intracellular signaling, leading to cell differentiation and activation. The presence of specific cytokines skews T-cell differentiation into Th1, Th2, or Th17 cells.

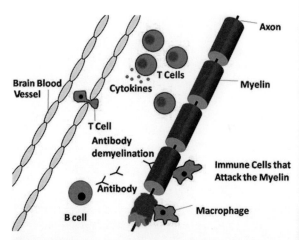

Figure 15.4 Activated T cells orchestrate damaging immune responses within the CNS. T cells migrate through the blood–brain barrier into the CNS and release cytokines inciting the activation of other cells, including B cells and macrophages, which act to damage myelin and axons.

patients age (less neutrophils, more lymphocytes, potential switch from IgG negative to IgG positive profile). This is consistent with previous limited cross-sectional data showing that positive CSF IgG findings in pediatric MS may be more common in patients undergoing lumbar puncture during their second or third attack compared with the first episode [11–13]. Thus, repeating the lumbar puncture in younger patients with atypical presentation may help elucidate the diagnosis.

Another study identified oligoclonal bands in only 8% of children with MS under the age of 10, and interestingly, the number rose to greater than 80% after five or more relapses, suggesting that repeated antigen exposure may enhance immune responses in the CNS. Oligoclonal IgG bands in the CSF have been reported to be positive in 64–92% of pediatric MS patients, and in 0–29% of pediatric ADEM cases followed for a variable number of years [27,32–34]. Within the KIDMUS cohort, 94% of children with positive oligoclonal bands went on to develop MS; however, only 40% of established MS patients in this study had oligoclonal bands, indicating that this test has a low sensitivity but high specificity for the development of MS [35].

Immunobiology of MS

Studies of immune responses in adult-onset MS, as well as lessons from therapeutic trials targeting various aspects of immune response, have lead to a simplified model of MS immune pathophysiology that invokes peripheral activation of immune cells during which the context of activation, including the profile of costimulatory signals and cytokines, influences the response profile of the activated immune cells (Figure 15.3). Subsequently, transmigration of the activated immune cells across the blood–brain barrier (BBB) involves steps of adhesion, chemoattraction, and active infiltration into the CNS; this leads to reactivation of infiltrating cells within the CNS, contributing to perivascular inflammation and injury (Figure 15.4). The immune responses contributing to the sub-pial pattern of demyelination, as well as to the more diffuse injury to the MS brain, are less well understood. Multiple immune cell subsets have been implicated as contributors to the disease process in adults with MS, including pro-inflammatory and anti-inflammatory/regulatory CD4 T cells, CD8 T cells, myeloid cell subsets, as well as subsets of B cells and NK cells [36].

Distinguishing features of the pediatric immune system

MS in children is rare, which may be in part due to key differences in the pediatric compared to adult immune system. Thymic involution which starts in puberty results in a decrease in circulating T cells in adults [37]. The ratio of naïve:memory T cells is highest in childhood and decreases with age [38].

T cell hyporesponsiveness is well described in aging models and in humans [39], and has been ascribed to both a change in effector populations as well as regulatory T cell function. A significant reduction in repertoire diversity of B and T cells is present in the elderly compared to the young [40–43]. An increase in the expression of natural killer cell (NK) receptors and killer cell immunoglobulin-like receptors (KIR) is found on T cells in adults compared to children [41]. A recent publication has studied the features in T- and B-cell populations in healthy children and adults from north and south Brazil [44]. Their findings parallel those observed in prior studies, and further detail the changes, which occur in the pediatric population. CD4+ T cells increase gradually from the neonatal period to age 40 years; following this period, there is a slow decline. CD8+ T cells decrease with advancing age. The proportion of HLA-DR+ CD4+ T cells is highest in the 6–10-year-old group and declines in puberty. NK cells are lowest in the neonatal period and increase steadily with age. Interestingly, in neonates, approximately 5% of peripheral blood mononuclear cells (PBMCs) were CD4+CD25hi, and this proportion significantly decreased in the 6–10 years age group, and re-increased in the pubertal and adult groups. Other studies have shown that CD8+CD28−CD122+ regulatory T cells increase with age; however, function remains the same in young and older adults [45]. Age-related features of the immune system may be relevant to overall protection from MS in children. Perturbations of these systems may result in autoimmune diseases in children. Identification of relevant differences between healthy children and those with MS may identify protective immune pathways.

T-cell responses and studies

Key changes in T-cell functions have been demonstrated in adults with MS, which is reviewed in recent publications [46–49].

It is generally thought that activated T cells with specificities to myelin antigens, including myelin basic protein (MBP), myelin oligodendrocyte glycoprotein (MOG), and proteolipid protein (PLP), are involved in the CNS inflammatory response of MS patients. There is considerable interest in the possibility that evaluation of myelin-directed T-cell responses at the time of pediatric MS will provide insights into the earliest events in the spectrum of human CNS demyelinating conditions. However, the mere

immunological recognition of CNS targets does not invariably lead to injury of CNS tissue, and could reflect the consequences of immune responses to injured tissue, rather than its cause.

A recent study of a large cohort of children with inflammatory demyelination and controls, demonstrated that children with inflammatory CNS demyelination as well as children with autoimmune diabetes (type 1 diabetes, T1D), exhibited heightened peripheral T-cell responses to a wide array of self-antigens [50]. However, it was also noted that children with inflammatory CNS demyelination and children with remote CNS injury exhibited similar abnormalities in their T-cell responses to myelin antigens, as compared to healthy controls [50]. A smaller study evaluating T cell responses to MBP and MOG epitopes in adult and pediatric MS found similar responses predominantly to MBP 83–102, 139–153, 146–162 and MOG 1–26, 38–60, and 63–87 in both groups to the same set of peptides [51]. Interestingly, T-cell responses to fetal MBP were minimal and similar in both children and adults with MS.

Pathologic immune responses thus do not merely reflect the presence of autoreactive immune cells, but rather the defective regulation of their responses. In the normal state, multiple immune regulatory mechanisms contribute to limiting the extent of inflammatory damage to self-tissue. In studies of adult MS, there is considerable evidence that cytokine responses are dysregulated both in the periphery and in the CNS [46,52]. Several studies have demonstrated enhanced production of the hallmark Th1 cytokine, interferon gamma (IFN-γ), from peripheral blood mononuclear cells (PBMCs) restimulated ex vivo in adult MS patients compared to controls [53,54]. Clinical attacks correlated with increased IFN-γ production in vitro [55]. Moreover, studies of Th_{17} cells suggest that these cells may play an important role in sub-types of demyelinating disease. In MS, upregulated IL-17 transcripts have been reported within lesions [56] and in both the CSF and blood of patients [57–59]. Recent immunological data suggest that Th_{17} cells are particularly adept at interacting with, and trafficking across, the human BBB [60,61]. Together, these findings implicate Th_{17} cells as important effectors in adult MS; however, whether this is true early in the ADS/MS spectrum is unknown.

It remains unclear whether overly proinflammatory T-cell responses represent a primary/initiating defect, or one that reflects chronic immune dysregulation later in the disease. The CD4+CD25^{hi} regulatory T cells that constitutively express the IL-2R alpha chain (CD25) and the intra-nuclear forkhead transcription factor *Foxp3* have been termed naturally occurring regulatory T cells (nTreg). Studies have demonstrated that CD4+CD25+Foxp3 regulatory T cells [62], as well as other populations of regulatory T cells including CD8+CD28−T cells [63,64], Tr1 cells [65,66] and TGF-β-producing Th3 cells [67] are dysregulated in adult MS. The presence and role of regulatory T-cell populations has yet to be elucidated in pediatric MS.

B cell and antibody responses

The field has generally considered that involvement of B cells in MS relates to their differentiation into plasma cells and the production of pathogenic CNS-reactive antibodies. There is ample evidence that antibodies are abnormally present in MS, both as elevated CSF immunoglobulin (Ig), as well as deposited within MS lesions in pathology studies [68–72]. Anti-myelin directed antibodies have been found within lesions of both MS and experimental autoimmune (allergic) encephalomyelitis (EAE), and there are suggestions that antibodies play particularly important roles in early/more aggressive forms of MS [73]. The role of circulating anti-myelin (including anti-MOG and anti-MBP) antibodies has been debated extensively in adult MS studies [36,74]. In contrast to studies in adults, where identification of inciting antigens may be obscured by epitope spread, pediatric-onset MS affords the unique opportunity to identify the earliest targets of the CNS-directed immune response. MOG is an attractive target since it is expressed on the outer myelin membrane and may be easily targeted by the immune response. Anti-MOG antibodies were higher in the serum of the younger children with MS and in children with an initial attack that was clinically indistinguishable from ADEM, whether or not they were subsequently found to have MS [72]. While MBP is not expressed on the outer surface of the intact myelin sheath, structural abnormalities in MBP may contribute to early disruption of myelin, resulting in immune targeting of exposed epitopes [75]. We have found that children can develop anti-myelin antibodies as part of their normal humoral immune repertoire (thus their presence is not in and of itself abnormal); however, their presence may modulate the expression of CNS inflammatory disease, as significantly more children with ADS and presence of anti-myelin

antibodies experience ADEM-like presentations (manuscript in preparation). While the role of antibodies in MS continues to be explored, the rapid reduction in new disease activity observed in the studies of B cell depletion in MS [76], without impacting CSF Ig levels or OCB [77], points to an unknown antibody-independent pro-inflammatory role of B cells in MS. Indeed, emerging animal and human studies are pointing to important antibody-independent roles of B cells – both in normal immune regulation, as well as in pathologic conditions [78,79]. For example, B cells of adult MS patients are deficient in their ability to produce the important down-regulatory cytokine IL-10 [78]. Whether such an abnormality is present in pediatric-onset MS remains to be determined.

Environment impacting pediatric MS disease biology

The etiology of MS is felt to reflect a complex interaction of host genetic factors with environmental exposures. Genetic contributions likely differ across ethnicities, and it is likely that the relative risk conveyed by individual host genes is differentially modified by the influence of environmental factors over time (detailed in Chapters 3 and 16).

Epidemiological studies have consistently implicated place of residence during childhood as a key determinant of pediatric MS risk [1,80,81]. Migration studies have consistently found that the risk of MS among migrants was influenced by the age at migration, with the critical period being prior to 15 years of age [82]. Of many environmental factors proposed as contributors to the MS disease process, several have been implicated in recent population-based studies of pediatric MS, and are of particular interest given their plausible impact on MS-relevant biology. These include particular infectious exposures and vitamin D status.

Responses to infectious agents

The inflammatory component of MS has been thought, at least in part, to relate to immune responses to environmental agents such as viruses, mostly encountered during the paediatric-age window of risk [20,83,84]. It appears likely that a viral trigger of the CNS inflammation observed in MS may entail one or more relatively common viruses affecting a predisposed individual.

Several studies examining viral exposures in pediatric MS, have consistently identified significantly increased frequencies of EBV seropositivity in children with MS compared to matched controls [20,83,85,86]. The differential seropositivity in pediatric patients and their controls was more pronounced than between adult MS patients and controls, emphasizing the fact that children are relatively environmentally naïve. From a biological perspective, it is intriguing to speculate how EBV may contribute to the early MS disease process. Possible mechanisms include "molecular mimicry", given the presence of EBV sequences that overlap with the myelin antigen MBP, as well the ability of EBV to transform and chronically activate B cells, which, as noted above, are increasingly implicated in MS pathophysiology. EBV is also known to express an IL-10-like molecule (viral IL-10, vIL-10), raising the possibility that this virus can impact on the ability of the human IL-10 to mediate its important immune regulatory functions. Further studies are required to elucidate the effects of EBV infection in pediatric MS.

Vitamin D

Early studies have suggested that increasing latitude in both the northern and southern hemispheres were associated with increased MS risk. This led to the hypothesis and demonstration of an inverse association between sunlight exposure and MS [87]. Vitamin D is metabolized in the skin by UV irradiation, and Munger et al. found that among Caucasian army recruits, 25-hydroxyvitamin D levels in the highest quintile (above 99.1 nmol/l) were associated with a lower risk of MS (OR = 0.38) [88].

Vitamin D has been shown to have immunomodulatory effects and decreases the incidence and severity of disease in the animal model of MS [89–97]. Calcitriol is the biologically active metabolite of vitamin D and functions via the nuclear vitamin D receptor (VDR). In-vitro and animal studies have demonstrated that calcitriol can down-regulate pro-inflammatory dendritic cells (DC) and reduce Th1 lymphocyte responses, while promoting anti-inflammatory Th2 lymphocyte responses [98–101]. Specific T-cell cytokines that tend to be suppressed by calcitriol include IFNγ, IL-2, and TNF-α, while production of IL-10 tends to be enhanced [102–105]. Calcitriol also suppresses expression of matrix metalloproteinase 9 (MMP-9), a molecule that is over-expressed during MS relapses and increases the permeability of the BBB to auto-reactive immune cells [106,107]. Prophylactic administration of calcitriol or calcitriol analogs can prevent the murine model of CNS demyelination, EAE, and calcitriol has also been shown to attenuate established EAE [89,108,109]. A calcitriol analog demonstrated dramatic synergism with interferon beta (IFNB) and additive effects with cyclosporine in the prevention of EAE [109]. Some of these observations in EAE were mediated via a reduction in monocyte activation [108] and macrophage accumulation within the CNS, and decreased proliferation of pro-inflammatory auto-reactive T lymphocytes in the CNS [95]. Support for a beneficial role of vitamin D in both the underlying immunological pathobiology and possibly to clinical disease manifestations in adults has been demonstrated [110,111].

A role for the VDR gene in increasing the risk of developing adult MS has been reported particularly for the progressive clinical sub-types of MS [112–114]. A significant interaction has recently been reported between winter sun exposure during childhood, a particular variant of the Cdx-2 VDR, and the risk to MS [115]. The "G" allele confers an increased risk of MS in the low sun exposure group ($\leq$2 h/day), supporting the involvement of the VDR gene in determining MS risk, and that such interaction is likely to be dependent on past sun exposure. Finally, a recent study has identified a link between the vitamin D response element (VDRE) region of the human leukocyte antigen [114] region (HLA DRB 1501) that is strongly associated with MS [116].

The need for biomarkers of inflammation and neurodegeneration

Clinically useful biological markers of inflammation are lacking in both adult- and pediatric-onset MS. Of particular utility would be early markers distinguishing between "monophasic" and "recurrent/chronic" disease, as well as markers that prognosticate disease severity and outcome, so as to guide early management decisions. Similarly, there is essentially no current information on serum or CSF biomarkers of neurodegeneration in pediatric MS, and insights from adult MS are also limited. Teunissen et al. found that neurofilament (NF) light chain levels were elevated in CIS and RRMS patients, as well as SPMS, and results correlated with disease state, EDSS scores and MRI results [117]. NF heavy chain was a less sensitive measure in the early stages of disease, but was increased in SPMS patients.

N-acetylaspartate (NAA)

NAA is selectively synthesized in neurons and is considered a marker of the functional integrity of neuronal mitochondrial metabolism. Decreases in NAA levels as measured by MR spectroscopy are seen early in MS lesion formation and correlate positively with axonal volume [118]. CSF NAA levels were decreased in SPMS, but not RRMS, compared with healthy controls [6]. Recent CSF studies examining markers of axonal damage found minimal changes in the majority of children with MS; however, a sub-group with prominent clinical symptoms at the time of CSF examination exhibited elevated levels of tau protein [119]. Further studies of biomarkers of neurodegeneration may help to identify children at high risk for severe or progressive damage, which would allow for early or more aggressive intervention.

Summary

In the past five years, there have been significant advances in the study of the immunopathogenesis of pediatric MS and demyelinating disorders of childhood. However, many unanswered questions remain. Studies characterizing the epidemiological, clinical, and MRI features have laid the groundwork for biological exploration. Clearly more research is needed to identify the underlying disease mechanisms of MS in children, and to explore the links between this and genetic and/or environmental triggers. Potent immunomodulatory and immunosuppressive therapies are being administered to children with MS, and there is therefore an imperative to understand underlying disease mechanisms and to identify disease- and disease state-specific biomarkers. Predictive biomarkers of MS in children suffering from an acute demyelinating syndrome and those with disease onset before the age of puberty will greatly facilitate management. Large national and multinational collaborative efforts are being developed to address these questions, and we expect there to be major advances in this field in the next five years.

References

1. Chitnis T, Glanz B, Jaffin S, Healy B. Demographics of pediatric-onset multiple sclerosis in an MS center population from the Northeastern United States. *Mult Scler* 2009;**15**: 627–631.

2. Boiko A, Vorobeychik G, Paty D, *et al.* Early onset multiple sclerosis: A longitudinal study. *Neurology* 2002;**59**:1006–1010.

3. Ghezzi A, Deplano V, Faroni J, *et al.* Multiple sclerosis in childhood: Clinical features of 149 cases. *Mult Scler* 1997;**3**:43–46.

4. Sindern E, Haas J, Stark E, Wurster U. Early onset MS under the age of 16: Clinical and paraclinical features. *Acta Neurol Scand* 1992;**86**:280–284.

5. Banwell B, Kennedy J, Sadovnick D, *et al.* Incidence of acquired demyelination of the CNS in Canadian children. *Neurology* 2009;**72**:232–239.

6. Teunissen CE, Iacobaeus E, Khademi E, *et al.* Combination of CSF *N*-acetylaspartate and neurofilaments in multiple sclerosis. *Neurology* 2009;**72**:1322–1329.

7. Trapp BD, Peterson J, Ransahoff RM, Rudick R, Mörk S, Bö L. Axonal transection in the lesions of multiple sclerosis. *N Engl J Med* 1998;**338**:278–285.

8. Lucchinetti C, Brück W, Parisi J, Scheithauer B, Rodriguez M, Lassmann H. Heterogeneity of multiple sclerosis lesions: Implications for the pathogenesis of demyelination. *Ann Neurol* 2000;**47**:707–717.

9. Kutzelnigg A, Lucchinetti CF, Stadelmann C, *et al.* Cortical demyelination and diffuse white matter injury in multiple sclerosis. *Brain* 2005;**128**:2705–2712.

10. Itoh T, Shimizu M, Kitami K, *et al.* Primary extranodal marginal zone B-cell lymphoma of the mucosa-associated lymphoid tissue type in the CNS. *Neuropathology* 2001;**21**:174–180.

11. Rangel-Moreno J, Hartson L, Navarro C, Gaxiola M, Selman R, Randall TD. Inducible bronchus-associated lymphoid tissue (iBALT) in patients with pulmonary complications of rheumatoid arthritis. *J Clin Invest* 2006;**116**:3183–3194.

12. Ishizu T, Osoegawa M, Mei F-J, *et al.* Intrathecal activation of the IL-17/IL-8 axis in opticospinal multiple sclerosis. *Brain* 2005;**128**:988–1002.

13. Inglese M, Salvi F, Iannucci G, Mancardi GL, Mascalchi M, Filippi M. Magnetization transfer and diffusion tensor MR imaging of acute disseminated encephalomyelitis. *Am J Neuroradiol* 2002;**23**: 267–272.

14. Anderson RC, Connolly ES Jr, Komotar RJ, *et al.* Clinicopathological review: Tumefactive demyelination in a 12-year-old girl. *Neurosurgery* 2005;**56**:1051–1057.

15. Dastgir J, DiMario FJ Jr. Acute tumefactive demyelinating lesions in a pediatric patient with known diagnosis of multiple sclerosis: Review of the literature and treatment proposal. *J Child Neurol* 2009;**24**:431–437.

16. McAdam LC, Blaser SI, Banwell BL. Pediatric tumefactive demyelination: Case series and review of the literature. *Pediatr Neurol* 2002;**26**:18–25.

17. Riva D, Chiapparini L, Pollo B, Balestrini MR, Massimino M, Milani N. A case of pediatric tumefactive demyelinating lesion misdiagnosed and treated as glioblastoma. *J Child Neurol* 2008;**23**:944–947.

18. Vanlandingham M, Hanigan W, Vedanarayanan V, Fratkin J. An uncommon illness with a rare presentation: Neurosurgical management of ADEM with tumefactive demyelination in children. *Childs Nerv Syst* 2010;**26**:655–661.

19. Tenembaum S, Chitnis T, Ness J, Hahn JS. Acute disseminated encephalomyelitis. *Neurology* 2007; **68**(16 Suppl 2):S23–36.

20. Banwell B, Krupp L, Kennedy J, et al. Clinical features and viral serologies in children with multiple sclerosis: A multinational observational study. *Lancet Neurol* 2007;**6**:773–781.

21. Young NP, Weinshenker BG, Parisi JE, et al. Perivenous demyelination: Association with clinically defined acute disseminated encephalomyelitis and comparison with pathologically confirmed multiple sclerosis. *Brain* 2010;**133**(Pt 2):333–348.

22. Polman CH, Reingold SC, Edan G, et al. Diagnostic criteria for multiple sclerosis: 2005 revisions to the "McDonald Criteria". *Ann Neurol* 2005;**58**:840–846.

23. Freedman MS, Thompson EJ, Deisenhammer F, et al. Recommended standard of cerebrospinal fluid analysis in the diagnosis of multiple sclerosis: A consensus statement. *Arch Neurol* 2005;**62**:865–870.

24. Tintore M, Rovira A, Brieva L, et al. Isolated demyelinating syndromes: Comparison of CSF oligoclonal bands and different MR imaging criteria to predict conversion to CDMS. *Mult Scler* 2001;**7**: 359–363.

25. Ghezzi A, Pozzilli C, Liguori M, et al. Prospective study of multiple sclerosis with early onset. *Mult Scler* 2002; **8**:115–118.

26. Ruggieri M, Polizzi A, Pavone L, Grimaldi LM. Multiple sclerosis in children under 6 years of age. *Neurology* 1999;**53**:478–484.

27. Pohl D, Rostasy K, Reiber H, Hanefeld F. CSF characteristics in early-onset multiple sclerosis. *Neurology* 2004;**63**:1966–1967.

28. Hanefeld F, Bauer HJ, Christen HJ, Kruse B, Bruhn H, Frahm J. Multiple sclerosis in childhood: Report of 15 cases. *Brain Dev* 1991;**13**:410–416.

29. Riikonen R. The role of infection and vaccination in the genesis of optic neuritis and multiple sclerosis in children. *Acta Neurol Scand* 1989;**80**:425–431.

30. Atzori M, Battistella PA, Perini P, et al. Clinical and diagnostic aspects of multiple sclerosis and acute monophasic encephalomyelitis in pediatric patients: A single centre prospective study. *Mult Scler* 2009;**15**:363–370.

31. Chabas D, Ness J, Belman A, et al. Younger children with MS have a distinct CSF inflammatory profile at disease onset. *Neurology* 2010;**74**:399–405.

32. Dale RC, de Sousa C, Chong WK, Cox TCS, Harding B, Neville BGR. Acute disseminated encephalomyelitis, multiphasic disseminated encephalomyelitis and multiple sclerosis in children. *Brain* 2000;**123**:2407–2422.

33. Hynson JL, Kornberg AJ, Coleman LT, Shield L, Harvey AS, Kean MJ. Clinical and neuroradiologic features of acute disseminated encephalomyelitis in children. *Neurology* 2001;**56**:1308–1312.

34. Tenembaum S, Chamoles N, Fejerman N. Acute disseminated encephalomyelitis: A long-term follow-up study of 84 pediatric patients. *Neurology* 2002;**59**:1224–1231.

35. Mikaeloff Y, Suissa S, Vallée L, et al. First episode of acute CNS inflammatory demyelination in childhood: Prognostic factors for multiple sclerosis and disability. *J Pediatr* 2004;**144**:246–252.

36. Bar-Or A. The immunology of multiple sclerosis. *Semin Neurol* 2008;**28**:29–45.

37. Taub DD, Longo DL. Insights into thymic aging and regeneration. *Immunol Rev* 2005;**205**:72–93.

38. Cossarizza A, Ortolani C, Paganelli R, et al. CD45 isoforms expression on CD4+ and CD8+ T cells throughout life, from newborns to centenarians: Implications for T cell memory. *Mech Ageing Dev* 1996;**86**:173–195.

39. Castle SC, Uyemura K, Crawford W, Wong W, Klaustermeyer WB, Makinodan T. Age-related impaired proliferation of peripheral blood mononuclear cells is associated with an increase in both IL-10 and IL-12. *Exp Gerontol* 1999; **34**:243–252.

40. Weksler ME. Changes in the B-cell repertoire with age. *Vaccine* 2000;**18**:1624–1628.

41. Vallejo AN. Age-dependent alterations of the T cell repertoire and functional diversity of T cells of the aged. *Immunol Res* 2006;**36**:221–228.

42. Goronzy JJ, Lee WW, Weyand CM. Aging and T-cell diversity. *Exp Gerontol* 2007;**42**:400–406.

43. Gorczynski RM, Kennedy M, MacRae S. Altered lymphocyte recognition repertoire during ageing. III. Changes in MHC restriction patterns in parental T lymphocytes and diminution in T suppressor function. *Immunology* 1984;**52**:611–620.

44. Faria AM, Monteiro de Moraes S, Ferreira de Freitas LH, *et al.* Variation rhythms of lymphocyte subsets during healthy aging. *Neuroimmunomodulation* 2008;**15**:365–379.

45. Simone R, Zicca A, Saverino D. The frequency of regulatory CD3+CD8+CD28- CD25+ T lymphocytes in human peripheral blood increases with age. *J Leukoc Biol* 2008;**84**:1454–1461.

46. Chitnis T. The role of CD4 T cells in the pathogenesis of multiple sclerosis. *Int Rev Neurobiol* 2007;**79**:43–72.

47. Chitnis T, Imitola J, Khoury SJ. Therapeutic strategies to prevent neurodegeneration and promote regeneration in multiple sclerosis. *Curr Drug Targets Immune Endocr Metabol Disord* 2005;**5**:11–26.

48. Chitnis T, Khoury SJ. Role of costimulatory pathways in the pathogenesis of multiple sclerosis and experimental autoimmune encephalomyelitis. *J Allergy Clin Immunol* 2003;**112**:837–849; quiz 850.

49. Costantino CM, Baecher-Allan C, Hafler DA. Multiple sclerosis and regulatory T cells. *J Clin Immunol* 2008;**28**:697–706.

50. Banwell B, Bar-Or A, Cheung R, *et al.* Abnormal T-cell reactivities in childhood inflammatory demyelinating disease and type 1 diabetes. *Ann Neurol* 2008;**63**: 98–111.

51. Correale J, Tenembaum SN. Myelin basic protein and myelin oligodendrocyte glycoprotein T-cell repertoire in childhood and juvenile multiple sclerosis. *Mult Scler* 2006;**12**:412–420.

52. Chitnis T, Khoury SJ. Cytokine shifts and tolerance in experimental autoimmune encephalomyelitis. *Immunol Res* 2003;**28**:223–239.

53. Balashov KE, Smith DR, Khoury SJ, Hafler DA, Weiner HL. Increased interleukin 12 production in progressive multiple sclerosis: Induction by activated CD4+ T cells via CD40 ligand. *Proc Natl Acad Sci USA* 1997;**94**:599–603.

54. Comabella M, Balashov K, Issazadeh S, Smith D, Weiner HL, Khoury SJ. Elevated interleukin-12 in progressive multiple sclerosis correlates with disease activity and is normalized by pulse cyclophosphamide therapy. *J Clin Invest* 1998;**102**:671–678.

55. Beck J, Rondot P, catinot L, Falcoff E, Kirchner H, Wietzerbin J. Increased production of interferon gamma and tumor necrosis factor precedes clinical manifestation in multiple sclerosis: Do cytokines trigger off exacerbations? *Acta Neurol Scand* 1988;**78**:318–323.

56. Lock C, Hermans G, Pedotti R, *et al.* Gene-microarray analysis of multiple sclerosis lesions yields new targets validated in autoimmune encephalomyelitis. *Nat Med* 2002;**8**:500–508.

57. Matusevicius D, Kivisäkk P, He B, *et al.* Interleukin-17 mRNA expression in blood and CSF mononuclear cells is augmented in multiple sclerosis. *Mult Scler* 1999;**5**:101–104.

58. Graber JJ, Allie SR, Mullen KM, *et al.* Interleukin-17 in transverse myelitis and multiple sclerosis. *J Neuroimmunol* 2008;**196**:124–132.

59. Frisullo G, Nociti V, Iorio R, *et al.* IL17 and IFNgamma production by peripheral blood mononuclear cells from clinically isolated syndrome to secondary progressive multiple sclerosis. *Cytokine* 2008;**44**:22–25.

60. Ifergan I, Kébir H, Bernard M, *et al.* The blood–brain barrier induces differentiation of migrating monocytes into Th17-polarizing dendritic cells. *Brain* 2008;**131**:785–799.

61. Kebir H, Kreymborg K, Ifergan I, *et al.* Human TH17 lymphocytes promote blood–brain barrier disruption and central nervous system inflammation. *Nat Med* 2007;**13**:1173–1175.

62. Viglietta V, Baecher-Allan C, Wiener HL, Hafler DA. Loss of functional suppression by CD4+CD25+ regulatory T cells in patients with multiple sclerosis. *J Exp Med* 2004;**199**:971–979.

63. Crucian B, Dunne P, Friedman H, Ragsdale R, Pross S, Widen R. Alterations in levels of CD28-/CD8+ suppressor cell precursor and CD45RO+/CD4+ memory T lymphocytes in the peripheral blood of multiple sclerosis patients. *Clin Diagn Lab Immunol* 1995;**2**:249–252.

64. Karaszewski JW, Reder AT, Anlar B, Kim WC, Arnason BG. Increased lymphocyte beta-adrenergic receptor density in progressive multiple sclerosis is specific for the CD8+, CD28– suppressor cell. *Ann Neurol* 1991;**30**:42–47.

65. Correale J, Gilmore W, McMillan M, *et al.* Patterns of cytokine secretion by autoreactive proteolipid protein-specific T cell clones during the course of multiple sclerosis. *J Immunol* 1995;**154**:2959–2968.

66. Pelfrey CM, Rudick RA, Cotleur AC, Lee JC, Tary-Lehmann M, Lehmann PV. Quantification of self-recognition in multiple sclerosis by single-cell analysis of cytokine production. *J Immunol* 2000;**165**:1641–1651.

67. Fukaura H, Kent SC, Pietrusewicz MJ, Khoury SJ, Hafler DA. Induction of circulating myelin basic protein and proteolipid protein-specific transforming growth factor-beta1-secreting Th3 T cells by oral administration of myelin in multiple sclerosis patients. *J Clin Invest* 1996;**98**:70–77.

68. Antel JP, Bar-Or A. Do myelin-directed antibodies predict multiple sclerosis? *N Engl J Med* 2003;**349**: 107–109.

69. Frohman EM, Racke MK, Raine CS. Multiple sclerosis – The plaque and its pathogenesis. *N Engl J Med* 2006; **354**:942–955.

70. Owens GP, Bennett JL, Lassmann H, *et al*. Antibodies produced by clonally expanded plasma cells in multiple sclerosis cerebrospinal fluid. *Ann Neurol* 2009;**65**: 639–649.

71. O'Connor KC, Chitnis T, Griffin DE, *et al*. Myelin basic protein-reactive autoantibodies in the serum and cerebrospinal fluid of multiple sclerosis patients are characterized by low-affinity interactions. *J Neuroimmunol* 2003;**136**:140–148.

72. O'Connor KC, McLaughlin KA, De Jager PL, *et al*. Self-antigen tetramers discriminate between myelin autoantibodies to native or denatured protein. *Nat Med* 2007;**13**:211–217.

73. Cross AH, Trotter JL, Lyons J. B cells and antibodies in CNS demyelinating disease. *J Neuroimmunol* 2001; **112**:1–14.

74. Antel J, Bar-Or A. Roles of immunoglobulins and B cells in multiple sclerosis: From pathogenesis to treatment. *J Neuroimmunol* 2006;**180**:3–8.

75. Moscarello MA, Mastronardi FG, Wood DD. The role of citrullinated proteins suggests a novel mechanism in the pathogenesis of multiple sclerosis. *Neurochem Res* 2007;**32**:251–256.

76. Hauser SL, Waubant E, Arnold DL, *et al*. B-cell depletion with rituximab in relapsing–remitting multiple sclerosis. *N Engl J Med* 2008;**358**:676–688.

77. Cross AH, Stark JL, Lauber J, Ramsbottom MJ, Lyons J-A. Rituximab reduces B cells and T cells in cerebrospinal fluid of multiple sclerosis patients. *J Neuroimmunol* 2006;**180**:63–70.

78. Duddy M, Niion M, Adatia F, *et al*. Distinct effector cytokine profiles of memory and naive human B cell subsets and implication in multiple sclerosis. *J Immunol* 2007;**178**:6092–6099.

79. Youinou P, Jamin C, Pers J-O, Berthou C, Saraux A, Renaudineau Y. B lymphocytes are required for development and treatment of autoimmune diseases. *Ann NY Acad Sci* 2005;**1050**:19–33.

80. Kennedy J, O'Connor P, Sadovnick AD, Perara M, Yee I, Banwell B. Age at onset of multiple sclerosis may be influenced by place of residence during childhood rather than ancestry. *Neuroepidemiology* 2006;**26**:162–167.

81. Bar-Or A, Smith D. Epidemiology of multiple sclerosis. In *Principles of Neuroepidemiology*, ed. T Batchelor and M Cudcowicz. St Louis, MO: Butterworh Heinemann, 2001.

82. Gale CR, Martyn CN. Migrant studies in multiple sclerosis. *Prog Neurobiol* 1995;**47**:425–448.

83. Alotaibi S, Kennedy J, Tellier R, Stephens D, Banwell B. Epstein–Barr virus in pediatric multiple sclerosis. *JAMA* 2004;**291**:1875–1879.

84. Ascherio A, Munger K. Epidemiology of multiple sclerosis: From risk factors to prevention. *Semin Neurol* 2008;**28**:17–28.

85. Lunemann JD, Huppke P, Roberts S, Brück W, Gärtner J, Münz C. Broadened and elevated humoral immune response to EBNA1 in pediatric multiple sclerosis. *Neurology* 2008;**71**:1033–1035.

86. Pohl D, Krone B, Rostasy K, *et al*. High seroprevalence of Epstein–Barr virus in children with multiple sclerosis. *Neurology* 2006;**67**:2063–2065.

87. van der Mei IA, Ponsonby A-L, Dwyer T, *et al*. Past exposure to sun, skin phenotype, and risk of multiple sclerosis: Case-control study. *BMJ* 2003;**327**:316.

88. Munger KL, Levin LI, Hollis BW, Howard NS, Ascherio A. Serum 25-hydroxyvitamin D levels and risk of multiple sclerosis. *JAMA* 2006;**296**:2832–2838.

89. Cantorna MT, Hayes CE, DeLuca HF. 1,25-dihydroxyvitamin D3 reversibly blocks the progression of relapsing encephalomyelitis, a model of multiple sclerosis. *Proc Natl Acad Sci USA* 1996;**93**:7861–7864.

90. Garcion E, Sindji L, Nataf S, Brachat P, Darcy F, Montero-Menei CN. Treatment of experimental autoimmune encephalomyelitis in rat by 1,25-dihydroxyvitamin D3 leads to early effects within the central nervous system. *Acta Neuropathol* 2003;**105**:438–448.

91. Mattner F, Smiroldo S, Galbiati F, *et al*. Inhibition of Th1 development and treatment of chronic-relapsing experimental allergic encephalomyelitis by a non-hypercalcemic analogue of 1,25-dihydroxyvitamin D(3). *Eur J Immunol* 2000;**30**:498–508.

92. Meehan TF, DeLuca HF. The vitamin D receptor is necessary for 1alpha,25-dihydroxyvitamin D(3) to suppress experimental autoimmune encephalomyelitis in mice. *Arch Biochem Biophys* 2002;**408**:200–204.

93. Meehan TF, DeLuca HF. CD8(+) T cells are not necessary for 1 alpha,25-dihydroxyvitamin D(3) to suppress experimental autoimmune encephalomyelitis in mice. *Proc Natl Acad Sci USA* 2002;**99**: 5557–5560.

94. Nashold FE, Hoag KA, Goverman J, Hayes CE. Rag-1-dependent cells are necessary for 1,25-dihydroxyvitamin D(3) prevention of experimental autoimmune encephalomyelitis. *J Neuroimmunol* 2001;**119**:16–29.

95. Nashold FE, Miller DJ, Hayes CE. 1,25-dihydroxyvitamin D3 treatment decreases macrophage accumulation in the CNS of mice with

experimental autoimmune encephalomyelitis. *J Neuroimmunol* 2000;**103**:171–179.

96. Nataf S, Garcion E, Darcy F, Chabannes D, Muller JY, Brachet P. 1,25-dihydroxyvitamin D3 exerts regional effects in the central nervous system during experimental allergic encephalomyelitis. *J Neuropathol Exp Neurol* 1996;**55**:904–914.

97. Spach KM, Hayes CE. Vitamin D3 confers protection from autoimmune encephalomyelitis only in female mice. *J Immunol* 2005;**175**:4119–4126.

98. Penna G, Amuchastegui S, Giarratana N, *et al.* 1,25-dihydroxyvitamin D3 selectively modulates tolerogenic properties in myeloid but not plasmacytoid dendritic cells. *J Immunol* 2007;**178**:145–153.

99. Adorini L, Penna G, Giarratana N, *et al.* Dendritic cells as key targets for immunomodulation by vitamin D receptor ligands. *J Steroid Biochem Mol Biol* 2004; **89–90**:437–441.

100. Penna G, Adorini L. 1 Alpha,25-dihydroxyvitamin D3 inhibits differentiation, maturation, activation, and survival of dendritic cells leading to impaired alloreactive T cell activation. *J Immunol* 2000;**164**: 2405–2411.

101. Griffin MD, Lutz W, Phan VA, Bachman LA, McKean DJ, Kumar R. Dendritic cell modulation by 1alpha,25-dihydroxyvitamin D3 and its analogs: A vitamin D receptor-dependent pathway that promotes a persistent state of immaturity in vitro and in vivo. *Proc Natl Acad Sci USA* 2001;**98**:6800–6805.

102. Alroy I, Towers TL, Freedman LP. Transcriptional repression of the interleukin-2 gene by vitamin D3: Direct inhibition of NFATp/AP-1 complex formation by a nuclear hormone receptor. *Mol Cell Biol* 1995;**15**:5789–5799.

103. Muller K, Bendtzen K. 1,25-dihydroxyvitamin D3 as a natural regulator of human immune functions. *J Investig Dermatol Symp Proc* 1996;**1**:68–71.

104. Muthian G, Raikwar HP, Rajasingh J, Bright JJ. 1,25-dihydroxyvitamin-D3 modulates JAK-STAT pathway in IL-12/IFNgamma axis leading to Th1 response in experimental allergic encephalomyelitis. *J Neurosci Res* 2006;**83**:1299–1309.

105. Cohen-Lahav M, Douvdevani A, Chaimovitz C, Shany S. The anti-inflammatory activity of 1,25-dihydroxyvitamin D3 in macrophages. *J Steroid Biochem Mol Biol* 2007;**103**:558–562.

106. Koli K, Keski-Oja J. 1alpha,25-dihydroxyvitamin D3 and its analogues down-regulate cell invasion-associated proteases in cultured malignant cells. *Cell Growth Differ* 2000;**11**:221–229.

107. Rahman A, Hershey S, Ahmed S, Nibbelink K, Simpson RU. Heart extracellular matrix gene expression profile in the vitamin D receptor knockout mice. *J Steroid Biochem Mol Biol* 2007;**103**:416–419.

108. Pedersen LB, Nashold FE, Spach KM, Hayes CE. 1,25-dihydroxyvitamin D3 reverses experimental autoimmune encephalomyelitis by inhibiting chemokine synthesis and monocyte trafficking. *J Neurosci Res* 2007; **85**:2480–2490.

109. Branisteanu DD, Waer M, Sobis H, Marcelis S, Vandeputte M, Bouillon R. Prevention of murine experimental allergic encephalomyelitis: Cooperative effects of cyclosporine and 1 alpha, 2 5-(OH)2D3. *J Neuroimmunol* 1995;**61**:151–160.

110. Goldberg P, Fleming MC, Picard EH. Multiple sclerosis: decreased relapse rate through dietary supplementation with calcium, magnesium, and vitamin D. *Med Hypotheses* 1986;**21**:193–200.

111. Wingerchuk DM, Lesaux J, Rice GP, Kremenchutzky M, Ebers GC. A pilot study of oral calcitriol (1,25-dihydroxyvitamin D3) for relapsing–remitting multiple sclerosis. *J Neurol Neurosurg Psychiatry* 2005;**76**:1294–1296.

112. Niino M, Fukazawa T, Yabe I, Kikuchi S, Sasaki H, Tashiro K. Vitamin D receptor gene polymorphism in multiple sclerosis and the association with HLA class II alleles. *J Neurol Sci* 2000;**177**:65–71.

113. Tajouri L, Ovcaric M, Curtain R, *et al.* Variation in the vitamin D receptor gene is associated with multiple sclerosis in an Australian population. *J Neurogenet* 2005;**19**:25–38.

114. Partridge JM, Weatherby SJ, Woolmore JA, *et al.* Susceptibility and outcome in MS: Associations with polymorphisms in pigmentation-related genes. *Neurology* 2004;**62**:2323–2325.

115. Dickinson JL, Perera DI, van der Mei AF, *et al.* Past environmental sun exposure and risk of multiple sclerosis: A role for the Cdx-2 vitamin D receptor variant in this interaction. *Mult Scler* 2009;**15**:563–570.

116. Ramagopalan SV, Maugeri NJ, Handunnetthi L, *et al.* Expression of the multiple sclerosis-associated MHC class II Allele HLA-DRB1*1501 is regulated by vitamin D. *PLoS Genet* 2009;**5**:e1000369.

117. Teunissen CE, Dijkstra C, Polman C. Biological markers in CSF and blood for axonal degeneration in multiple sclerosis. *Lancet Neurol* 2005;**4**:32–41.

118. Rigotti DJ, Inglese M, Gonen O. Whole-brain N-acetylaspartate as a surrogate marker of neuronal damage in diffuse neurologic disorders. *Am J Neuroradiol* 2007;**28**:1843–1849.

119. Rostasy K, Withut E, Pohl D, *et al.* Tau, phospho-tau, and S-100B in the cerebrospinal fluid of children with multiple sclerosis. *J Child Neurol* 2005;**20**:822–825.

Chapter 16

Genetics of pediatric multiple sclerosis

A. D. Sadovnick and R. Q. Hintzen

The etiology of multiple sclerosis (MS) remains unclear. However, as with almost all common complex traits, genetic and environmental components have important roles, both independently and interactively, in disease susceptibility. Stochastic and epigenetic effects cannot be overlooked [1–3] – see Figure 16.1.

In MS, much of the work on molecular genetics (e.g. linkage studies, candidate genes, genome wide association studies (GWAS)) [4] and genetic epidemiology ("a science which deals with the aetiology, distribution, and control of disease in groups of relatives and with inherited causes of disease in populations" [2,5]) has focused on adults. Nevertheless, it is reasonable to expect, at least to some extent, overlap with the pediatric MS population, as defined in this textbook by Chabas and Waubant. This is not to say that pediatric-onset MS cases have been specifically excluded from molecular genetic studies. Rather, in

most instances, all ascertained patients have been included, but identification has been through adult-orientated neurologists and clinics [6–8]. With the increasing recognition of pediatric MS as a distinct entity [9,10], it is now becoming very clear that genetic/genetic epidemiological data must be compared and contrasted for the following groups.

1. **Group 1: Pediatric MS** – clearly diagnosed <18 years and ascertained through pediatric sources.
2. **Group 2: Pediatric/Adult MS** – onset in retrospect <18 years but diagnosed at a later age and ascertained through adult-oriented resources.
3. **Group 3: Adult MS** – onset at age 18 years and older and ascertained through adult oriented resources.

It is yet to be determined whether the etiology and natural history differ in any way among these three groups. One obvious question to be answered is the severity of the onset symptoms and rate of progression for Group 1 (Pediatric MS) that bring these individuals to attention so early compared to Group 2. It is possible that genetic, environmental, stochastic, and epidemiological factors act (or interact) differently to result in this early disease manifestation. With respect to genes, it remains to be seen whether these act similarly in terms of susceptibility/resistance and disease course for all three groups.

Many of the studies reported here are based on persons with MS who were ascertained in adulthood (Groups 2 and 3). It is very rare that Groups 2 and 3 are separated in report methodologies.

Thus, in this chapter, our objectives are (1) to discuss what is suspected about the genetics/genetic epidemiology of pediatric MS as largely derived from information on adults (as defined in Groups 2 and 3), and (2) to draw attention to needed areas of research on pediatric MS, including etiology, pathogenesis,

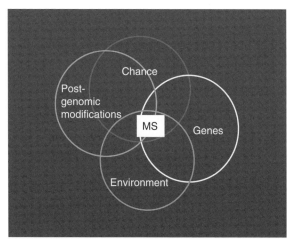

Figure 16.1 The complexity arises from the fact that one cannot accurately predict the expression of the phenotype from knowledge of the individual effects of individual factors considered alone.

Demyelinating Disorders of the Central Nervous System in Childhood, ed. Dorothée Chabas and Emmanuelle L. Waubant. Published by Cambridge University Press. © Cambridge University Press 2011.

natural history, response to therapy (disease-modifying, symptomatic), recovery from relapse, cognition, activities of daily living, etc., as defined in Group 1).

Genes versus family environment

Eichhorst, in 1913 [11], labeled MS as an "inherited, transmissible disease". By 1950, there were 85 reports of families with two or more members having disseminated sclerosis [12]. However, the first direct evidence for a relationship between genes and MS susceptibility came in 1972, when Jersild *et al.* [13] reported an association between human leukocyte antigen (HLA) system alleles and MS. A decade later, Ebers *et al.* provided insight into the familial nature of MS with a report of typing sibling pairs affected with MS for HLA [14]. However, finding a familial aggregation of MS [15,16] did not answer the question of "nature" versus "nurture". It has only been through a series of genetic epidemiological studies on special family pairs including twins [17–19], adoptees [20], half siblings [21,22], and stepsiblings [23] that it was shown that the familial aggregation of MS is due to the sharing of genetic material (DNA) rather than the shared family environment. In general, as the amount of DNA identical by descent ("IBD") rather than identical by state ("IBS") sharing increases, the familial recurrence risk increases for MS – monozygotic (MZ) twins with 100% DNA sharing > dizygotic (DZ) twins and non-twin siblings with 50% DNA sharing > half siblings with 25% DNA sharing > 1st cousins with 12.5% DNA sharing > general population with no or very little DNA IBD sharing.

Nevertheless, ubiquitous, population-based environmental factors are also deemed important in MS susceptibility. Evidence comes from several sources, including the following.

1. Twin concordance: the MZ twin concordance rate does not approach 100% [19].
2. Migration studies: migration (low- to high-risk regions for MS; high- to low-risk regions for MS) can alter the risk to develop MS, even in adulthood [24].
3. Timing of birth: timing (month) of birth studies [25].
4. Gender ratio: temporal changes in the gender ratio as an indicator of increasing MS rates occur too fast to be accredited to genetic mutations [26–28].

Migration data are very interesting with respect to pediatric MS, although these have not specifically

focused on pediatric-onset MS (as defined for Group 1). Initially, it was believed that puberty was the critical stage to change MS risk upon migration [29], but this is no longer the case [24]. Data on MS in first-generation born offspring of immigrants from "low to high MS risk regions" [30] indicate that these offspring had a greater MS risk than their parents for adult onset MS. Parental ethnicity was also recognized as an important risk factor, especially in mixed matings where the risk to develop MS was higher for offspring of "high-risk" mothers (e.g. Caucasian) × "low-risk" (e.g. "Asian") fathers compared to "high-risk" fathers × "low-risk" mothers [31,32] – *vide infra* for parent of origin effect.

Recently, we specifically looked at the issue of migration and ethnicity with respect to parental status ("high-risk" versus "low-risk") and place of birth for a group of adult and pediatric MS patients seen at one adult and one pediatric clinic in Toronto, Ontario, a multicultural region of Canada [33]. Country of birth, residence during childhood, and ancestry were compared for 44 children and 573 adults with MS. Our results demonstrate that although both the pediatric and adult cohorts were essentially born and raised in the same region of Ontario, Canada, children with MS were more likely to report Caribbean, Asian, or Middle Eastern ancestry, and were less likely to have European heritage compared to individuals with adult MS cases. The difference in ancestry between the pediatric and adult MS cohorts can be explained in several ways.

(1) Individuals raised in a region of high MS prevalence, but whose ancestors originate from regions in which MS is rare, have an earlier age of MS onset;
      or
(2) Place of residence during childhood, irrespective of ancestry, determines lifetime MS risk – a fact that will be reflected in a change in the demographics of the adult MS cohort in our region as Canadian-raised children of recent immigrants reach the typical age of adult-onset MS.

Familial risks of MS

MS is not a monogenic disease and thus recurrence risk data for relatives of patients are based on empiric (observed) data rather than strict theoretical models. The data do not fit the polygenic threshold model

Table 16.1 Transmission of MS to offspring by an affected parent

Affected offspring				
	Affected daughters	Affected sons	Total affected	F:M
Mothers with MS	404 (71.13%)	164 (28.87%)	568 (100%)	2.46
Fathers with MS	159 (70.67%)	66 (29.33%)	225 (100%)	2.41
Unaffected offspring				
	Unaffected daughters	Unaffected sons	Total unaffected	F:M
Mothers with MS	2558 (48.69%)	2696 (51.31%)	5254 (100%)	0.95
Fathers with MS	1034 (47.76%)	1131 (52.24%)	2165 (100%)	0.91

(adapted from [36])

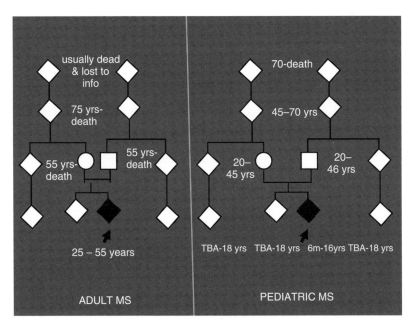

Figure 16.2 Adult and pediatric MS.

(equal and additive genes) [34] or the Carter effect [35,36] which predicts that offspring of the rarer affected sex (males in MS) will have more affected children than the more commonly affected sex (females in MS). In a large Canadian data set, in contrast to an earlier, smaller report by others [37], equal transmission of MS was seen from affected fathers and from affected mothers (9.41% vs. 9.76%), even after stratifying by sex of affected offspring [36] – see Table 16.1. There were no cases of paediatric-onset MS in the offspring listed in Table 16.1.

To calculate familial recurrence risks, age correction is used when a disease has a wide range of onset to account for "remaining risk" for unaffected relatives, incorporating their age at the time the family history was taken and other risk factors such as gender and ethnicity. Historically, this method has been used in MS families [15,16] and validated by longitudinal data [38], but the usual context is with reference to adults with MS.

Recurrence risk data are collected by taking a family history and documenting affected and unaffected statuses among family members of index cases (e.g. see [15,16,19–23]). For adult MS, as illustrated in Figure 16.2, this is relatively straightforward, since the index case and most of his/her "same

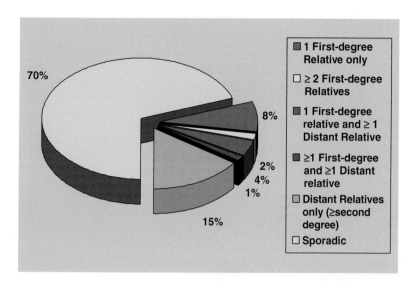

generation" relatives (siblings, first cousins, half siblings) are of a similar age and usually have some remaining risk to develop MS, based on age and gender. Family history information collected on earlier generations (e.g. parents, aunts and uncles; grandparents) tends to not need age-correction, since most of these individuals will have passed the usual upper limit of the age risk for MS. However, as shown in Figure 16.2, this is not the case for pediatric MS. Same-generation relatives of index cases are still very young and some are yet to be born. Parents, aunts, uncles, and grandparents can still be well within the "at-risk" age range to develop MS. Thus, trying to calculate familial rates for a pediatric population is very difficult.

Preliminary data from a longitudinal cohort of pediatric patients with CNS demyelination of various etiologies [10] have, as of January 2008, identified 96 cases of MS, of whom 9 (9.4%) have a family member with MS. Using the same definition across different cohorts, in no case did the additionally affected family member(s) have "pediatric" MS. This is in contrast to the approximately 30% of adult MS patients identified to have a family history through a large, population-based longitudinally followed cohort of Canadian adults with MS [39] which is now in its fifth phase – see Figure 16.3.

The family information on pediatric MS is of interest for several reasons including:

1. there must be a link of risk factors between adult and pediatric MS as these observed nine additional cases in a small pediatric cohort are still more frequent than expected compared to the general population. Given these data, we cannot assume that adult relatives of pediatric cases (e.g. parents) who are still well within the age range to develop MS will not become affected over time; and

2. the absence of familial pediatric-onset MS suggests that genetic changes, if any, which influence this very early onset may be somatic rather than germline, i.e. may have a lower genetic load.

Obviously much more work is needed in this area once large population-based longitudinal cohorts are collected. However, based on data to date, it appears unlikely that pediatric MS will occur more than once in a sibship and perhaps even in a family.

Autoimmune diseases in families

MS in Northern Europeans has been associated with extended major histocompatibility complex (MHC) haplotypes, especially those containing *HLA-DRB1*1501* [40,41]. This association, taken together with indirect evidence from animal models [42], the female preponderance in MS [26], reports that the MS relapse rate decreases during gestation [43], and the presence of T and B cells reactive to myelin basic protein (MBP) antigens [44] is interpreted by some to suggest an autoimmune etiology for MS, although complexities identified within the HLA belie such a simple mechanism for MS susceptibility [45–48]. Nevertheless, despite clinical and serological features unique to a specific autoimmune disease, it has been suggested that different autoimmune disorders, including MS, share susceptibility genes [49,50]. Taken further, it has been reported that biological relatives of MS patients have a greater risk of auto-immune disease compared to the general population (e.g. [51–53]).

Recent work on the longitudinal, population-based Canadian study [54] found that after correcting for age and sex (key confounders in collecting this type of data), MS patients had no increased risk over spousal controls for autoimmune disease (OR = 1.07, 95% CI 0.86–1.23, $\chi^2 = 0.47$, $p = $ ns) nor did their first-degree relatives (OR = 0.89, 95% CI 0.63–1.17, $\chi^2 = 1.11$, $p = $ ns). A modest, selective increase in thyroid disease and pernicious anemia in MS patients could be taken to cohere to MHC co-associations. However, similar risks among controls, MS patients and first-degree relatives of MS patients for rheuma-toid arthritis, type 1 diabetes, ulcerative colitis, and Crohn's disease refute suggestions of autoimmune genetic loading. In fact, differences in reported auto-immune disease frequency based on the gender of the MS interviewee were much larger than differences between cases and controls. Multiplex families (with two or more cases of MS) were not more likely to report autoimmune diseases than simplex families (with one case of MS). Thus, this study did not sup-port a general propensity to autoimmune disease in MS families and clearly highlighted the importance of controlling for gender in such studies.

Very preliminary data on autoimmune disease in family members of 76 children presenting with their first demyelinating episode of various etiologies, including NMO, recurrent optic neuritis (ON), ADEM, acute complete transverse myelitis, and MS [10] found that an autoimmune disease was reported in 33 families (43%). At this time, no controls have been assessed and no correction for gender bias has been made. However, in this small sample, a positive family history of auto-immune disease was more likely if the presenting child was male, very young (e.g. under age 12) and of Euro-pean ancestry.

Molecular genetic studies in pediatric MS (Group 1)

Studies on the molecular genetic contribution to pediatric-onset MS are scarce. Therefore, we can only briefly touch upon them here. The focus of this section again must largely be on what has been learned from adults with MS (i.e. Groups 2 and 3 as earlier described).

A Russian study showed that HLA-DR15 was overrepresented in children with MS when compared with the general population [55], as was the TNFα 7 allele [56]. By contrast, a study of 24 children with MS in Turkey did not detect MS-specific TNFα mutations [57]. Genetic studies on the gene encoding myelin oligodendrocyte glycoprotein (MOG), located in close proximity to the HLA region, did not show any disease-specific associations in a study of 75 German children with MS [58], although the sample size was very small.

The major histocompatibility complex
MHC class II

As stated earlier in this chapter, the association between MS and MHC on chromosome 6 has long been recognized [13,14,59–61]. The strongest signal in this area comes from the MHC class II region. The originally serologically defined markers of this region have been refined as the DR15 sub-type of DR2 and DQ6. The corresponding genotypes are *DRB1*1501*, *DRB5*0101*, *DQA1*0102*, and *DQB2*0602*. The asso-ciation is strongest in northern Europeans but is seen in virtually all populations, with a notable exception being some Mediterranean populations, where MS is associated with DR4.

The main locus *HLA DRB1*15* is clearly not acting on its own. It is now well recognized that complex gene–gene interactions exist in this highly poly-morphic area, a phenomenon that is called "epistasis" [62,63]. Synergistic interactions can be observed. The relative risk of getting MS for an individual who carries the *HLA-DRB1*15* allele is about 3 [63]. This risk is more than doubled when the same individual also carries the *HLA-DRB1*08* allele. This strong increase is only observed in conjunction with *HLA-DRB1*15*, as on its own, *HLA-DRB1*08* has only a modest effect – see Figure 16.4.

Conversely, protective interactions take place. The *HLA DRB1*14* carries such a protective effect that it

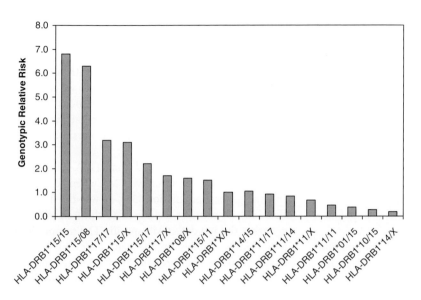

Figure 16.4 Epistasis in the HLA class II region in MS. Used with permission from Ramagopalan and Ebers [3].

completely abrogates the increased risk of *HLA-DRB1*15* (see Figure 16.4). Epistatic interactions also appear to play a role in disease course. For example, *HLA-DRB1*15* and *HLA-DRB1*01* separately do not influence the clinical phenotype, but when present they produce a milder disease course [64].

Epigenetic interactions within the HLA locus

Recent evidence suggests that the HLA locus is an important site where epigenetic interactions take place. Using the large Canadian database, it has been possible to study affected aunt/uncle/niece/nephew (AUNN) pairs. It was found somewhat unexpectedly that in these pairs, the allele frequencies for *HLA-DRB1*1501* were different between the first and second generations affected [65]. Affected aunts had significantly lower *HLA-DRB1*15* frequency compared with their affected nieces. However, *HLA-DRB1*15* frequency in affected males remained the same over the two generations.

The risk carried by *HLA-DRB1*15* was increased in families with affected second-degree relatives (AUNN: OR 4) when compared with those comprising only first-degree relatives (ASP: OR 2). This demonstrates heterogeneity of risk among *HLA-DRB1*15* haplotypes based on whether collateral parental relatives are affected. This study implicates gene–environment interactions in susceptibility [65]. It appears that that epigenetic modifications differentiate among HLA class II risk haplotypes and play a role in the gender bias in MS.

The HLA class II MS risk area has been demonstrated to be under control of vitamin D responsive elements. Ramagopalan and colleagues sought responsive regulatory elements in the MHC class II region [66]. Sequence analysis localized a single MHC vitamin D response element (VDRE) to the promoter region of *HLA-DRB1*. Sequencing of this promoter in greater than 1000 chromosomes from *HLA-DRB1* homozygotes showed absolute conservation of this putative VDRE on *HLA-DRB1*15*.

Using a luciferase reporter assay, a functional role for this VDRE was demonstrated [66]. B cells transiently transfected with the *HLA-DRB1*15* gene promoter showed increased expression on stimulation with 1,25-dihydroxyvitamin D3 ($p = 0.002$) that was lost either on deletion of the VDRE or with the homologous "VDRE" sequence found in non-MS-associated *HLA-DRB1* haplotypes [66]. Flow cytometric analysis showed a specific increase in the cell surface expression of *HLA-DRB1* upon addition of vitamin D only in *HLA-DRB1*15*-bearing lymphoblastoid cells.

Finally, class II interactions may exist with EBV induced infectious mononucleosis (IM). In a Danish study, IM-naïve individuals, *DRB1*15* carried a 2.4-fold (95% CI 2.0–3.0) increased MS risk [67]. In contrast, among persons with IM history, *DRB1*15* was associated with a 7.0-fold (95% CI 3.3–15.4) increased MS risk. Thus, the MS risk conferred by *HLA-DRB1*15* was 2.9 (95% CI 1.3–6.5) fold stronger in the presence than in the absence of a history with IM.

MHC class I

There is also evidence for a (weaker) role of MHC class I. Whether this is independent of the class II effect remains controversial [68–70]. In this respect, it is of interest to note that recently identified polymorphisms in the class I area are associated with IM [71]. These single nucleotide polymorphisms (SNPs), rs2530388 and rs6457110, are in significant linkage disequilibrium with the HLA-A locus. Carriers of the allele A of SNP rs253088 and allele T of rs6457110 have an enhanced risk to get this EBV-mediated infectious disease. It remains to be shown whether this region is also active in the risk of getting MS.

Immune genes

It has been estimated that the HLA locus accounts for 20–60% of the genetic susceptibility in MS. This implicates that a large portion of the genetic component of MS remains to be explained. This has prompted researchers to start genome-wide analyses approaches to identify additional risk genes (see Table 16.2). The International MS Genetics Consortium (IMSGC) performed a study using 500 000 SNP arrays. Association with MS was found with 17 SNPs located in 14 regions [72]. Only two regions, *HLA-DR* and *IL2RA*, initially achieved genome-wide significance ($p < 5 \times 10^{-8}$). For a third gene, *IL7R*, convincing functional support was obtained [72], and genome-wide significance was established in a joint analysis on 15 000 patients [73]. Follow-up studies have now provided support for 6 out of the original 17 SNPs [74–77]. The overall ORs of these non-HLA SNPs were modest, all below 1.30.

In summary, GWAS have reported significant findings for SNPs in the following non-HLA immune genes: *IL2RA*, *IL7R*, *CLEC16A*, *CD226*, *CD58* and the area around *EVI5*. It should be stressed that the associations are at the SNP level. Sometimes they are situated in intronic areas. Whether these SNPs are causative remains to be determined in most cases.

Although the identification of these risk genes certainly helps to understand the biological pathways involved in MS, their individual contribution is at present of no clinical value. For example, the frequency of the risk allele in the *IL7R* gene lies around 70% in the normal population. Individuals who carry this gene increase their risks for MS by a factor of 1.2. The allele is estimated to increase the risk of the disease by a factor of just 1.2. Practically, this means

Table 16.2 Validated non-HLA MS risk SNPs

Gene	Function	Chromosome	OR
IL2RA	Cytokine receptor	10p15	1.25
IL7RA	Cytokine receptor	5p13	1.20
CLEC16A	C-type lectin	16p13	1.2
CD226	Cytokine receptor	18q22	1.13
CD58	Adhesion	1p13	1.24
EVI5	Unknown	1p22	1.14
KIF1B	Axonal transport	1p36	1.34

Note:
GWA significance reached in at least one study or independently replicated in at least 1 additional study.

that the overall population risk for MS of 1 per 1000 changes to approximately 1 per 833. In other words, the chance not to develop MS in the presence of the risk allele *IL7R* gene is still 832 per 833 individuals.

It is worthwhile to spend a few words on the possible biological links between the MS risk genes and pathogenesis.

IL7R encodes for the receptor for interleukin-7, which is expressed on T- and B-lymphocytes. The signal transduced by this receptor is crucial for lymphocyte survival and immune homeostasis. There are indications that the exonic *IL7R* SNP associated with MS leads to less membrane expressed but more soluble receptor protein, therefore influencing receptor signaling [78].

IL2RA encodes for the alpha chain of the interleukin-2 receptor (IL2R). The involvement of the *IL2R* chain in the pathogenesis of MS might also be related to the important role that the IL2–IL2R pathway plays in adaptive immune regulation. It is of note that the IL2R-mediated susceptibility effect is shared with type 1 diabetes (T1D), Graves' disease, and rheumatoid arthritis [79].

A SNP in the *CLEC16A* gene (intron 21) was found to be significantly associated with MS when combining an Australian study and the IMSGC screen ($p = 3 \times 10^{-8}$) for a GWAS [77]. A study in Sardinia [76], again exploring the contribution of GWA significant T1D genes to MS risk, found significance also for another SNP in intron 19. A third autoimmune disorder that has been associated with *CLEC16A* is autoimmune Addison's disease [79]. To date, these data indicate that in this single gene, different SNPs are involved in different autoimmune disorders.

It remains to be determined to what extent the different genetic variants within the *CLEC16A* area contribute to susceptibility for certain autoimmune disorders. *CLEC16A* is a sugar-binding C-type lectin receptor, a family of receptors that provide signals for a decision between tolerance and immunity. They can bind bacterial products as well as endogenous ligands and their signal can counteract the signal of Toll-like receptors, therewith influencing T-helper cell function. It has been suggested that there may be a role for C-type lectin receptors in MS pathogenesis as well as a link with infections [80].

The lead for testing CD226 does in fact not come from GWA screens in MS but from genetic studies in T1D [81,82]. In T1D, a SNP in this gene enhances the risk for the disease with an OR of 1.3. CD226 (also known as DNAX accessory molecule 1, DNAM-1) is a membrane protein involved in the adhesion and co-stimulation of T cells. Furthermore, in an experimental model of MS, experimental autoimmune encephalomyelitis, anti-CD226 monoclonal antibody treatment delayed the onset and reduced the severity of experimental autoimmune encephalomyelitis [83]. It has been suggested that the genetic variant could alter the expression or signaling of CD226, as it occurs in the molecule's cytoplasmic tail.

The SNP associated with CD58 lies in intron 1 of the gene. CD58 is the ligand for the T cell-specific CD2 membrane molecule, an adhesion molecule that transduces important signals for T cell proliferation and differentiation [84]. A role for the CD58 molecules has been suggested in chronic inflammatory polyneuropathies [85].

Ecotropic viral integration site 5 (*EVI-5*) has been given this name because it can serve as an integration site for retroviral elements in mice. This ubiquitous gene further plays a role in the end phase of mitosis, and has been linked to lymphomagenesis [86]. Although the area around *EVI-5* has been found associated with MS in several studies, the signal in this area seems broad and there is room for the possibility that other genes may be involved.

Most recently, strong evidence has been presented for the association of the following genes with MS: *STAT3* [87], *CD6, IRF8, TNFRSF1A* [88], *TYK2* [89], plus new loci at chromosomes 12 and 20 [90].

The first neuronal risk genes

Another recent GWAS was performed in a genetic isolate in the Netherlands [91]. While only 45 MS cases and 195 controls were included, it was believed that the relative genetic homogeneity of this small population would nevertheless be advantageous. Affymetrix 500K SNP arrays were used and a new MS risk SNP was identified, rs10492972, located in the *KIF1B* gene. Replication studies in three populations from The Netherlands, Canada, and Sweden including a total of 2679 cases and 3125 controls showed similar frequencies of the risk allele, around 0.34, and yielded an overall OR for MS of 1.34 [92]. This is the highest OR observed to date for a non-HLA risk allele. *KIF1B* encodes a kinesin superfamily member believed to be responsible for axonal transport of mitochondria and synaptic vesicle precursors. It has an ATPase binding domain and is enriched in motor neurons. Recently, dysregulation of ATPases and mitochondrial mislocalization have been shown to have a role in several neurodegenerative diseases. *KIF1B* knockout mice have been reported to have CNS abnormalities such as atrophy [93]. Although the SNP lies in intron 5 of the gene and may not be the true causative variant, this finding draws attention to a neuronal pathway. It should be acknowledged that a large consortium could not replicate the association of *KIF1B* with MS (S. Sawcer *et al.* personal communication). However, this same consortium did report evidence of the association of another kinesin, *KIF21B* [94].

Single gene disorders that mimick MS

There are several monogenetic disorders which may give a MS-like phenotype [95]. Of interest, these can have onset either during childhood or adulthood, despite having the same pathogenic causal gene (see Table 16.2). This can be interpreted as evidence that the same situation may exist in complex diseases. Thus, in MS, it is possible that the same biological mechanisms may lead to disease manifestation in either childhood or adulthood. The genes that cause the monogenetic MS-mimicking diseases do not play a role in MS itself.

Mitochondrial monogenetic diseases take a special position here as several can be associated with often subclinical white matter abnormalities [96]. Although mitochondrial genes do not contribute generally to MS susceptibility, mutations of mitochondrial DNA are responsible for a rare illness similar to MS that is characterized by predominant involvement of the anterior visual pathway, called Harding's disease [97]. It is of note that neuropathological studies of MS tissue

Table 16.3 Monogenetic diseases that may mimick multiple sclerosis

Disease	Gene	Inheritance
Leukodystrophies		
MLD	Arylsulphatase	Recessive
X-ALD		Recessive
Fabry	Alpha-galactosidase	Recessive
Mitochondrial diseases		
LHON	Mt DNA	Maternal
MELAS	Mt DNA	Maternal
MERFF	Mt DNA	Maternal
Macrophage activation syndrome		
Hemophagocytic lymphohistiocytosis	HPLH1, PRF1, UNC13D, STX11	Autosomal recessive
Chediak–Higashi	LYST	Autosomal recessive
Griscelli	Rab27	Autosomal recessive
X-linked proliferative syndrome	SAP	X-linked

indicate a role for mitochondrial dysfunction [98,99]. This has prompted research into a role for mitochondrial DNA in MS, although no clear gene variant has been identified [100,101]. However, recent findings suggest that super-haplogroup U may be a risk factor in MS. A trend was found towards an association with the *NDUFS2* gene in the Complex I pathway, providing further support that this may be disrupted in MS.

Summary

Much is still needed to be known about the molecular genetics and genetic epidemiology of MS. Large scale collaborative studies are needed. It is of particular interest that, to date, no recurrence of pediatric MS, as earlier defined as Group 1, has been reported, although adult MS does exist in relatives of pediatric cases. It is currently impossible to state with certainty whether there is a recurrence risk for pediatric MS in families. One key to looking at this topic is to remember the three groups previously defined and to determine similarities and differences with respect to genetics and genetic epidemiology. Group 2 may in fact be the most informative if long-term follow-up is not available for Group 1.

References

1. Ebers GC. Enviromental factors and multiple sclerosis. *Lancet Neurol* 2008;**7**:268–277.

2. Ramagopalan RV, Dyment DA, Ebers GC. Genetic epidemiology: The use of old and new tools for multiple sclerosis. *Trends Neurosci* 2008;**31**:645–652.

3. Ramagopalan RV, Ebers GC. Epistasis: Multiple sclerosis and the major histocompatibility complex. *Neurology* 2009;**72**:566–567.

4. Mullen SA, Crompton DE, Carney PW, Helbig I, Berkovic SF. A neurologist's guide to genome-wide association studies. *Neurology* 2009;**72**:558–565.

5. Morton N. *Outline of Genetic Epidemiology*. Basel: E. Karger; 1982.

6. Duquette P, Murray TJ, Pleines J, *et al*. Multiple sclerosis in childhood: Clinical profile in 125 patients. *J Pediatr* 1987;**111**:359–363.

7. Boiko A, Vorobeychik G, Paty D, Sadovnick D, and the UBC MS Clinic Neurologists. Early onset multiple sclerosis: a longitudinal study. *Neurology* 2002;**59**:1006–1010.

8. Renoux C, Vukusic S, Mikaeloff Y, *et al*. Natural history of multiple sclerosis with childhood onset. *N Engl J Med* 2007;**356**:2603–2613.

9. Ness JN, Chabas D, Sadovnick AD, Pohl D, Banwell B, Weinstock-Guttman B. Clinical features of children and adolescents with multiple sclerosis. *Neurology* 2007;**68**(Suppl 2):S37–S45.

10. Banwell B, Kennedy J, Sadovnick AD, *et al*. The incidence of acquired demyelination of the central nervous system in Canadian children. *Neurology* 2009;**72**:232–239.

11. Eichhorst H. Multiple Sklerose und spastiche spinalparalyse. *Med Klin* 1913;**9**:1617–1619.

12. Pratt RTC, Compston ND, McAlpine D. The familial incidence of disseminated sclerosis and its significance. *Brain* 1951;**74**:191–232.

13. Jersild C, Svejgaard A, Fog T. HL-A antigens and multiple sclerosis. *Lancet* 1972;**1**:1240–1241.

14. Ebers GC, Paty DW, Stiller CR, Nelson RF, Seland TP, Larsen B. HLA-typing in multiple sclerosis sibling pairs. *Lancet* 1982;**2**:88–90.

15. Sadovnick AD, MacLeod PM. The familial nature of multiple sclerosis: Empiric recurrence risks for first, second, and third degree relatives of patients. *Neurology* 1981;**31**:1039–1041.

16. Sadovnick AD, Baird PA, Ward RH. Multiple sclerosis: Updated risks for relatives. *Am J Med Genet* 1988;**29**:533–541.

17. Ebers GC, Bulman DE, Sadovnick AD, *et al.* A population based study of multiple sclerosis in twins. *New Engl J Med* 1986;**315**:1638–1642.

18. Sadovnick AD, Armstrong H, Rice GP, *et al.* A population-based study of multiple sclerosis in twins: Update. *Ann Neurol* 1993;**33**:281–285.

19. Willer CJ, Dyment DA, Risch NJ, Sadovnick AD, Ebers GC. Twin concordance and sibling recurrence rates in multiple sclerosis. *Proc Natl Acad Sci* 2003;**100**:12877–12882.

20. Ebers GC, Sadovnick AD, Risch NJ, and the Canadian Collaborative Study Group. A genetic basis for familial aggregation in multiple sclerosis. *Nature* 1995;**377**:150–151.

21. Sadovnick AD, Ebers GC, Dyment D, Risch NJ, and the Canadian Collaborative Study Group. Evidence for genetic basis of multiple sclerosis. *Lancet* 1996;**347**:728–730.

22. Ebers GC, Sadovnick AD, Dyment DA, Yee IML, Willer CJ, Risch N. Parent of origin effect in multiple sclerosis: Observations in half siblings. *Lancet* 2004;**363**:1773–1774.

23. Dyment DA, Yee IM, Ebers GC, Sadovnick AD, for the Canadian Collaborative Study Group. Multiple sclerosis in stepsiblings: Recurrence risk and ascertainment. *J Neurol Neurosurg Psychiatry* 2006;**77**:258–259.

24. Hammond SR, English DR, McLeod JG. The age-range of risk of developing multiple sclerosis: Evidence from a migrant population in Australia. *Brain* 2000;**123**:968–974.

25. Willer CJ, Dyment DA, Sadovnick AD, Rothwell PM, Murray TJ, Ebers GC. Timing of birth and risk of multiple sclerosis: A population based study. *Br Med J* 2005;**330**:120–124.

26. Orton SM, Herrrera BM, Yee IM, *et al.* Sex ratio of multiple sclerosis in Canada: A longitudinal study. *Lancet Neurol* 2006;**5**:932–936.

27. Alonso A, Hernan MA. Temporal trends in the incidence of multiple sclerosis: A systematic review. *Neurology* 2008;**71**:129–135.

28. Grytten N, Glad SB, Aarseth JH, Nyland H, Midgard R, Myhr KM. A 50-year follow-up of the incidence of multiple sclerosis in Hordaland County, Norway. *Neurology* 2006;**66**:182–186.

29. Dean G, Kurtzke JF. On the risk of multiple sclerosis according to age at immigration to South Africa. *Br Med J* 1971;**3**:725–729.

30. Elian M, Nightingale S, Dean G. Multiple sclerosis among United Kingdom-born children of immigrants from the Indian subcontinent, Africa and the West Indies. *J Neurol Neurosurg Psychiatry* 1990;**53**:906–911.

31. Kurtzke JF, Bui Q-H. Multiple sclerosis in a migrant population: 2. Half-orientals immigrating in childhood. *Ann Neurol* 1980;**8**:256–260.

32. Ramagopalan SV, Yee IM, Dyment DA, *et al.* Parent-of-origin effects in multiple sclerosis: Observations from interracial matings. *Neurology* 2009;**73**:602–605.

33. Kennedy J, O'Connor P, Sadovnick AD, Perara M, Yee I, Banwell B. Age at onset of multiple sclerosis may be influenced by place of residence during childhood rather than ancestry. *Neuroepidemiology* 2006;**26**: 162–167.

34. Sadovnick AD, Spence MA, Tideman S. A goodness-of-fit test for the polygenic threshold model: Application to multiple sclerosis. *Am J Med Genet* 1981;**8**:355–361.

35. Carter CO. The inheritance of congenital pyloric stenosis. *Br Med Bull* 1961;**15**:251–254.

36. Herrera M, Ramagopalan SV, Orton S, *et al.* Parental transmission of MS in a population-based Canadian cohort. *Neurology* 2007;**69**:1208–1212.

37. Kantarci OH, Barcellos LF, Atkinson EJ, *et al.* Men transmit MS more often to their children vs. women: The Carter effect. *Neurology* 2006;**67**:305–310.

38. Ebers GC, Koopman WJ, Hader W, *et al.* The natural history of multiple sclerosis: A geographically based study. 8. Familial multiple sclerosis. *Brain* 2000;**123**:641–649.

39. Sadovnick AD, Risch NJ, Ebers GC, and the Canadian Collaborative Study Group. Canadian Collaborative Project on Genetic Susceptibility to MS, phase 2: Rationale and method. *Can J Neurol Sci* 1998;**25**: 216–221.

40. Fogdell A, Hillert J, Sachs C, Olerup O. The multiple sclerosis- and narcolepsy-associated HLA class II haplotype includes the DRB5*0101 allele. *Tissue Antigens* 1995;**46**:333–336.

41. Dyment DA, Ebers GC, Sadovnick AD. Genetics of multiple sclerosis. *Lancet Neurol* 2004;**3**:104–110.

42. Lassmann H. Neuropathology in multiple sclerosis: New concepts. *Mult Scler* 1998;**4**:93–98.

43. Vukusic S, Hutchinson M, Hours M, *et al.* Pregnancy and multiple sclerosis (the PRIMS study): Clinical predictors of post-partum relapse. *Brain* 2004;**127**:1353–1360.

44. Olsson T, Zhi WW, Höjeberg B, *et al.* Autoreactive T lymphocytes in multiple sclerosis determined by antigen-induced secretion of interferon-gamma. *J Clin Invest* 1990;**86**:981–985.

45. Dyment DA, Herrera BM, Cader MZ, *et al.* Complex interactions among MHC haplotypes in multiple sclerosis: Susceptibility and resistance. *Hum Mol Genet* 2005;**14**:2019–2026.

46. Chao MJ, Barnardo MC, Lincoln MR, *et al.* HLA class I alleles tag HLA-DRB1*1501 haplotypes for differential risk in multiple sclerosis susceptibility. *Proc Natl Acad Sci* 2008;**105**:13069–13074.

47. Chao MJ, Ramagopalan SV, Herrera BM, *et al.* Epigenetics in multiple sclerosis susceptibility: Difference in transgenerational risk localizes to the major histocompatibility complex. *Hum Mol Genet* 2009;**18**:261–266.

48. Ramagopalan SV, McMahon R, Dyment DA, Sadovnick AD, Ebers GC, Wittkowski KM. An extended statistical approach provides insights into genetic risk factors for multiple sclerosis in the HLA-DRB1 Gene. *BMC Med Genet* 2009;**10**:10.

49. Bias WB, Reveille JD, Beaty TH, Meyers DA, Arnett FC. Evidence that autoimmunity in man is a Mendelian dominant trait. *Am J Hum Genet* 1986;**39**:584–602.

50. Becker KG, Simon RM, Bailey-Wilson JE, *et al.* Clustering of non-major histocompatibility complex susceptibility candidate loci in human autoimmune diseases. *Proc Natl Acad Sci* 1998;**95**:9979–9984.

51. Heinzlef O, Alamowitch S, Sazdovitch V, *et al.* Autoimmune diseases in families of French patients with multiple sclerosis. *Acta Neurol Scand* 2000;**101**:36–40.

52. Barcellos LF, Kamdar BB, Ramsay PP, *et al.* Clustering of autoimmune diseases in families with a high risk for multiple sclerosis: A descriptive study. *Lancet Neurol* 2006;**5**:924–931.

53. Henderson RD, Bain CJ, Pender MP. The occurrence of autoimmune diseases in patients with multiple sclerosis and their families. *J Clin Neurosci* 2000;**7**: 434–437.

54. Ramagopalan SV, Valdar W, Dyment DA, *et al.* Asssociation of infectious Mononucleosis with multiple sclerosis: A population-based study. *Neuroepidemiology* 2009;**32**:257–262.

55. Boiko AN, Gusev EI, Sudomoina MA, *et al.* Association and linkage of juvenile MS with HLA-DR2 (15) in Russians. *Neurology* 2002;**58**:658–860.

56. Boiko AN, Guseva ME, Guseva MR, *et al.* Clinico-immunogenetic characteristics of multiple sclerosis with optic neuritis in children. *J Neurovirol* 2000; **6**(Suppl 2):S152–5.

57. Anlar B, Alikasifoglu M, Kose G, Guven A, Gurer Y, Yakut A. Tumor necrosis factor-alpha gene polymorphisms in children with multiple sclerosis. *Neuropediatrics* 2001;**32**:214–216.

58. Ohlenbusch A, Pohl D, Hanefeld F. Myelin oligodendrocyte gene polymorphisms and childhood multiple sclerosis. *Pediatr Res* 2002;**52**:175–179.

59. Compston DA, Batchelor JR, McDonald WI. B-lymphocyte alloantigens associated with multiple sclerosis. *Lancet* 1976;**308**:1261–1265.

60. Terasaki PI, Park MS, Opelz G, Ting A. Multiple sclerosis and high incidence of a B lymphocyte antigen. *Science* 1976;**193**:1245–1247.

61. Compston A, Coles A. Multiple sclerosis. *Lancet* 2008;**372**:1502–1517.

62. Ramagopalan SV, Ebers GC. Epistasis: Multiple sclerosis and the major histocompatibility complex. *Neurology* 2009;**72**:566–567.

63. Dyment DA, Herrera BM, Cader MZ, *et al.* Complex interactions among MHC haplotypes in multiple sclerosis: Susceptibility and resistance. *Hum Mol Genet* 2005;**14**:2019–2026.

64. DeLuca GC, Ramagopalan SV, Herrera BM, *et al.* An extremes of outcome strategy provides evidence that multiple sclerosis severity is determined by alleles at the HLA-DRB1 locus. *Proc Natl Acad Sci* 2007;**104**:20896–20901.

65. Chao MJ, Ramagopalan SV, Herrera BM, *et al.* Epigenetics in multiple sclerosis susceptibility: Difference in transgenerational risk localizes to the major histocompatibility complex. *Hum Mol Genet* 2009;**15**:261–266.

66. Ramagopalan SV, Maugeri NJ, Handunnetthi L, *et al.* Expression of the multiple sclerosis-associated MHC class II Allele HLA-DRB1*1501 is regulated by vitamin D. *PLoS Genet* 2009 Feb 6 [Epub ahead of print].

67. Nielsen T, Rostgaard K, Askling J, *et al.* Effects of infectious mononucleosis and HLA-DRB1*15 in multiple sclerosis. *Mult Scler* 2009 Jan 19 [Epub ahead of print].

68. Haines JL, Terwedow HA, Burgess K, *et al.* Linkage of the MHC to familial multiple sclerosis suggests genetic heterogeneity. The Multiple Sclerosis Genetics Group. *Hum Mol Genet* 1998;**7**:1229–1234.

69. Yeo TW, De Jager PL, Gregory SG, *et al.* A second major histocompatibility complex susceptibility locus for multiple sclerosis. *Ann Neurol* 2007;**61**: 228–236.

70. Chao MJ, Barnardo MC, Lincoln MR, *et al.* HLA class I alleles tag HLA-DRB1*1501 haplotypes for differential risk in multiple sclerosis susceptibility. *Proc Natl Acad Sci* 2008;**105**:13069–13074.

71. McAulay KA, Higgins CD, Macsween KF, *et al.* HLA class I polymorphisms are associated with development of infectious mononucleosis upon primary EBV infection. *J Clin Invest* 2007;**117**: 3042–3048.

72. International Multiple Sclerosis Genetics Consortium, Hafler DA, Compston A, *et al.* Risk alleles for multiple sclerosis identified by a genomewide study. *N Engl J Med* 2007;**357**:851–862.

73. Lundmark F, Duvefelt K, Iacobaeus E, *et al.* Variation in interleukin 7 receptor alpha chain (IL7R) influences risk of multiple sclerosis. *Nature Genet* 2007;**39**: 1108–1113.

74. International Multiple Sclerosis Genetics Consortium (IMSGC). Refining genetic associations in multiple sclerosis. *Lancet Neurol* 2008;**7**:567–569.

75. International Multiple Sclerosis Genetics Consortium (IMSGC). The expanding genetic overlap between multiple sclerosis and type I diabetes. *Genes Immun* 2009;**10**:11–14.

76. Zoledziewska M, Costa G, Pitzalis M, *et al.* Variation within the *CLEC16A* gene shows consistent disease association with both multiple sclerosis and type 1 diabetes in Sardinia. *Genes Immun* 2008;**10**:15–17.

77. Rubio JP, Stankovich J, Field J, *et al.* Replication of *KIAA0350, IL2RA, RPL5* and *CD58* as multiple sclerosis susceptibility genes in Australians. *Genes Immun* 2008;**9**:624–630.

78. Gregory SG, Schmidt S, Seth P, *et al.* Interleukin 7 receptor alpha chain (IL7R) shows allelic and functional association with multiple sclerosis. *Nat Genet* 2007;**39**:1083–1191.

79. Skinningsrud B, Husebye ES, Pearce SH, *et al.* Polymorphisms in *CLEC16A* and *CIITA* at 16p13 are associated with primary adrenal insufficiency. *J Clin Endocrinol Metab* 2008;**93**:3310–3317.

80. 't Hart BA, Laman JD, Bauer J, Blezer E, van Kooyk Y, Hintzen RQ. Modelling of multiple sclerosis: Lessons learned in a non-human primate. *Lancet Neurol* 2004;**3**:588–597.

81. Hafler JP, Maier LM, Cooper JD, *et al.* CD226 Gly307Ser association with multiple autoimmune diseases. *Genes Immun* 2009;**10**:5–10.

82. Seldin MF, Amos CI. Shared susceptibility variations in autoimmune diseases: A brief perspective on common issues. *Genes Immun* 2009;**10**:1–4.

83. Dardalhon V, Schubart AS, Reddy J, *et al.* CD226 is specifically expressed on the surface of Th1 cells and regulates their expansion and effector functions. *J Immunol* 2005;**175**:1558–1565.

84. van Kemenade FJ, Tellegen E, Maurice MM, *et al.* Simultaneous regulation of CD2 adhesion and signaling functions by a novel CD2 monoclonal antibody. *J Immunol* 1994;**152**:4425–4432.

85. Van Rhijn I, Van den Berg LH, Bosboom WM, Otten HG, Logtenberg T. Expression of accessory molecules for T-cell activation in peripheral nerve of patients with CIDP and vasculitic neuropathy. *Brain* 2000;**123**:2020–2029.

86. Liao X, Buchberg AM, Jenkins MA, Copeland NG. Evi-5, a common site of retroviral integration in AKXD T-cell lymphomas, maps near Gfi-1 on mouse chromosome 5. *J Virol* 1995;**69**:7132–7137.

87. Jakkula E, Leppä V, Sulonen AM, *et al.* Genome-wide association study in a high-risk isolate for multiple sclerosis reveals associated variants in *STAT3* gene. *Am J Hum Genet* 2010;**86**:285–291.

88. De Jager PL, Jia X, Wang J, *et al.* 2. Meta-analysis of genome scans and replication identify CD6, IRF8 and TNFRSF1A as new multiple sclerosis susceptibility loci. *Nat Genet* 2009;**41**:776–782.

89. Ban M, Goris A, Lorentzen AR, *et al.* 3. Replication analysis identifies TYK2 as a multiple sclerosis susceptibility factor. *Eur J Hum Genet* 2009;**17**: 1309–1313.

90. Australia and New Zealand Multiple Sclerosis Genetics Consortium. Genome-wide association study identifies new multiple sclerosis susceptibility loci on chromosomes 12 and 20. (ANZgene). *Nat Genet* 2009;**41**:824–828.

91. Hoppenbrouwers IA, Aulchenko YS, Ebers GC, *et al. EVI5* is a risk gene for multiple sclerosis. *Genes Immun* 2008;**9**:334–337.

92. Aulchenko YS, Hoppenbrouwers IA, Ramagopalan SV, *et al.* Genetic variation in the KIF1B locus influences susceptibility to multiple sclerosis. *Nat Genet* 2008;**40**:1402–1403.

93. Zhao C, Takiat J, Tanaka Y, *et al.* Charcot–Marie–Tooth disease type 2A caused by mutation in a microtubule motor KIF1B. *Cell* 2001;**105**: 587–597.

94. International Multiple Sclerosis Genetics Consortium (IMSGC). Comprehensive follow-up of the first genome-wide association study of multiple sclerosis identifies KIF21B and TMEM39A as susceptibility loci. *Hum Mol Genet* 2010;**19**:953–962.

95. Hahn JS, Pohl D, Rensel M, Rao S, International Pediatric MS Study Group. Differential diagnosis and evaluation in pediatric multiple sclerosis. *Neurology* 2007;**68**(16 Suppl 2):S13–22.

96. Valanne L, Ketonen L, Majander A, Suomalainen A, Pihko H. Neuroradiologic findings in children with mitochondrial disorders. *Am J Neuroradiol* 1998;**19**:369–377.

97. Harding AE, Sweeney MG, Miller DH, *et al.* Occurrence of a multiple sclerosis-like illness in women who have a Leber's hereditary optic neuropathy mitochondrial DNA mutation. *Brain* 1992;**115**: 979–989.

98. Riordan-Eva P, Sanders MD, Govan GG, Sweeney MG, Da Costa J, Harding AE. The clinical features of Leber's hereditary optic neuropathy defined by the presence of a pathogenic mitochondrial DNA mutation. *Brain* 1995;**118**:319–337.

99. Trapp BD, Stys PK. Virtual hypoxia and chronic necrosis of demyelinated axons in multiple sclerosis. *Lancet Neurol* 2009;**8**:280–291.

100. Mahad DJ, Ziabreva I, Campbell G, *et al.* Mitochondrial changes within axons in multiple sclerosis. *Brain* 2009;**69**:214–216.

101. Ban M, Elson J, Walton A, *et al.* Investigation of the role of mitochondrial DNA in multiple sclerosis susceptibility. *PLoS* 2008;**3**:e2891.

Clinical and biological features of acute disseminated encephalomyelitis

Jin S. Hahn and Silvia Tenembaum

Acute disseminated encephalomyelitis (ADEM) is an acute inflammatory and demyelinating disorder of the central nervous system that is immune-mediated. ADEM is also known as "post-infectious," "post-exanthematous," or "post-vaccinal" encephalomyelitis [1,2]. The term ADEM started to be used clinically in the 1960s [3], and has become more widely used since the 1970s [4,5]. In most patients it is preceded by a viral illness, but may also occur after bacterial infections and vaccinations. ADEM presents with acute mental status changes (encephalopathy) and other various focal or multi-focal neurological signs. ADEM is traditionally considered a monophasic illness, and the neurological symptoms and signs resolve over time. However, recurrent and multiphasic courses may occur, raising diagnostic challenges in distinguishing these forms from multiple sclerosis (MS).

This chapter focuses on the clinical features and our current understanding of the pathophysiology of ADEM in children. Since there are no prospectively validated diagnostic criteria for ADEM (see Chapter 2), the current understanding of the clinical presentation of ADEM is based on retrospective series of patients using non-standardized criteria. The proposed consensus diagnostic criteria for ADEM published in 2007 by the International Study Group on Pediatric MS [6] and the expanded spectrum of ADEM that include recurrent and multiphasic forms will also be discussed in this chapter. The neuroimaging and treatment aspects of ADEM will be discussed in the following two chapters (Chapters 18 and 19).

Clinical features

Epidemiology

ADEM can occur at any age, but is more common in pediatric patients than in adults. Few systematic population-based studies have been performed that address the incidence and geographic distribution of ADEM. In a study conducted in San Diego County, USA the estimated mean incidence of ADEM was 0.4 per 100 000 per year among persons less than 20 years of age living in that region [7]. A population-based study from southern Japan found that the incidence of childhood ADEM under the age of 15 years was 0.64 per 100 000 person per year with a mean age of onset of 5.7 years [8]. In comparison, the mean age at onset of MS was 9.3 years, which was significantly higher than that of ADEM [8]. The overall incidence of ADEM was much higher than childhood MS, with more than three times the number of cases of ADEM identified compared to MS during the five-year study period. Large, nationwide survey studies of ADEM in Germany [9] and Canada [10] have yielded lower incidences (0.07 and 0.2 per 100 000 per year, respectively).

The median age of presentation in childhood ADEM ranges from five to eight years of age [7,8, 11–14]. The youngest age of onset of ADEM ranges from 10 to 11 months depending on the series [7,8]. The mean onset ages of vaccine-associated ADEM was younger (3.2 years) than infection-associated ADEM (6.2 years) [8].

Unlike MS in which there is a clear female predominance (with F:M ratio of 2:1), in ADEM there does not appear to be a particular gender predominance [7,12]. In fact, a slight male predominance has been described in four pediatric cohorts (M:F ratios of 1.2 to 1.3) [13–16]. In the Japanese study, the male:female ratio was 2.3:1 [8].

ADEM appears to be a disorder that is seen throughout the world and affects all ethnicities. Case series have been reported from countries in North America [7,10], South America [14], Europe [9,12,17,18], the Middle

Demyelinating Disorders of the Central Nervous System in Childhood, ed. Dorothée Chabas and Emmanuelle L. Waubant. Published by Cambridge University Press. © Cambridge University Press 2011.

East [13], Asia [8], South Asia [16,19], Oceania [11], and Africa [20].

In children with ADEM, the presence of associated diseases is low. In the German study, only 2 of the 28 children had associated diseases: one, an idiopathic thrombocytopenic purpura, and one, a nephrotic syndrome [9].

Antecedents

The diagnosis of ADEM is often made in the setting of a defined viral illness or vaccination: signs of recent preceding infection were reported in 88–93% of the patients, while 5–15% of these patients had received a vaccination within one month before the ADEM event [7,8]. However, in some cases (approximately 10%), no clear antecedent history of either is present. Nevertheless, in ADEM there is a presumed trigger for immune-mediated process, but its manifestations may be too subtle or subclinical to be noted in the history.

A seasonal peak of incidence during the winter and spring months has been found in several studies [7,12,21], but not in others [8,10]. The seasonal variation has suggested the role of infectious agents in the pathogenesis of ADEM.

Post-infectious forms of ADEM typically begin within 2–21 days after an infection. The mean latency between the onset of neurological symptoms and antecedent illness or vaccination was 17.7 days [8]. Viral infections commonly associated with ADEM include influenza virus, enterovirus, measles, mumps, rubella, varicella-zoster, Epstein–Barr virus, cytomegalovirus, herpes simplex virus, human herpesvirus-6, hepatitis A, and coxsackievirus.

In the pre-vaccine era, ADEM was more frequently associated with pediatric exanthematous infections. Post-measles ADEM has an incidence of 1–2 per 1000 infections and is more common in children over 5 years of age [22]. The neurological symptoms begin as the rash and fever are resolving. Neurological complications of acute varicella-zoster virus infection are much less common (less than 1 per 10 000 infections). Post-varicella encephalomyelitis with similar pathology to that of post-measles encephalomyelitis is rare and typically starts 1–2 weeks after the onset of rash [23]. Neurological complications of rubella are even less common than varicella with incidence of approximately 1 per 20 0000 infections, but with high mortality rate of approximately 20% [24]. Survivors, however, rarely have any neurological sequelae.

Mumps frequently causes acute viral meningitis and mild encephalitis that may be difficult to distinguish from ADEM. ADEM following exanthematous viral infections (e.g. measles, mumps, rubella) are less common in developed countries where rates of childhood immunizations are high.

In the post-vaccine era, upper respiratory tract infections are more frequently associated with ADEM. Influenza virus A and B, have been associated rarely with ADEM, although acute encephalitis is more common than ADEM [24].

Bacterial triggers include *Mycoplasma pneumoniae* [25,26], *Borrelia burgdorferi* [27], *Leptospira* [28], and beta-hemolytic *Streptococcus* [29]. ADEM affecting bilateral thalami may occur after Japanese B encephalitis vaccination [30–34]. Other organisms include *Legionella, Chlamydia, Rickettsia rickettsii, Salmonella typhi*, and *Plasmodium falciparum* (reviewed in [24,35]).

Acute hemorrhagic leukoencephalomyelitis (AHLE) typically follows influenza or upper respiratory infection [36]. The latency between the infection and the neurological symptoms does not differ significantly from ADEM. However, in this hyperacute form of demyelination, when the neurological manifestations ensue, there is a very rapid and fulminant progression, often resulting in death [37].

Vaccinations associated with ADEM include hepatitis B, pertussis, diphtheria, measles, mumps, rubella, pneumococcus, varicella, influenza, Japanese B encephalitis, small pox, and poliomyelitis (reviewed in [38]). The latency may be longer than that seen in post-infectious ADEM [24]. The rate of post-measles vaccine encephalomyelitis is 10–20 per million doses, which is much lower than the incidence following natural measles infection (1–2 per 1000 infections) [39]. The rate of post-mumps vaccine-related encephalitis (Jeryl-Lynn strain) is very low at 1 per 1.8 million doses [40]. Rubella vaccine has been associated with rare reports of optic neuritis (ON) and transverse myelitis [39].

Vaccines produced in CNS tissue have been shown to carry a higher risk of ADEM, in particular the Semple form of the rabies vaccine [14,41]. The Semple form of the vaccine is no longer used and has been replaced by non-neural vaccine. Immunization with Japanese encephalitis virus vaccine (which is prepared from mouse brain-derived virus) has been associated with encephalomyelitis [42]. In general, vaccination forms with high rates of complications are no longer in use.

It is not clear whether live-attenuated vaccines have a higher incidence of developing ADEM compared to non-live vaccines. Encephalomyelitis has been reported after administration of live-attenuated oral polio vaccine [43]. However, most neurological complications due to oral polio vaccine are due to paralytic poliomyelitis from the vaccine rather than an immune-mediated encephalomyelitis. The inactivated polio vaccine does not cause paralytic poliomyelitis.

Rare cases of ADEM have been described in adults following solid organ [44,45] and bone marrow transplantations [46–48]. ADEM confirmed by brain biopsy has also been reported in children after hematopoietic stem cell transplantation [49]. These patients were being treated with immunosuppressive agents after transplantation. In some cases, the ADEM occurred months [48] or years [45] after the transplantation. Although an antecedent infectious agent has rarely been isolated, it is thought to be the trigger. The pathogenetic mechanism is unknown, but it is thought that the altered immune status after transplantation may predispose the patient to ADEM.

Clinical presentation

Since there are no specific biomarkers in ADEM, the diagnosis of ADEM is still based on clinical and neuroimaging characteristics. ADEM is usually a monophasic illness presenting with neurological symptoms and signs within 2 days to 4 weeks after an antecedent event (such as infection or vaccination). The antecedent event is reported in approximately 90% of case [7,8], although some studies report lower rates [11,14]. This may be due to the fact that many viral illnesses produce non-specific symptoms or may be completely asymptomatic. The presence of a preceding infection is helpful but not required in making the diagnosis of ADEM [6].

Several large studies have described the symptoms and signs of ADEM [7,12,14]. Typically, ADEM presents with a prodromal phase consisting of fever, malaise, headaches, nausea, and vomiting. Subsequently, neurological symptoms and signs, such as weakness, ataxia, headaches, mental status changes (encephalopathy), and seizures, rapidly develop, often within several hours. The maximum deficits usually occur within a few days (mean 4.5 days) [14].

The distribution of the CNS lesions determines the neurological signs and symptoms. Children with ADEM typically have mental status changes (encephalopathy). The degree of encephalopathy ranges from mild (irritability or lethargy) to more severe grade (obtundation or coma). Encephalopathy is thought to be due to the diffuse involvement of cortex and white matter. In addition, children with ADEM present with multiple neurological findings (polysymptomatic presentation), which include seizures (13–35%), cranial nerve palsies (22–45%), visual loss due to optic neuritis (7–23%), speech impairment or aphasia (5–21%), unilateral or bilateral pyramidal tract signs (60–95%), acute hemiplegia (76%), hemiparesthesia (2–3%), and ataxia (18–65%) [7,11,13,14,21]. Signs of myelopathy can also be seen in up to one-quarter of the cases [14]. Dystonic extrapyramidal movement disorders and behavioral changes are particularly common in the post-Group A streptococcal form of ADEM [29].

Given the multi-focal nature of lesions in typical ADEM, patients usually present with multiple symptoms. In fact, the International Pediatric MS Study Group (IPMSSG) proposed definition requires ADEM to be a polyfocal, polysymptomatic disease [6,71]. The "polysymptomatic" criterion was specified to help differentiate ADEM patients from MS patients who typically present with symptoms that can be explained by a single CNS lesion. The active MS lesions are usually more limited in size and do not flare up altogether at the same time. The proposed definitions also include a "polyfocal" criterion, usually referring to the involvement of two or more regions of the CNS (spinal cord/optic nerve/cerebral/brainstem/cerebellum) on MRI studies. This latter criterion helps differentiate it from CIS or initial demyelinating event of MS (see Chapter 2 for definitions of ADEM and MS).

The range of the severity of the neurological manifestations is wide and the clinical phenotype is highly variable. Occasionally ADEM may present in a subtle manner with irritability, headaches, and somnolence. At other times, it may display a rapid progression of symptoms and signs to coma and decerebrate rigidity. Respiratory failure due to brainstem/cervical cord involvement or severe suppression of consciousness occurs in 11–16% of cases [72].

Neuroimaging findings

Neuroimaging studies are useful and essential tools in establishing the diagnosis of ADEM. MRI imaging with and without gadolinium injection is the imaging modality of choice for the brain and spinal cord since it is more sensitive than computerized tomography in detecting demyelinating lesions. Detailed neuroimaging findings can be found in Chapter 18.

Laboratory tests

There are very few systematic studies on laboratory investigation of ADEM [12,14,21]. Furthermore, there are no specific biomarkers of ADEM, so none of the tests are diagnostic of ADEM. Cerebrospinal fluid (CSF) analysis in ADEM shows evidence of inflammation (either pleocytosis or high protein) in 70–75% of patients [12,21]. The CSF shows mild pleocytosis in 40–81% of patients with ADEM (0–137 with a mean of 41 [12,17,21]) that predominantly consists of mononuclear cells [7,12]. Elevated CSF protein occurs in 36–60% of the patients (range 45–120 mg/dl with a mean of 74 mg/dl [12,17,21]). Occasionally in ADEM, there will be elevation of the myelin basic protein, total IgG, and presence of CSF-restricted IgG oligoclonal bands (OCB) [12,14,21]. The presence of myelin basic protein (MBP) in the CSF is of unknown clinical relevance. The presence of intrathecal synthesis of OCB may be found in ADEM as an acute manifestation and ranges from 4 to 29% of the patients [12,17]; however, CSF OCBs are usually absent in the convalescent phase [14,73]. OCBs are more frequently and consistently observed in MS (see Chapter 15).

CSF cultures for viruses and other pathogens are rarely positive. With newer PCR techniques, there may be a greater sensitivity for pathogens such as herpes simplex virus, HIV, human herpesvirus-6, enterovirus, EBV, varicella-zoster virus, *Mycoplasma*, and *Chlamydia*. These tests are done to help identify the presumed antecedent infection, but are not a necessary component in making the diagnosis of ADEM.

The peripheral white blood cell (WBC) count may be elevated in 39–64% of the patients [12,21]. In one series the range was 3200 to 25 100/mm^3 with a mean of 11 300/mm^3 [21]. The erythrocyte sedimentation rate was elevated in 42–46% of patients [12,21]. C-reactive protein was elevated in about a third of the patients [12]. Other laboratory tests looking for evidence of autoimmune disorders (such as anti-nuclear antibody, serum complement (C3, C4), LE cell test, anticardiolipin antibodies, and lupus anticoagulant) are normal [14].

Acute hemorrhagic leukoencephalitis

Acute hemorrhagic leukoencephalitis (AHLE), acute hemorrhagic encephalomyelitis (AHEM), and acute necrotizing hemorrhagic leukoencephalitis (ANHLE) of Weston Hurst are rare hyperacute variants of ADEM. The clinical course is acute and rapidly progressive and frequently causes fulminant inflammatory hemorrhagic demyelination of CNS white matter. Lesions on MRI tend to be large, with perilesional edema and mass effect [74,75]. AHLE is usually triggered by upper respiratory tract infections. Death from brain edema is common within one week of onset of the encephalopathy. However, case reports of favorable outcomes with the use of early and aggressive treatments including various combinations of high-dose corticosteroids, immunoglobulin, cyclophosphamide, and plasma exchange have been published [76–79].

Differential diagnosis

Fever, encephalopathy, and neurological signs and symptoms are by nature frequent presenting features of ADEM. Many inflammatory and non-inflammatory disorders of the CNS may have similar clinical and neuroimaging presentation. Due to the acute therapeutic implications, the exclusion of CNS infections should be the first diagnostic step in every child with a first episode of CNS symptoms. Meningitis, encephalitis, and brain abscesses must be excluded. Furthermore, a broad range of viral, bacterial, and parasitical diseases that could cause signs and symptoms mimicking ADEM should be considered.

A lumbar puncture should be performed if there are no contraindications. The work-up for the initial demyelinating event should include CSF cell count with differential, protein, glucose, IgG index and isofocalization of IgG in the CSF and matched serum. CSF and matching serum should be sent for CSF-restricted IgG oligoclonal bands, and if possible, cytology. If there is evidence of an inflammatory process (CSF pleocytosis, elevated CSF protein), or gadolinium-enhancing lesions on MRI, screening for infectious agents, such as viruses, bacteria, and fungi, should be carried out.

Neuroimaging studies of both the brain and spinal cord should be performed, as these imaging findings may be useful in differentiating ADEM from other diseases. Many of the MRI patterns seen in ADEM may be mimicked by other disorders. When the MRI shows large focal tumor-like lesions, one should consider brain tumors, Shilder's disease, Marburg's variant of MS, and brain abscess [80,81]. A lesion pattern with posterior cerebral white matter involvement may develop in children with acute hypertensive encephalopathy associated with renal disease or under immunosuppressive therapy [82]. An MRI pattern of symmetric bithalamic involvement may be seen in children with acute necrotizing encephalopathy, deep cerebral venous thrombosis, hypernatremia, and extrapontine myelinolysis. Bilateral basal ganglia involvement may be seen with organic acidurias, post-streptococcal ADEM, infantile bilateral striatal necrosis, *Mycoplasma pneumoniae*, and voltage-gated potassium channel antibody associated encephalitis [29,83–85]. The presence of complete ring-enhancing lesions in the cerebral white matter is unusual in ADEM, and should evoke consideration of brain abscess, tuberculomas, neurocysticercosis, toxoplasmosis and histoplasmosis.

Lesions restricted to one hemisphere, or showing a predominant cortical–subcortical distribution, are unlikely in ADEM and should evoke consideration of vascular conditions such as moyamoya disease or vasculitis. A cerebral angiography should be performed as well when a primary angiitis of the CNS is suspected in a child with multi-focal neurological deficits, acquired demyelination and persistent headache [86,87]. Recurrent episodes of CNS demyelination should raise the potential diagnosis of MS (see below), but may represent neurologic manifestations in the setting of systemic vasculitides of childhood or collagen vascular diseases, such as systemic lupus erythematosus, Behçet syndrome, neurosarcoidosis, and Sjögren's disease [86,88]. The association of silent or symptomatic brain lesions and recurrent demyelinating attacks with prominent involvement of optic nerves and spinal cord should raise the diagnosis of neuromyelitis optica (NMO) [89,90]. The detection of NMO-IgG in serum distinguishes NMO from other demyelinating disorders.

In children with a progressive leukoencephalopathy and neurologic decline despite aggressive corticosteroid treatment, diagnosis such as leukodystrophies, mitochondrial disorders, and CNS malignancies should be considered, in addition to progressive multi-focal leukoencephalopathy, primary hemophagocytic lymphohistiocytosis (HLH), or macrophage activation syndrome (MAS), and sub-acute sclerosing panencephalitis.

More details regarding the differential diagnosis of pediatric CNS demyelination are provided in Chapter 6.

Outcome in ADEM and further episodes of demyelination

ADEM has traditionally been considered a monophasic illness. Therefore, the symptoms and signs usually resolve over time, although residual neurologic deficits may occur. The most common neurological sequelae following ADEM are focal motor dysfunction ranging from mild ataxia to hemiparesis [24]. The natural course of ADEM without treatment seems to be that of gradual improvement over several weeks with 50–70% of the patients achieving full recovery [19,91,92]. Subtle neuropsychological abnormalities have been reported in children after ADEM years after the disease, particularly if the onset of ADEM was before 5 years of age [93].

Mortality rates seem to be relatively low (~5–7% in a population study [7,26]), although higher rates have been seen in the past when ADEM was associated with exanthematous disease such as measles [24]. The deaths are due to fulminant disease causing cerebral edema and elevated intracranial pressure. The outcome in ADEM in the era of corticosteroid and other immunologic treatments are similar, with 57–89% of patients attaining recovery without significant sequelae 1–12 weeks after the clinical onset [7,11,12,14,21].

Several series have consistently reported a proportion of patients that have further attacks of demyelination [7,11,12,14,17,21]. Estimates of relapses from studies using restrictive criteria for ADEM range from 10 to 18% [14,17]. The variability may in part be due to the different diagnostic criteria used to define relapses and the duration of follow-up.

Monophasic ADEM, recurrent ADEM, and multiphasic ADEM

A variety of definitions and terminology have been used to describe patients with ADEM who relapse. Consistency is crucial if we are to advance in our understanding of ADEM and its outcomes and therapeutic options. To improve the diagnosis and develop a uniform classification, the IPMSSG developed proposed criteria to be applied to ADEM and variants

Table 17.1 Infectious pathogens and vaccines associated with ADEM

Source	Pathogen or vaccine	Study and prevalence
Viral		
Yeh *et al.* [50]	Coronavirus	CR, 15-year-old boy, CSF-PCR and serum titers positive
David *et al.* [51]	Coxsackie B	CR, 8-year-old boy
Yamamoto *et al.* [52]	Dengue virus	CR, 58-year-old man
Fujimoto *et al.* [53]	Epstein–Barr virus	Case studies of ADEM in Epstein–Barr virus
Tan *et al.* [54]; Sacconi *et al.* [55]	Hepatitis virus (A and C)	CRs, children and adults
Kaji *et al.* [56]	Herpes simplex virus	Case series; ~10% developed ADEM after herpes simplex virus CNS infections
Silver *et al.* [57]	HIV	CRs, bioptic neuropathologic abnormalities discussed
Kamei *et al.* [58]	Human herpesvirus 6	CR, 19-month-old boy
Fenichel [39]	Measles	100/100 000 with high mortality
Sonmez *et al.* [59]	Mumps	CRs with parainfectious myelitis and brainstem encephalitis
Voudris *et al.* [60]	Parainfluenza viruses	CRs, 1 after bone-marrow transplant
Fenichel [39]	Rubella virus	1/10 000–1/20 000
Miller *et al.* [61]	Varicella-zoster virus	1/10 000–1/20 000
Bacterial		
van Assen *et al.* [62]	*Borrelia burgdorferi*	CR, 45-year-old man, post-mortem neuropathologic abnormalities discussed
Heick and Skriver [63]	*Chlamydia*	CR, 18-year-old woman; tracheal swab PCR and serum IgM positive
Spieker *et al.* [64]	*Legionella*	CRs
Riedel *et al.* [25]	*Mycoplasma pneumoniae*	CRs, children and adults
Wei and Baumann [65]	*Rickettsia rickettsii*	CR, 7-year-old boy with Rocky Mountain spotted fever after tick bite
Dale *et al.* [29]	*Streptococcus*	Case series with basal ganglia involvement and specific auto-antibodies
Other		
Koibuchi *et al.* [66]	*Plasmodium vivax*	CRs
Vaccinations		
Hynson *et al.* [11]	Hepatitis B	2 cases of 31 patients were vaccinated 3–6 weeks prior to onset of ADEM
Plesner *et al.* [42]	Japanese B encephalitis	Certain vaccines propagated in mouse brains; incidences up to 0.2/100 000

Table 17.1 *(cont.)*

Source	Pathogen or vaccine	Study and prevalance
Fenichel [39]	Measles	0.1/100 000 for live measles vaccination; this is compared with 0.2–0.3/100 000 background encephalitis*
Nalin [40]	Mumps	Strain-dependent 0.06–1.4/100 000*
Fenichel [39]	Pertussis	0.9/100 000 for DPT-triple vaccine*
Ozawa *et al.* [67]	Polio	CR, 6-year-old girl; oral vaccination 4 years prior; at onset, polio virus culture positive from pharyngeal swap and CSF
Hemachudha *et al.* [68]	Rabies	Semple-type (attenuated live virus, propagated in rabbit or goat CNS tissue cultures): up to 1/600 No complications reported for newer vaccines produced in human diploid cells
Fenichel [39]	Rubella	Reports of isolated myelitis and optic neuritis
Bolukbasi and Ozmenoglu [69]	Tetanus	CR, 43-year-old man
Schattenfroh [70]	Tick-borne encephalitis	CR, 35-year-old man

Abbreviations: ADEM, acute disseminated encephalomyelitis; CSF, cerebrospinal fluid; CNS, central nervous system; CR, case report; DPT, diphtheria, pertussis, and tetanus; PCR, polymerase chain reaction.
Note:
* Acute disseminated encephalomyelitis was not explicitly stated; mostly the clinical terms *encephalopathy* or *encephalitis* were used. Most of these studies were conducted before the advent of magnetic resonance imaging. Hence, the actual ADEM incidence may be even lower. Reproduced with permission from [35].

(Table 17.2) [6,71]. Here we provide a discussion of these proposed definition criteria focusing on ADEM. A broader discussion of these criteria is included in Chapter 2. In these definitions, ADEM is characterized by a transitory and self-limiting, acute or subacute multi-focal inflammatory demyelinating process accompanied by encephalopathy. The proposed criteria also define various relapsing forms, including "recurrent" and "multiphasic" ADEM. In brief, in "recurrent" ADEM, a subsequent attack is stereotypical of the first attack and there is no evidence of involvement of a different part of the CNS clinically or by MRI. In "multiphasic" ADEM, there must be new symptoms or involvement of a different part of the CNS than that of the initial attack. The criteria for the duration between attacks are detailed in Table 17.2. Whether children who have multiphasic forms of ADEM will eventually develop into MS is not known, but multiphasic ADEM seems to be a self-limited demyelinating process and not a lifelong disease like MS. Studies with considerable follow-up have identified a subset of children with ADEM who

have one relapse of ADEM-like episodes usually within 1–2 years after the initial episode, and then no further attacks [7,11–14,21].

The outcome in children with the final diagnosis of multiphasic ADEM is also favorable. Recovery without sequelae was found in 86% of children in the UK study [12]. In 8 children with multiphasic ADEM the median Disability Status Score was 1 (range 0–2.5) at the last follow-up (mean 8.2 years, range 3–16) [14].

Distinguishing ADEM from CIS and MS

When a first-time demyelinating attack of the CNS occurs, there is often a concern that the child may develop MS. The concern is further heightened if the child has recurrent or multiphasic ADEM. Since MS and ADEM may present with symptoms and signs that are indistinguishable, the differentiation of MS from ADEM is often difficult. The distinction between ADEM and MS may be important since the

Table 17.2 Proposed IPMSSG definition of ADEM, recurrent ADEM, and multiphasic ADEM

Sub-type	Clinical characteristics	MRI findings	Duration between events
ADEM	• A first clinical event with a presumed inflammatory or demyelinating cause, with acute or sub-acute onset that affects multi-focal areas of the CNS. The clinical presentation must be polysymptomatic and must include encephalopathy, which is defined as one or more of the following:	• Neuroimaging shows focal or multi-focal lesion(s), predominantly involving white matter, without radiologic evidence of previous destructive white matter changes:	• If a relapse takes place within 4 weeks of tapering steroid treatment or within the first 3 months from the initial event, this early relapse is considered temporally related to the same acute monophasic condition.
	• Behavioral change, e.g. confusion, excessive irritability	• Brain MRI, with FLAIR or T2-weighted images, reveals large (>1–2 cm in size) lesions that are multi-focal, hyperintense, and located in the supratentorial or infratentorial white matter regions; gray matter, especially basal ganglia and thalamus, is frequently involved	• New or fluctuating symptoms, signs, or MRI findings occurring within 3 months of the inciting ADEM event are considered part of the acute event
	• Alteration in consciousness, e.g. lethargy, coma	• In rare cases, brain MR images show a large single lesion ($\geq$1–2 cm), predominantly affecting white matter	
	• Event should be followed by improvement, either clinically, on MRI or both, but there may be residual deficits	• Spinal cord MRI may show confluent intramedullary lesion(s) with variable enhancement, in addition to abnormal brain MRI findings above specified.	
	• No history of a clinical episode with features of a prior demyelinating event		
	• No other etiologies can explain the event		
Recurrent ADEM	• New event of ADEM with recurrence of the initial symptoms and signs without involvement of new clinical areas by history, examination, or neuroimaging	• MRI shows no new lesions; original lesions may have enlarged	• Subsequent event must occur $\geq$3 months after the first ADEM event and $\geq$1 month after completing steroid therapy
	• No better explanation exists		
Multiphasic ADEM	• ADEM followed by a new clinical event also meeting criteria for ADEM, but involving new anatomic areas of the CNS as confirmed by history, neurologic examination, and neuroimaging	• The brain MRI must show new areas of involvement but also demonstrate complete or partial resolution of those lesions associated with the first ADEM event	• Subsequent event must occur $\geq$3 months after initial ADEM event and $\geq$1 month after completing steroid therapy
	• The subsequent event must include a polysymptomatic presentation including encephalopathy, with neurologic symptoms or signs that differ from the initial event		

Modified from [6].

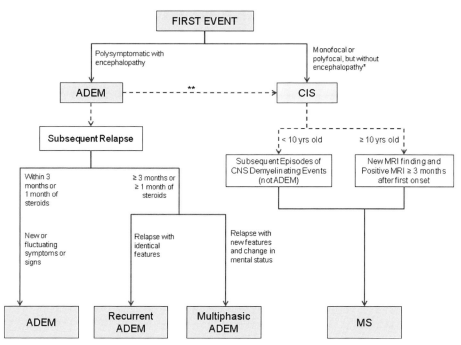

Figure 17.1 Flow diagram to aid diagnosis of ADEM and MS. Modified from [6]. Dotted lines indicate that the subsequent pathway are not obligatory. *Encephalopathy is usually absent in CIS cases, although it may be present in brainstem syndrome. **This pathway indicates after a patient with ADEM may develop MS. However, according to the Study Group proposed definition, the initial ADEM episode is not considered the first attack of MS unless the patient has a new non-ADEM demyelinating event (second event), followed by a subsequent episode (third event) or new lesions on MRI, to meet the criteria for pediatric MS.

advent of MS disease-modifying treatments are available and are being used more frequently in children with MS.

Definitions of CIS and MS

The IPMSSG proposed that for a diagnosis of ADEM, there must be a polyfocal, polysymptomatic disease plus encephalopathy [6,71]. Patients who do not have encephalopathy are categorized as having a clinical isolated syndrome (CIS). Therefore, CIS is defined as a first acute-clinical episode for CNS symptoms with a presumed inflammatory demyelinating cause for which there is no prior history of a demyelinating event [6]. This clinical event may either be monofocal or multi-focal, but usually does not include encephalopathy (except in cases of brainstem syndromes) or fever. Examples include optic neuritis, transverse myelitis, hemispheric dysfunction, and/or brainstem/cerebellar dysfunction. This distinction is important because of a hypothesis that children who present with CIS are more likely to develop MS than those who present with ADEM.

The IPMSSG also proposed definition for pediatric MS [6]: pediatric MS requires multiple episodes of CNS demyelination separated in time and space as specified for adults. The MRI can be used to meet the dissemination in space requirement if the McDonald criteria for a "positive MRI" are applied [94]. An episode consistent with ADEM cannot be considered as the first event of MS. Therefore, when a child has an initial event consistent with ADEM, a second non-ADEM demyelinating event alone is not sufficient for the diagnosis of MS. There would have to be additional evidence of dissemination in time and space, i.e. either a new (third) non-ADEM event occurring at least 3 months from after the second event or new T2 MRI lesions developing at least 3 months from the second event. The IPMSSG provided a flow diagram to aid diagnosis (Figure 17.1).

Clinical and neuroimaging distinctions

The clinical distinction between ADEM and the first attack of MS presents challenges, especially in young children. There are several features that have been

Table 17.3 Comparison of typical features of acquired demyelinating disorders: ADEM and MS

Typical features	ADEM	MS
Age	Occurs in children and adults. In children typically younger age group (<10 years)	Uncommon in children and >50 years. In pediatric population, more frequent in adolescents
Gender	No gender or slight male predilection (F:M = 1:1.2)	Female predilection (F:M = 2:1)
Antecedent infection/immunization	Very frequent	Variable (may trigger relapse)
Clinical presentation	Polysymptomatic	Usually monosymptomatic
Encephalopathy	Present	Rare but possible early in the disease
Seizures	Variable; more common in younger children	Rare
Clinical course	A single event may wax and wane over the course, up to 12 weeks; rare "recurrent" or "multiphasic" forms	Relapses common with discrete events separated by ≥4 weeks
MRI lesions of deep gray matter (basal ganglia and thalamus)	Frequent	Rare
MRI lesions of corpus callosum	Variable	Common
MRI course	Lesions typically either resolve or show only residual findings	Typically associated with development of new lesions
CSF pleocytosis	Variable	Rare, usually <50 WBC/µl
CSF oligoclonal bands	Variable (0–29%)	Frequent (85%)

A proportion of patients with ADEM may experience additional relapses and accumulate lesions on neuroimaging studies. These patients are subsequently reclassified as MS based on clinical events, laboratory findings, and MRI changes.
Modified from [6,103].

proposed to help distinguish ADEM from MS [11,95]. Some of these features are shown in Table 17.3. Encephalopathy is required by definition in ADEM, and has been emphasized as a key distinguishing factor in pediatric ADEM when compared with MS. In pediatric MS, the presence of encephalopathy is uncommon during the initial presentation. However, the severity of mental status changes that constitutes encephalopathy is not well specified, leaving some room for variability in diagnosis of ADEM. Irritability and lethargy, which are included in criteria for encephalopathy, may also occur non-specifically with childhood illnesses.

ADEM is also by definition polysymptomatic at presentation (multi-focal neurological signs and findings), indicative of a widespread involvement of the brain, brainstem, spinal cord, and optic nerves.

However, polysymptomatic presentation may not be specific for ADEM, as it was found in 67% (113/168) of children who developed a second attack consistent with MS [18]. It should be noted that in this series, the Poser Criteria for MS were used and a first episode of ADEM was counted as a demyelinating event.

The 2000 UK study compared the clinical and neuroradiologic characteristics of children with demyelinating conditions: 28 with ADEM (monophasic CNS demyelination), 7 had multiphasic disseminated encephalomyelitis (MDEM, relapse occurring during the initial immunological event), and 13 with MS (disease disseminated in space and time) with a mean follow-up of 5.6 years [12]. ADEM/MDEM was more likely if the patient had a preceding illness, polysymptomatic presentation, encephalopathy, pyramidal signs, or bilateral ON. MS was more likely if unilateral optic neuritis or periventricular lesions on MRI were present [12]. In patients with MS new lesions appeared on subsequent imaging, while in ADEM/MDEM patients the old lesions resolved (complete resolution in 37%) without the appearance of new ones.

Laboratory Distinctions

Significant CSF pleocytosis is more common in ADEM. Some children with ADEM present with a meningoencephalitis picture, which when present may be more indicative of ADEM. Intrathecal synthesis of OCB in CSF may be present in 65–95% of patients with MS [96], but are found less frequently in ADEM. In the 2000 UK study, patients ultimately diagnosed with MS were more likely to have CSF OCB (64% in MS versus 29% in the ADEM group), but this difference was not significant [12]. Since there are no biological markers for ADEM, diagnosis of ADEM in lieu of MS cannot be made alone based on CSF studies.

Risk of developing MS after an initial acute demyelinating event

Some studies suggest that children with an initial ADEM event have a variable risk for the eventual development of MS ranging from approximately 8 to 30% [7,12,17,18,97–99]. The wide range in rates of conversion to MS may be due to varying criteria used to define pediatric MS and the duration of follow-up. The studies also suggest that children with initial demyelinating event with a CIS presentation, in contrast to ADEM presentation, have higher rates of developing MS.

In the 2004 French study of 296 children with first-time demyelinating episode, Mikaeloff *et al.* found that 29% (34/119) of children who had an initial diagnosis of ADEM (polysymptomatic onset, mental status changes, and suggestive brain MRI) developed a relapse (new symptoms lasting more than 24 h, occurring >1 month of initial episode) and were diagnosed with MS [18]. In comparison, 75% (134/177) of children with an initial episode of CIS developed a second attack. Overall, positive predictive factors for the development of a second attack were: (1) age at onset 10 years or older (Hazard Ratio (HR) = 1.67), (2) MS-suggestive initial MRI

(HR = 1.54), and (3) optic nerve lesion (HR = 2.59). A lower risk of developing a second attack was found in patients with myelitis (HR = 0.23) and severe mental status change (HR = 0.59) at initial presentation.

In the 2007 French cohort study of 132 children presenting with ADEM, Mikaeloff *et al.* used homogeneous, stringent criteria for ADEM similar to those used by IPMSSG including mental status changes [17]. Thus they excluded patients with no change in mental status at onset and with symptoms occurring at an isolated CNS site (CIS). They followed the children for mean of 5.4 years for any episodes of further occurrences. Of the patients, 18% (24/132) had a second attack (although the authors did not mention whether this group qualified as having MS). Multivariate survival analysis identified risk factors for relapse that included ON during the first attack (HR = 7.8), family history of CNS inflammatory demyelination (HR = 5.2), Barkhof MS criteria on MRI (HR = 3.8), and no neurological sequelae after the first attack (HR = 2.5). The rate of relapse after initial episode of ADEM in the 2004 French study was higher (29%), which the authors attributed to the different period of study inclusion and slight differences in the definition of ADEM. Not all of the 24 children with second attack may have MS, as 5 of them had mental status changes during their second attack, and thus fit better with a diagnosis of multiphasic ADEM according to the proposed definitions of the international pediatric MS study group [6].

In a recent UK study, Dale and Pillai applied the IPMSSG criteria of ADEM, CIS, and MS to a new cohort of 40 pediatric patients with presumed initial inflammatory demyelinating event [98]. The presenting diagnosis was ADEM in 12 and CIS in 28. Although the mean follow-up period was short (2.2 years, range 6 months to 5.4 years), only 1 of 12 patients (8%) with ADEM converted to MS, whereas 13 of 28 (46%) with CIS relapsed and fulfilled the criteria of MS. Although the follow-up period was modest, the IPMSSG criteria appeared to perform well in terms of predicting risk of early relapses. A longer follow-up period will be needed to see if more patients with CIS relapse and are reclassified with MS. In addition, none of the patients diagnosed initially with ADEM had intrathecal synthesis of OCB, as compared to 9/24 in the CIS group [98]. Patients with ADEM were more likely to be young and male, whereas patients with CIS were more likely to be older and female.

Pathology and immunopathology of ADEM

The pathophysiology of ADEM has historically been attributed to an immune-mediated injury to the white matter. Pathologic and radiographic findings identify changes predominantly in the white matter and occasionally in the deep gray matter where myelinated tracts run through the deep nuclei. The etiology has historically been attributed to infectious, post-infectious and post-vaccinal sources.

Pathological features

The pathology samples in ADEM have been obtained from autopsy studies of post-viral (measles, rubella, mumps) ADEM [100] and brain biopsies (Figure 17.2) [7]. The hallmark feature of ADEM is perivenular inflammatory infiltrates of T cells and macrophages, associated with perivenular demyelination [100,101]. The lesions of similar age are usually present bilaterally, although not necessarily symmetrically, within the cerebral white matter, brainstem, and sometimes the cerebellum and spinal cord [101]. Small veins and venules in the affected white matter are surrounded by lymphocytes and macrophages. A sleeve of adjacent white matter is edematous and demyelinated. The arteries and arterioles are relatively spared. In more fulminant and often fatal cases, the brain shows in addition diffuse brain edema with uncal and tonsillar herniation and fibrin deposition within vascular lumens [7]. The demyelination may also be more extensive.

In the hemorraghic variants of ADEM (i.e. AHEM, AHLE, and ANHLE), the affected brain areas show edema and contain blood vessels that have undergone fibrinoid necrosis [101]. Zones of demyelination and acutely hemorrhagic or necrotic tissue containing neutrophils and mononuclear inflammatory cells surround the vessels.

Although ADEM is typically described as demyelination with relative preservation of axons, axonal damage and fragmentation has been identified in the brains of some adult patients with acute demyelinating events [102]. Lesions predominate in the white matter, but can also involve the cortex and deep gray matter structures. No evidence of direct viral, bacterial, fungal or parasitic infection is found in pathological samples.

Small active plaques of MS that are centered around venules may have an appearance similar to demyelinating lesions of ADEM. However, in ADEM the demyelination is usually confined to a much narrower perivenous or perivenular zone that extends in a sleeve-like fashion along the blood vessels [101]. Furthermore, in ADEM the lesions are likely to be of uniform age, whereas in MS the lesions are likely to be at different stages (i.e. active plaques, inactive plaques, chronic active plaques, and shadow plaques) [101].

Immunopathogenesis

The immunopathogenesis of ADEM is not well developed compared to that of MS (reviewed in [103,104]). The animal model of experimental autoimmune encephalomyelitis (EAE) is likely a good model for ADEM, given its histological features and typically monophasic course of disease. In EAE mice or rats are inoculated with a combination of either homogenized CNS tissue or encephalitogenic myelin peptides with Freund's adjuvant. This results in an autoimmune demyelinating syndrome of weakness with diffuse CNS demyelination that is often monophasic [5]. The post-vaccinal form of ADEM may be related to contamination with myelin antigens from CNS culture tissue in which the virus was propagated. This is thought to be the case of ADEM following the Semple rabies vaccine, which contains rabies virus-infected neural tissue from the host animal [68].

The molecular mimicry hypothesis in ADEM suggests that due to partial structural or amino-acid sequence homologies, antigenic epitopes are shared between certain pathogens or vaccines and a host CNS myelin antigens (reviewed in [104]). The pathogens have the capacity to activate the immune system, and in particular myelin-reactive T-cell clones [105]. Such activated T cells are capable of entering the CNS during the course of routine immune surveillance. When they encounter the homologous myelin protein antigen, an inflammatory immune reaction against the presumed foreign antigen is elicited. An initial physiological immune response leads to a harmful CNS-specific autoimmune response distant from the original site of inoculation of the pathogens. Thus, microbial infections or vaccinations preceding ADEM may elicit a cross-reactive anti-myelin response through molecular mimicry. Alternatively, ADEM may be caused by the re-activation of existing myelin-reactive T cell clones through a non-specific inflammatory process.

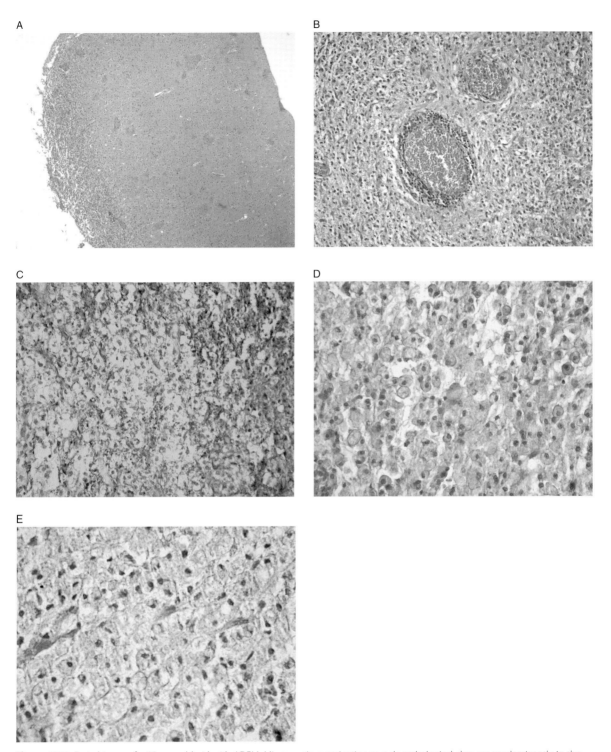

Figure 17.2 Brain biopsy of a 12-year old girl with ADEM. Microscopic examination reveals pathological changes predominantly in the white matter (A, hematoxylin–eosin). The diffuse inflammatory process is characterized by a perivascular infiltration of mononuclear cells, typically around veins and venules (B, hematoxylin–eosin), and reactive astroglial proliferation (C, GFAP). Infiltration of mononuclear cells comprises mainly macrophages (D, hematoxylin–eosin) containing punctate myelin debris (E, Luxol fast blue–PAS staining). Courtesy of Drs. F. Lubieniecki and A.L. Taratuto, Neuropathology Department, National Pediatric Hospital Dr. J. P. Garrahan, Buenos Aires, Argentina. (See plate section for color version).

Supporting the molecular mimicry hypothesis of ADEM, various sequences in myelin have been shown to resemble various viral sequences. With some viruses, cross-reactive T-cell responses with MBP antigens have been demonstrated including HHV-6 [106], coronavirus [107], influenza virus [108], and Epstein–Barr virus [109]. Proteolipid protein shares common sequences with *Haemophilus influenza* [110]. Semliki Forest Virus (SFV) peptides mimic myelin oligodendrocyte glycoprotein (MOG) [111]. MBP-reactive T cells are also found in patients with post-infectious ADEM [112], including the post-Group A streptococcal form [113].

Another hypothesis is that direct CNS infection with a secondary inflammatory cascade may be involved in ADEM [103]. The resulting tissue damage is then thought to disrupt the blood–brain barrier, causing leakage of CNS-confined autoantigens into the circulation where they are processed by the peripheral immune system. This leads to a breakdown of tolerance, resulting in a self-directed autoimmune attack against the CNS driven by encephalitogenic T cells. Theiler's murine encephalomyelitis virus-induced demyelinating disease (TMEV-IDD) may be a good model for post-infectious etiology. TMEV-IDD is induced in genetically susceptible mice by direct CNS infection with the neurotropic TMEV, inducing diffuse CNS inflammation and demyelination [114]. Initially an immune-mediated reaction primarily involves TMEV-specific CD4+ and CD8+ T cells [115,116]. During the chronic stages of the disease, T-cell reactivity to host myelin peptides have been observed.

The role of autoantibodies directed against the various CNS myelin antigens have been studied in ADEM. In the post-rabies vaccine form of ADEM, studies have demonstrated enhanced anti-MBP antibody titers in patients [117]. In the post-Group A streptococcal variant of ADEM, anti-basal ganglia antibodies were found in the sera of patients [29]. Elevated titers of anti-myelin antibodies in sera from ADEM patients have recently been demonstrated as compared to patients with MS or viral encephalitis. Autoantibodies directed against a folded tetrameric form of MOG have been identified in a subset of ADEM patients, only rarely in pediatric- and adult-onset MS patients, and were absent in individuals with viral encephalitis [118,119]. Collectively, these studies suggest that enhanced T- and B-cell myelin responses play a role in the pathogenesis of both post-infectious and post-vaccinal ADEM; however, further studies are required to determine a causal relationship.

Studies of cytokines and chemokines in ADEM have shown various up-regulation patterns, but no specific pattern or biomarker that helps differentiate it from MS. One study found that IL-4, but not interferon gamma, was the predominant cytokine secreted by MBP-reactive T-cell lines in patients with ADEM [112]. Other studies have shown elevated CSF levels of IL-6, IL-10, and TNF-α [120,121]. Production of interferon gamma, but not IL-4, by T cells was elevated in four patients with ADEM during the acute phase but not in controls with other neurologic disorders [122]. Another study of CSF reported a predominant Th1 cytokine profile, with decreased IL-17 levels (a cytokine associated with the pathogenesis of MS) in 14 children with ADEM and 20 controls. The results suggest that various cytokines related to activation of macrophasges/microglias and of Th1 and Th2 cells are up-regulated in CSF in patients with ADEM [123].

Genetic susceptibility for ADEM seems to exist based on a few small studies. ADEM was associated with the MHC class II alleles HLA-DRB1*01 and HLA-DRB*03(017) in a Russian study [91]. A similar study from Korea showed that the frequency of HLA-DRB1*15 was increased in children with ADEM; in comparison, the frequency of HLA-DRB5*06 was higher in other neuroinflammatory disorders, including MS and CIS [124]. In populations studies, HLA class II *DR2* haplotype has been associated with MS susceptibility [125]. Similar associations have been found in the pediatric MS population [126]. Thus, class II alleles may play a role in MS as well as in ADEM; however, there may be differences between alleles associated with the two demyelinating diseases.

Conclusions

ADEM is characterized as a transient and self-limited, acute or sub-acute polyfocal inflammatory demyelinating process typically accompanied by encephalopathy. In the past few years there has been progress in defining the diagnostic criteria for ADEM. Although the IPMSSG criteria are stringent, there might be increased specificity gained at the expense of sensitivity. The application of the criteria will under-diagnose the occasional patient with polysymptomatic presentation and polyfocal demyelinating lesions who does not have encephalopathy (that some would consider to have ADEM) [127]. However, increased specificity and consistency will allow better understanding of the natural course and outcome in ADEM in future longitudinal studies.

The hallmarks of ADEM are polysymptomatic presentation with encephalopathy, large polyfocal MRI lesions involving white matter as well as deep gray matter, and CSF pleocytosis without CSF OCBs. Consideration should be given to other disorders that can mimic ADEM. Rarely, a brain biopsy is needed in some patients when the diagnosis is uncertain and clinical and neuroimaging suggest an alternative diagnosis such as neoplasm. One caveat is that ADEM can also present with large tumor-like lesions [81].

There are many clinical and neuroimaging features that allow determination of ADEM versus first attack of MS; however, none of these are fully discriminating. Being able to determine whether a patient will experience a monophasic or relapsing course is important for prognosis, counseling, and therapeutic planning. Even the most stringent criteria of ADEM do not reliably predict a monophasic course. There will be a small percentage of children who will have a relapse and convert to MS [98]. Some series have found a higher relapse rate (up to 30% in pediatric series), but this may be due to the use of less stringent criteria for ADEM and variability in study patient ascertainment and follow-up duration.

Overall, the prognosis for a final diagnosis of monophasic ADEM is typically good, although long-lasting cognitive behavioral problems have been noted in some. Prolonged follow-up MRI studies should be performed to monitor the patient and assess the risk of developing MS.

References

1. Johnson RT. The pathogenesis of acute viral encephalitis and postinfectious encephalomyelitis. *J Infect Dis* 1987;**155**:359–364.

2. Scott TF. Postinfectious and vaccinal encephalitis. *Med Clin North Am* 1967;**51**:701–717.

3. Sood SC, Singh H. Acute disseminated encephalomyelitis complicating smallpox. *Indian Pediatr* 1967;**4**:361–363.

4. Behan PO, Moore MJ, Lisak RP. Acute disseminated encephalomyelitis. *Br J Clin Pract* 1974;**28**:243–245.

5. Alvord EC. Acute disseminated encephalomyelitis and "allergic" neuroencephalopathies: Multiple sclerosis and other demyelinating diseases. In *Handbook of Clinical Neurology*, ed. PJ Vinken and GW Bruyn. Amsterdam: North Holland Publishing Company; 1970:500–571.

6. Krupp LB, Banwell B, Tenembaum S. Consensus definitions proposed for pediatric multiple sclerosis and related disorders. *Neurology* 2007;**68**:S7–12.

7. Leake JA, Albani S, Kao AS, *et al.* Acute disseminated encephalomyelitis in childhood: Epidemiologic, clinical and laboratory features. *Pediatr Infect Dis J* 2004;**23**:756–764.

8. Torisu H, Kira R, Ishizaki Y, *et al.* Clinical study of childhood acute disseminated encephalomyelitis, multiple sclerosis, and acute transverse myelitis in Fukuoka Prefecture, Japan. *Brain Dev* 2010;**32**:454–462. Epub 2009/11/28.

9. Pohl D, Hennemuth I, von Kries R, Hanefeld F. Paediatric multiple sclerosis and acute disseminated encephalomyelitis in Germany: Results of a nationwide survey. *Eur J Pediatr* 2007;**166**:405–412.

10. Banwell B, Kennedy J, Sadovnick D, *et al.* Incidence of acquired demyelination of the CNS in Canadian children. *Neurology* 2009;**72**:232–239.

11. Hynson JL, Kornberg AJ, Coleman LT, Shield L, Harvey AS, Kean MJ. Clinical and neuroradiologic features of acute disseminated encephalomyelitis in children. *Neurology* 2001;**56**:1308–1312.

12. Dale RC, de Sousa C, Chong WK, Cox TC, Harding B, Neville BG. Acute disseminated encephalomyelitis, multiphasic disseminated encephalomyelitis and multiple sclerosis in children. *Brain* 2000;**123**:2407–2422.

13. Anlar B, Basaran C, Kose G, *et al.* Acute disseminated encephalomyelitis in children: Outcome and prognosis. *Neuropediatrics* 2003;**34**:194–199.

14. Tenembaum S, Chamoles N, Fejerman N. Acute disseminated encephalomyelitis: A long-term follow-up study of 84 pediatric patients. *Neurology* 2002;**59**:1224–1231.

15. Murthy JM. Acute disseminated encephalomyelitis. *Neurol India* 2002;**50**:238–243.

16. Singhi PD, Ray M, Singhi S, Kumar Khandelwal N. Acute disseminated encephalomyelitis in North Indian children: Clinical profile and follow-up. *J Child Neurol* 2006;**21**:851–857.

17. Mikaeloff Y, Caridade G, Husson B, Suissa S, Tardieu M. Acute disseminated encephalomyelitis cohort study: Prognostic factors for relapse. *Eur J Paediatr Neurol* 2007;**11**:90–95.

18. Mikaeloff Y, Suissa S, Vallee L, *et al.* First episode of acute CNS inflammatory demyelination in childhood: Prognostic factors for multiple sclerosis and disability. *J Pediatr* 2004;**144**:246–252.

19. Murthy JM, Yangala R, Meena AK, Jaganmohan Reddy J. Acute disseminated encephalomyelitis: Clinical and MRI study from South India. *J Neurol Sci* 1999;**165**:133–138.

20. Govender R, Wieselthaler NA, Ndondo A, Wilmshurst JM. Acquired demyelinating disorders of childhood in the Western Cape, South Africa. *J Child Neurol* 2010;**25**:48–56.

21. Murthy SN, Faden HS, Cohen ME, Bakshi R. Acute disseminated encephalomyelitis in children. *Pediatrics* 2002;**110**:e21.

22. Gibbons JL, Miller HG, Stanton JB. Para-infectious encephalomyelitis and related syndromes; a critical review of the neurological complications of certain specific fevers. *Q J Med* 1956;**25**:427–505.

23. Johnson R, Milbourn PE. Central nervous system manifestations of chickenpox. *Can Med Assoc J* 1970;**102**:831–834.

24. Noorbakhsh F, Johnson RT, Emery D, Power C. Acute disseminated encephalomyelitis: Clinical and pathogenesis features. *Neurol Clin* 2008;**26**:759–780, ix.

25. Riedel K, Kempf VA, Bechtold A, Klimmer M. Acute disseminated encephalomyelitis (ADEM) due to *Mycoplasma pneumoniae* infection in an adolescent. *Infection* 2001;**29**:240–242.

26. Samile N, Hassan T. Acute disseminated encephalomyelitis in children. A descriptive study in Tehran, Iran. *Saudi Med J* 2007;**28**:396–399.

27. Belman AL, Coyle PK, Roque C, Cantos E. MRI findings in children infected by *Borrelia burgdorferi*. *Pediatr Neurol* 1992;**8**:428–431.

28. Alonso-Valle H, Munoz R, Hernandez JL, Matorras P. Acute disseminated encephalomyelitis following *Leptospira* infection. *Eur Neurol* 2001;**46**:104–105.

29. Dale RC, Church AJ, Cardoso F, *et al.* Poststreptococcal acute disseminated encephalomyelitis with basal ganglia involvement and auto-reactive antibasal ganglia antibodies. *Ann Neurol* 2001;**50**:588–595.

30. Ohtaki E, Murakami Y, Komori H, Yamashita Y, Matsuishi T. Acute disseminated encephalomyelitis after Japanese B encephalitis vaccination. *Pediatr Neurol* 1992;**8**:137–139.

31. Cusmai R, Bertini E, Di Capua M, *et al.* Bilateral, reversible, selective thalamic involvement demonstrated by brain MR and acute severe neurological dysfunction with favorable outcome. *Neuropediatrics* 1994;**25**:44–47.

32. Mizuguchi M, Abe J, Mikkaichi K, *et al.* Acute necrotising encephalopathy of childhood: A new syndrome presenting with multifocal, symmetric

33. Ruggieri M, Polizzi A, Pavone L, Musumeci S. Thalamic syndrome in children with measles infection and selective, reversible thalamic involvement. *Pediatrics* 1998;**101**:112–119.

34. Hartfield DS, Loewy JA, Yager JY. Transient thalamic changes on MRI in a child with hypernatremia. *Pediatr Neurol* 1999;**20**:60–62.

35. Menge T, Hemmer B, Nessler S, *et al.* Acute disseminated encephalomyelitis: An update. *Arch Neurol* 2005;**62**:1673–1680.

36. An SF, Groves M, Martinian L, Kuo LT, Scaravilli F. Detection of infectious agents in brain of patients with acute hemorrhagic leukoencephalitis. *J Neurovirol* 2002;**8**:439–446.

37. Lann MA, Lovell MA, Kleinschmidt-DeMasters BK. Acute hemorrhagic leukoencephalitis: A critical entity for forensic pathologists to recognize. *Am J Forensic Med Pathol* 2010;**31**:7–11.

38. Huynh W, Cordato DJ, Kehdi E, Masters LT, Dedousis C. Post-vaccination encephalomyelitis: Literature review and illustrative case. *J Clin Neurosci* 2008;**15**:1315–1322.

39. Fenichel GM. Neurological complications of immunization. *Ann Neurol* 1982;**12**:119–128.

40. Nalin DR. Mumps, measles, and rubella vaccination and encephalitis. *BMJ* 1989;**299**:1219.

41. Hemachudha T, Phanuphak P, Johnson RT, Griffin DE, Ratanavongsiri J, Siriprasomsup W. Neurologic complications of Semple-type rabies vaccine: Clinical and immunologic studies. *Neurology* 1987;**37**:550–556.

42. Plesner AM, Arlien-Soborg P, Herning M. Neurological complications to vaccination against Japanese encephalitis. *Eur J Neurol* 1998;**5**:479–485.

43. Shibazaki K, Murakami T, Kushida R, Kurokawa K, Terada K, Sunada Y. Acute disseminated encephalomyelitis associated with oral polio vaccine. *Intern Med* 2006;**45**:1143–1146.

44. Horowitz MB, Comey C, Hirsch W, Marion D, Griffith B, Martinez J. Acute disseminated encephalomyelitis (ADEM) or ADEM-like inflammatory changes in a heart-lung transplant recipient: A case report. *Neuroradiology* 1995;**37**:434–437.

45. Aboagye-Kumi M, Yango A Jr, Fischer S, *et al.* Acute disseminated encephalomyelitis in a renal transplant recipient: A case report. *Transplant Proc* 2008;**40**:1751–1753.

46. Re A, Giachetti R. Acute disseminated encephalomyelitis (ADEM) after autologous peripheral blood stem cell transplant for non-Hodgkin's

brain lesions. *J Neurol Neurosurg Psychiatry* 1995;**58**:555–561.

lymphoma. *Bone Marrow Transplant* 1999;**24**: 1351–1354.

47. Au WY, Lie AK, Cheung RT, *et al.* Acute disseminated encephalomyelitis after para-influenza infection post bone marrow transplantation. *Leuk Lymphoma* 2002;**43**:455–457.

48. Tomonari A, Tojo A, Adachi D, *et al.* Acute disseminated encephalomyelitis (ADEM) after allogeneic bone marrow transplantation for acute myeloid leukemia. *Ann Hematol* 2003;**82**:37–40.

49. Woodard P, Helton K, McDaniel H, *et al.* Encephalopathy in pediatric patients after allogeneic hematopoietic stem cell transplantation is associated with a poor prognosis. *Bone Marrow Transplant* 2004;**33**:1151–1157.

50. Yeh EA, Collins A, Cohen ME, Duffner PK, Faden H. Detection of coronavirus in the central nervous system of a child with acute disseminated encephalomyelitis. *Pediatrics* 2004;**113**:e73–76.

51. David P, Baleriaux D, Bank WO, *et al.* MRI of acute disseminated encephalomyelitis after coxsackie B infection. *J Neuroradiol* 1993;**20**:258–265.

52. Yamamoto Y, Takasaki T, Yamada K, *et al.* Acute disseminated encephalomyelitis following dengue fever. *J Infect Chemother* 2002;**8**:175–177.

53. Fujimoto H, Asaoka K, Imaizumi T, Ayabe M, Shoji H, Kaji M. Epstein–Barr virus infections of the central nervous system. *Intern Med* 2003;**42**:33–40.

54. Tan H, Kilicaslan B, Onbas O, Buyukavci M. Acute disseminated encephalomyelitis following hepatitis A virus infection. *Pediatr Neurol* 2004;**30**:207–209.

55. Sacconi S, Salviati L, Merelli E. Acute disseminated encephalomyelitis associated with hepatitis C virus infection. *Arch Neurol* 2001;**58**:1679–1681.

56. Kaji M, Kusuhara T, Ayabe M, Hino H, Shoji H, Nagao T. Survey of herpes simplex virus infections of the central nervous system, including acute disseminated encephalomyelitis, in the Kyushu and Okinawa regions of Japan. *Mult Scler* 1996;**2**:83–87.

57. Silver B, McAvoy K, Mikesell S, Smith TW. Fulminating encephalopathy with perivenular demyelination and vacuolar myelopathy as the initial presentation of human immunodeficiency virus infection. *Arch Neurol* 1997;**54**:647–650.

58. Kamei A, Ichinohe S, Onuma R, Hiraga S, Fujiwara T. Acute disseminated demyelination due to primary human herpesvirus-6 infection. *Eur J Pediatr* 1997;**156**:709–712.

59. Sonmez FM, Odemis E, Ahmetoglu A, Ayvaz A. Brainstem encephalitis and acute disseminated encephalomyelitis following mumps. *Pediatr Neurol* 2004;**30**:132–134.

60. Voudris KA, Vagiakou EA, Skardoutsou A. Acute disseminated encephalomyelitis associated with parainfluenza virus infection of childhood. *Brain Dev* 2002;**24**:112–114.

61. Miller DH, Kay R, Schon F, McDonald WI, Haas LF, Hughes RA. Optic neuritis following chickenpox in adults. *J Neurol* 1986;**233**:182–184.

62. van Assen S, Bosma F, Staals LM, *et al.* Acute disseminated encephalomyelitis associated with *Borrelia burgdorferi*. *J Neurol* 2004;**251**:626–629.

63. Heick A, Skriver E. *Chlamydia pneumoniae*-associated ADEM. *Eur J Neurol* 2000;**7**:435–438.

64. Spieker S, Petersen D, Rolfs A, *et al.* Acute disseminated encephalomyelitis following Pontiac fever. *Eur Neurol* 1998;**40**:169–172.

65. Wei TY, Baumann RJ. Acute disseminated encephalomyelitis after Rocky Mountain spotted fever. *Pediatr Neurol* 1999;**21**:503–505.

66. Koibuchi T, Nakamura T, Miura T, *et al.* Acute disseminated encephalomyelitis following *Plasmodium vivax* malaria. *J Infect Chemother* 2003;**9**:254–256.

67. Ozawa H, Noma S, Yoshida Y, Sekine H, Hashimoto T. Acute disseminated encephalomyelitis associated with poliomyelitis vaccine. *Pediatr Neurol* 2000;**23**:177–179.

68. Hemachudha T, Griffin DE, Giffels JJ, Johnson RT, Moser AB, Phanuphak P. Myelin basic protein as an encephalitogen in encephalomyelitis and polyneuritis following rabies vaccination. *N Engl J Med* 1987;**316**:369–374.

69. Bolukbasi O, Ozmenoglu M. Acute disseminated encephalomyelitis associated with tetanus vaccination. *Eur Neurol* 1999;**41**:231–232.

70. Schattenfroh C. Acute disseminated encephalomyelitis after active immunization against early summer encephalitis. *Nervenarzt* 2004;**75**:776–779.

71. Tenembaum S, Chitnis T, Ness J, Hahn JS. Acute disseminated encephalomyelitis. *Neurology* 2007;**68**: S23–36.

72. Wingerchuk DM. The clinical course of acute disseminated encephalomyelitis. *Neurol Res* 2006;**28**:341–347.

73. Marchioni E, Ravaglia S, Piccolo G, *et al.* Postinfectious inflammatory disorders: Subgroups based on prospective follow-up. *Neurology* 2005;**65**:1057–1065.

74. Mader I, Wolff M, Niemann G, Kuker W. Acute haemorrhagic encephalomyelitis (AHEM): MRI findings. *Neuropediatrics* 2004;**35**:143–146.

75. Kuperan S, Ostrow P, Landi MK, Bakshi R. Acute hemorrhagic leukoencephalitis vs ADEM: FLAIR MRI

and neuropathology findings. *Neurology* 2003;**60**: 721–722.

76. Rosman NP, Gottlieb SM, Bernstein CA. Acute hemorrhagic leukoencephalitis: Recovery and reversal of magnetic resonance imaging findings in a child. *J Child Neurol* 1997;**12**:448–454.

77. Klein CJ, Wijdicks EF, Earnest FT. Full recovery after acute hemorrhagic leukoencephalitis (Hurst's disease). *J Neurol* 2000;**247**:977–979.

78. Ryan LJ, Bowman R, Zantek ND, *et al*. Use of therapeutic plasma exchange in the management of acute hemorrhagic leukoencephalitis: A case report and review of the literature. *Transfusion* 2007;**47**: 981–986.

79. Payne ET, Rutka JT, Ho TK, Halliday WC, Banwell BL. Treatment leading to dramatic recovery in acute hemorrhagic leukoencephalitis. *J Child Neurol* 2007;**22**:109–113.

80. Poser CM, Goutieres F, Carpentier MA, Aicardi J. Schilder's myelinoclastic diffuse sclerosis. *Pediatrics* 1986;**77**:107–112.

81. Kepes JJ. Large focal tumor-like demyelinating lesions of the brain: Intermediate entity between multiple sclerosis and acute disseminated encephalomyelitis? A study of 31 patients. *Ann Neurol* 1993;**33**:18–27.

82. Alehan F, Erol I, Agildere AM, *et al*. Posterior leukoencephalopathy syndrome in children and adolescents. *J Child Neurol* 2007;**22**:406–413.

83. Goutières F, Aicardi J. Acute neurological dysfunction associated with destructive lesions of the basal ganglia in children. *Ann Neurol* 1982;**12**: 328–332.

84. Green C, Riley DE. Treatment of dystonia in striatal necrosis caused by *Mycoplasma pneumoniae*. *Pediatr Neurol* 2002;**26**:318–320.

85. Hiraga A, Kuwabara S, Hayakawa S, *et al*. Voltage-gated potassium channel antibody-associated encephalitis with basal ganglia lesions. *Neurology* 2006;**66**:1780–1781.

86. Benseler S, Schneider R. Central nervous system vasculitis in children. *Curr Opin Rheumatol* 2004;**16**:43–50.

87. Lanthier S, Lortie A, Michaud J, Laxer R, Jay V, deVeber G. Isolated angiitis of the CNS in children. *Neurology* 2001;**56**:837–842.

88. Cikes N. Central nervous system involvement in systemic connective tissue diseases. *Clin Neurol Neurosurg* 2006;**108**:311–317.

89. Banwell B, Tenembaum S, Lennon VA, *et al*. Neuromyelitis optica-IgG in childhood inflammatory demyelinating CNS disorders. *Neurology* 2008;**70**: 344–352.

90. Pittock SJ, Lennon VA, Krecke K, Wingerchuk DM, Lucchinetti CF, Weinshenker BG. Brain abnormalities in neuromyelitis optica. *Arch Neurol* 2006;**63**:390–396.

91. Idrissova ZR, Boldyreva MN, Dekonenko EP, *et al*. Acute disseminated encephalomyelitis in children: Clinical features and HLA-DR linkage. *Eur J Neurol* 2003;**10**:537–546.

92. Kimura S, Nezu A, Ohtsuki N, Kobayashi T, Osaka H, Uehara S. Serial magnetic resonance imaging in children with postinfectious encephalitis. *Brain Dev* 1996;**18**:461–465.

93. Jacobs RK, Anderson VA, Neale JL, Shield LK, Kornberg AJ. Neuropsychological outcome after acute disseminated encephalomyelitis: Impact of age at illness onset. *Pediatr Neurol* 2004;**31**:191–197.

94. McDonald WI, Compston A, Edan G, *et al*. Recommended diagnostic criteria for multiple sclerosis: Guidelines from the International Panel on the diagnosis of multiple sclerosis. *Ann Neurol* 2001;**50**:121–127.

95. Brass SD, Caramanos Z, Santos C, Dilenge ME, Lapierre Y, Rosenblatt B. Multiple sclerosis vs acute disseminated encephalomyelitis in childhood. *Pediatr Neurol* 2003;**29**:227–231.

96. Orrell RW. Grand rounds – Hammersmith Hospitals. Distinguishing acute disseminated encephalomyelitis from multiple sclerosis. *BMJ* 1996;**313**:802–804.

97. Morimatsu M. Recurrent ADEM or MS? *Intern Med* 2004;**43**:647–648.

98. Dale RC, Pillai SC. Early relapse risk after a first CNS inflammatory demyelination episode: Examining international consensus definitions. *Dev Med Child Neurol* 2007;**49**:887–893.

99. Alper G, Heyman R, Wang L. Multiple sclerosis and acute disseminated encephalomyelitis diagnosed in children after long-term follow-up: Comparison of presenting features. *Dev Med Child Neurol* 2009;**51**:480–486.

100. Hart MN, Earle KM. Haemorrhagic and perivenous encephalitis: A clinical–pathological review of 38 cases. *J Neurol Neurosurg Psychiatry* 1975;**38**:585–591.

101. Love S. Demyelinating diseases. *J Clin Pathol* 2006;**59**:1151–1159.

102. Ghosh N, DeLuca GC, Esiri MM. Evidence of axonal damage in human acute demyelinating diseases. *J Neurol Sci* 2004;**222**:29–34.

103. Wingerchuk DM, Lucchinetti CF. Comparative immunopathogenesis of acute disseminated encephalomyelitis, neuromyelitis optica, and multiple sclerosis. *Curr Opin Neurol* 2007;**20**:343–350.

104. Menge T, Kieseier BC, Nessler S, Hemmer B, Hartung HP, Stuve O. Acute disseminated encephalomyelitis: An

acute hit against the brain. *Curr Opin Neurol* 2007;**20**:247–254.

105. Wucherpfennig KW, Strominger JL. Molecular mimicry in T cell-mediated autoimmunity: Viral peptides activate human T cell clones specific for myelin basic protein. *Cell* 1995;**80**:695–705.

106. Tejada-Simon MV, Zang YC, Hong J, Rivera VM, Zhang JZ. Cross-reactivity with myelin basic protein and human herpesvirus-6 in multiple sclerosis. *Ann Neurol* 2003;**53**:189–197.

107. Talbot PJ, Paquette JS, Ciurli C, Antel JP, Ouellet F. Myelin basic protein and human coronavirus 229E cross-reactive T cells in multiple sclerosis. *Ann Neurol* 1996;**39**:233–240.

108. Markovic-Plese S, Hemmer B, Zhao Y, Simon R, Pinilla C, Martin R. High level of cross-reactivity in influenza virus hemagglutinin-specific CD4+ T-cell response: Implications for the initiation of autoimmune response in multiple sclerosis. *J Neuroimmunol* 2005;**169**:31–38.

109. Lang HL, Jacobsen H, Ikemizu S, *et al.* A functional and structural basis for TCR cross-reactivity in multiple sclerosis. *Nat Immunol* 2002;**3**:940–943.

110. Olson JK, Croxford JL, Miller SD. Virus-induced autoimmunity: Potential role of viruses in initiation, perpetuation, and progression of T-cell-mediated autoimmune disease. *Viral Immunol* 2001;**14**:227–250.

111. Mokhtarian F, Zhang Z, Shi Y, Gonzales E, Sobel RA. Molecular mimicry between a viral peptide and a myelin oligodendrocyte glycoprotein peptide induces autoimmune demyelinating disease in mice. *J Neuroimmunol* 1999;**95**:43–54.

112. Pohl-Koppe A, Burchett SK, Thiele EA, Hafler DA. Myelin basic protein reactive Th2 T cells are found in acute disseminated encephalomyelitis. *J Neuroimmunol* 1998;**91**:19–27.

113. Jorens PG, VanderBorght A, Ceulemans B, *et al.* Encephalomyelitis-associated antimyelin autoreactivity induced by streptococcal exotoxins. *Neurology* 2000;**54**:1433–1441.

114. Fuller KG, Olson JK, Howard LM, Croxford JL, Miller SD. Mouse models of multiple sclerosis: Experimental autoimmune encephalomyelitis and Theiler's virus-induced demyelinating disease. *Methods Mol Med* 2004;**102**:339–361.

115. Clatch RJ, Lipton HL, Miller SD. Characterization of Theiler's murine encephalomyelitis virus (TMEV)-

specific delayed-type hypersensitivity responses in TMEV-induced demyelinating disease: Correlation with clinical signs. *J Immunol* 1986;**136**:920–927.

116. Rodriguez M, Pavelko KD, Njenga MK, Logan WC, Wettstein PJ. The balance between persistent virus infection and immune cells determines demyelination. *J Immunol* 1996;**157**:5699–5709.

117. Ubol S, Hemachudha T, Whitaker JN, Griffin DE. Antibody to peptides of human myelin basic protein in post-rabies vaccine encephalomyelitis sera. *J Neuroimmunol* 1990;**26**:107–111.

118. O'Connor KC, Chitnis T, Griffin DE, *et al.* Myelin basic protein-reactive autoantibodies in the serum and cerebrospinal fluid of multiple sclerosis patients are characterized by low-affinity interactions. *J Neuroimmunol* 2003;**136**:140–148.

119. O'Connor KC, McLaughlin KA, De Jager PL, *et al.* Self-antigen tetramers discriminate between myelin autoantibodies to native or denatured protein. *Nat Med* 2007;**13**:211–217.

120. Dale RC, Morovat A. Interleukin-6 and oligoclonal IgG synthesis in children with acute disseminated encephalomyelitis. *Neuropediatrics* 2003;**34**:141–145.

121. Ichiyama T, Shoji H, Kato M, *et al.* Cerebrospinal fluid levels of cytokines and soluble tumour necrosis factor receptor in acute disseminated encephalomyelitis. *Eur J Pediatr* 2002;**161**:133–137.

122. Yoshitomi T, Matsubara T, Nishikawa M, *et al.* Increased peripheral blood interferon gamma-producing T cells in acute disseminated encephalomyelitis. *J Neuroimmunol* 2000;**111**:224–228.

123. Ishizu T, Minohara M, Ichiyama T, *et al.* CSF cytokine and chemokine profiles in acute disseminated encephalomyelitis. *J Neuroimmunol* 2006;**175**:52–58.

124. Oh HH, Kwon SH, Kim CW, *et al.* Molecular analysis of HLA class II-associated susceptibility to neuroinflammatory diseases in Korean children. *J Korean Med Sci* 2004;**19**:426–430.

125. McElroy JP, Oksenberg JR. Multiple sclerosis genetics. *Curr Top Microbiol Immunol* 2008;**318**:45–72.

126. Boiko A, Vorobeychik G, Paty D, Devonshire V, Sadovnick D. Early onset multiple sclerosis: A longitudinal study. *Neurology* 2002;**59**:1006–1010.

127. Suppiej A, Vittorini R, Fontanin M, *et al.* Acute disseminated encephalomyelitis in children: Focus on relapsing patients. *Pediatr Neurol* 2008;**39**:12–17.

MRI features of acute disseminated encephalomyelitis

Russell C. Dale and Esther Tantsis

Overview

Acute disseminated encephalomyelitis (ADEM) is an inflammatory demyelinating central nervous system disorder. Unlike multiple sclerosis (MS), ADEM is considered to be a monophasic inflammatory disorder (although early relapses are possible). Whether ADEM and MS are immunopathologically related or distinct has not been established.

ADEM is an important model of hyperacute, post-infectious inflammatory demyelination. As there is increasing emphasis on early treatment of MS in children, it is increasingly important to discriminate between monophasic ADEM and chronic relapsing MS. As a consequence, there have been a number of studies attempting to differentiate ADEM from MS. This chapter will discuss the characteristic MRI features of ADEM, with particular emphasis on distinguishing it from the typical MRI of clinically isolated syndromes (CIS) and MS.

MRI of ADEM: lessons from early reports

Early reports were flawed due to the variable and inconsistent clinical definitions of ADEM, CIS, and MS. Indeed, ADEM was previously diagnosed when any child presented with acute polysymptomatic encephalitis with evidence of MRI disseminated hyperintense lesions [1–5]. Despite these limitations, these studies were able to describe features characteristic of monophasic demyelination (ADEM) and how it differed from MS. The features that were validated by at least two reports from these important early studies are presented in Table 18.1. Many of these characteristics are still considered typical of ADEM and are discussed in more detail later.

In 2007, the International Pediatric MS Study Group proposed the first consensus definitions of ADEM, CIS, and MS [6]. The essential inclusion criteria were clinical, rather than radiological. The most important discriminating feature of ADEM when compared to CIS and MS was the presence of encephalopathy in ADEM. This is discussed in more detail in Chapters 2 and 17. According to the consensus definitions, the MRI lesions in ADEM should be large (>1 cm in size), multi-focal, hyperintense lesions (using T2-weighted imaging) and should involve the supratentorial and infratentorial white matter, and gray matter (particularly the basal ganglia and thalamus) [6]. The consensus definitions note that MRI findings of ADEM are insufficient grounds for a diagnosis, and that an ADEM diagnosis must "rest on clinical features first" [6]. It is very likely that the consensus definitions will be modified with time.

Overview of MRI in ADEM

As discussed above, a diagnosis of ADEM is predominantly clinical, and is thought to include an acute polysymptomatic illness with encephalopathy. However, MRI is fundamental in ADEM, as it demonstrates the presence of hyperintense demyelinating lesions. Although the characteristic features of ADEM are disseminated asymmetrical white matter lesions, the lesion size, characteristics, and distribution of these lesions are highly variable [1,3,4]. Similarly, there are MRI features more commonly seen in ADEM compared to CIS and MS. However, there are no absolute differentiating features of ADEM compared to CIS and MS. It is notable that there may be a lag time in the visualization of MRI lesions: early in the course of ADEM, the MRI may be normal; however, with time the MRI lesions may emerge [7]. Likewise, even though the patient's clinical state may improve rapidly after treatment, the improvements in the MRI lesions

Demyelinating Disorders of the Central Nervous System in Childhood, ed. Dorothée Chabas and Emmanuelle L. Waubant. Published by Cambridge University Press. © Cambridge University Press 2011.

Table 18.1 Typical MRI features of ADEM identified in early cohorts, before 2007 International consensus definitions [1–5]

MRI characteristics	Characteristic or typical features of ADEM
Lesion characteristics	Poorly demarcated lesions with edema
	Variable size (large and small)
	Spinal cord lesions are multi-segmental, confluent and edematous
	Gadolinium enhancement uncommon
Lesion distribution	Bilateral, but asymmetrical lesions
	Relative sparing of periventricular white matter*
	Relative sparing of corpus callosum*
	Cortical gray matter lesions common*
	Deep gray matter lesions common*
Frequent ADEM variants	Bithalamic or bistriatal variants
	Mass-like lesions (tumor-like or tumefactive)
Outcome of lesions	Variable resolution of original lesions
	No new lesions on repeat MRI >6 months after ADEM

Note:
*Compared to MS.

may be delayed or absent. It is therefore important not to repeat the MRI too early during convalescence, unless there are clinical concerns of new lesions (personal practice).

Lesion characteristics of ADEM

ADEM is a disseminated demyelinating disorder. The general MRI characteristics of ADEM are asymmetrical, hyperintense, usually disseminated, lesions of the central nervous system (CNS). The MRI of ADEM and CIS both demonstrate hyperintense demyelinating lesions, although there are certain characteristics more commonly seen in ADEM. The general and specific features of ADEM MRI are described as follows.

Lesion size

ADEM lesions are variable in size, and can be both small and large (and often both) [3,8]. However, ADEM is typically characterized by large lesions often >1 cm, and sometimes >4 cm in size (Figure 18.1) [9–11]. Dale *et al.* reported that 82% of ADEM patients had a lesion >1 cm compared to 58% of MS patients at presentation [1]. Neuteboom *et al.* further reported small lesions more commonly in MS than ADEM (74% vs. 25%) [11]. In addition, the lesion load is often larger in monophasic ADEM compared to the first episode of MS. Mikaeloff *et al.* noted a lesion load >50% in 13% (8/64) of monophasic patients compared to 0% (0/52) patients with relapsing disease [12]. Ghassemi *et al.* reported supratentorial T2-weighted lesion volume to be an order of magnitude greater in ADEM compared to CIS [13]. Sometimes the lesions are so large and associated with edema to be confused with tumors, termed "tumefactive" or "mass-like" lesions because of their large size and surrounding edema. Kepes reported 31 patients with focal tumor-like demyelinating lesions that were initially thought to be tumors and biopsied. Most of the patients did not relapse during variable follow-up and were thought to be more reminiscent of ADEM than MS [14]. However, Mikaeloff *et al.* found tumor-like lesions with equal frequency in monophasic and relapsing patients, and therefore, like many MRI features in demyelinating disorders, this feature cannot discriminate ADEM from CIS or MS with absolute certainty [12].

Lesion number

Although the lesion load in ADEM is typically larger than in CIS and MS, this is due to the lesion *size* rather than the *number* of lesions. Indeed, CIS and MS more commonly have a higher lesion *number* compared to ADEM. In the four significant studies that have reported the lesion number in detail, all have reported a higher lesion number in CIS/MS compared to ADEM [10–12,15]. Specifically, CIS/MS patients more commonly have >9 T2 lesions than ADEM patients (54–66% vs. 17–34%) [11,12].

Lesion margins

The lesion margins in ADEM are generally "poorly defined", "poorly marginated", or "poorly demarcated", meaning that the lesion edges are not clearly

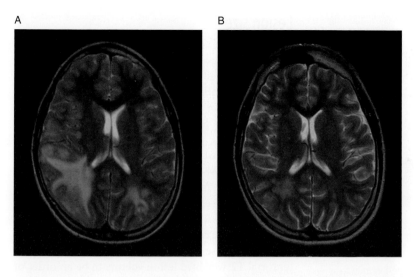

Figure 18.1 MRI in 6-year-old with ADEM (A), and follow-up MRI 4 years later (B). MRI demonstrates very large, poorly marginated white matter lesions involving the deep white matter and juxtacortical white matter (A). There is partial resolution and no new lesions on follow-up imaging (B).

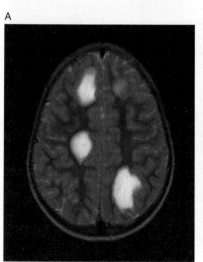
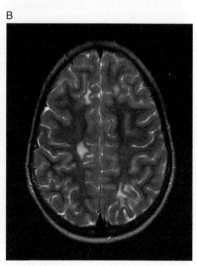

Figure 18.2 MRI of 5-year-old with ADEM (A) and follow-up MRI 6 years later (B). MRI shows large globular, poorly defined lesions (A). There is partial resolution of the lesions, and no new lesions (B).

defined, they are "blurry", "diffuse", or "indistinct". This finding has been described as being typical of ADEM, in contrast to CIS/MS (Figures 18.1 and 18.2) [1,8,9,12]. This feature has been introduced into the French KIDMUS MRI criteria: the sole presence of well-defined lesions is typical of MS (in contrast to ADEM) [12], and also in the new Callen criteria for differentiating ADEM from MS (discussed later) [10]. It should be noted, however, that the definition of a "well-defined lesion" is subjective, and may have a poor inter-rater correlation.

Lesion shape

There is no typical shape of ADEM lesions on MRI. The ADEM lesions have variable shape including both round and irregular [9]. Periventricular lesions that are ovoid and orientate perpendicular to the corpus callosum are termed "Dawson's fingers" and are characteristic of adult and pediatric MS (Figure 18.3) [9]. However, they are not absolutely specific. This latter feature has been given two definitions in the pediatric demyelination literature.

Periventricular perpendicular ovoid lesions (PVPOL) have similar characteristics to Dawson's fingers and have been described more commonly in pediatric MS than ADEM (Figure 18.3). Alper found PVPOLs only in MS (15/26) compared to 0/24 with ADEM [16]. Indeed, Alper suggested that the presence of PVPOL even in a patient with clinical ADEM (encephalopathy) should be highly suspicious of MS, rather than monophasic ADEM [16].

A 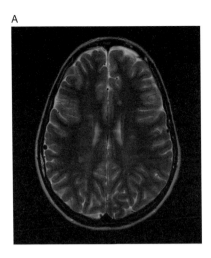 B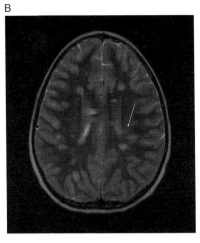

Figure 18.3 Two patients with MS. A 9-year-old with two episodes of CNS demyelination. There are small, well-demarcated white matter lesions with corpus callosum and periventricular white matter involvement (A). A separate patient with MS demonstrates Dawson's fingers (PVPOL or well-defined ovoid lesions) perpendicular to corpus callosum (arrow) (B). Note the large number of lesions in MS.

Well-defined ovoid lesions perpendicular to the long axis of the corpus callosum (defined in KIDMUS criteria) [12]. These well-defined lesions are similar to PVPOL and Dawson's fingers but do not need to abut the periventricular margin. This criterion was proposed by Mikaeloff as a feature more commonly seen in pediatric MS compared with ADEM, and have been incorporated into the French KIDMUS MRI criteria for pediatric MS [12]. Three separate studies have tested this characteristic and found it to be suggestive of MS (38–60% of MS, compared to 0–5% of ADEM) [10,11,17].

T1-weighted characteristics (black holes)

For some time, it has been established that T2-weighted MR imaging including fluid-attenuated inversion recovery (FLAIR) is the best way of visualizing CNS demyelinating lesions. T1-weighted MR imaging is often normal in acute or chronic demyelination. When T1-weighted imaging is abnormal, the presence of hypodense lesions on T1-weighted MR imaging is also termed "black holes" and may suggest a more substantial injury or degeneration (although this is contentious) [10]. It is recognized that black holes are commonly seen in chronic demyelination such as adult MS. Callen *et al.* recently noted black holes significantly more frequently in MS than ADEM (58% vs. 5%) and have proposed the "presence of black holes" as one of three MR characteristics that can differentiate MS from ADEM in children (Figure 18.4) [10]. Although some investigators agree with this trend, there is some controversy around the definition of black holes, as the presence of black holes can be dependent upon the T1

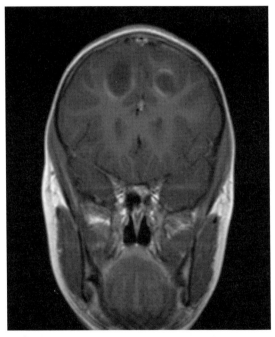

Figure 18.4 A 7-year-old with ADEM. T1-weighted images show hypo dense large lesions (black hole) with gadolinium open-ring" enhancement.

protocol parameters. Black holes which enhance are certainly reported in acute demyelination, including ADEM [10,12,18].

Gadolinium enhancement

Gadolinium enhancement infers disruption of the blood–brain barrier. Gadolinium enhancement occurs in acute demyelinating lesions with a variable

Table 18.2 Lesion regional distribution of ADEM lesions in different studies

Study	[16]	[1]	[9]	[12]	[3]	[20]	[2]	[8]
White matter	68%	91%	–	–	90%	–	–	–
PV white matter	18%	44%	67%	41%	–	46%	60%	20%
Subcortical or juxtacortical white matter	50%	91%	80%	53%	–	79%	93%	60%
Cortical gray matter	–	12%	67%	21%	–	–	80%	15%
Basal ganglia	–	28%	40%	–	39%	42%	20%	–
Thalamic	–	41%	27%	–	32%	58%	27%	–
Cerebellum	50%	31%	27%	30%	–	37%	13%	–
Spine	–	28%	47%	11%	16%	–	–	–
Brainstem	41%	56%	47%	38%	42%	54%	47%	60%
Corpus callosum	9%	–	7%	27%	29%	37%	7%	5%

Pv: periventricular; SC or JC: subcortical or juxtacortical.

pattern: homogenous, nodular, gyral, or sometimes an "open-ring" pattern (Figure 18.4) [4,19]. Gadolinium enhancement is evident in ~10–30% of ADEM scans [3,4,12,15,20], although higher rates have been reported, possibly related to the dosage of gadolinium given [8]. Gadolinium enhancement has been described more frequently in MS compared to ADEM in one study (24% vs. 13%) [12]. As gadolinium enhancement does not appear to give much additional information regarding prognosis or severity, it is not routinely administered, unless the MRI is performed in follow-up and the presence of new active lesions may influence treatment options (Figure 18.4).

Lesion distribution

Lesion symmetry

Acquired demyelinating and inflammatory disorders typically have an asymmetrical lesion distribution within the white matter, in contrast to genetic and metabolic leuodystrophies when the pattern is typically more symmetrical. The minor exception to this rule is in the ADEM variant where there is bithalamic or bistriatal lesion involvement (described below).

Lesion regional involvement

It is classically taught that ADEM is a white matter disorder. However, rather than being a pure white matter disorder, it is clear that ADEM lesions are disseminated throughout the CNS. Although white matter lesions are virtually universally present, cortical, cerebellar, brainstem, thalamic, and striatal gray matter lesions are also common. Table 18.2 shows the regional distribution of ADEM lesions in different studies. As can be seen, there is variability between studies, most notably for the cortical gray lesions, which may be related to the differing sensitivity of T2 acquisition in different studies.

As demonstrated in the table, lesions affect white matter most commonly, but also frequently involve cortical gray matter, deep gray matter, and brainstem. The following features regarding lesion site were seen in these studies (Table 18.2).

- White matter lesions occur in deep, subcortical or juxtacortical white matter more commonly in ADEM than in MS.
- There are less periventricular white matter lesions in ADEM compared to MS.
- There are less corpus callosum lesions (unless part of large lesion) in ADEM compared to MS.
- There are more lesions involving the cortical gray matter, and deep gray matter (basal ganglia and thalami) in ADEM compared to MS.

Although none of these lesion sites can absolutely differentiate ADEM from MS, these trends have been repeatedly described [21]. Many of these trends have been introduced into diagnostic criteria to discriminate ADEM from MS (see later) [10].

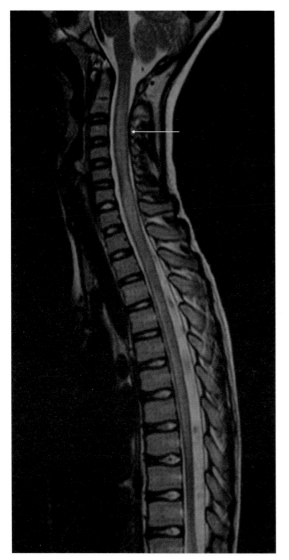

Figure 18.5 Spinal involvement in 8-year-old with ADEM. Edematous spinal cord enlargement over long cervical and thoracic cord segments.

Spinal involvement in ADEM

Typically spinal cord lesions in ADEM are large and extend over long segments of the spinal cord (often thoracic). The spinal lesions in ADEM are often edematous, and the margins are ill-defined (Figure 18.5) [2,9,21]. This is in contrast to the MS spinal lesions which usually involve the cervical cord, are non-edematous, small lesions that extend only over short segments [9]. Spinal cord MRI has been less studied than brain MRI and its importance in differentiating ADEM from MS may be underestimated. In

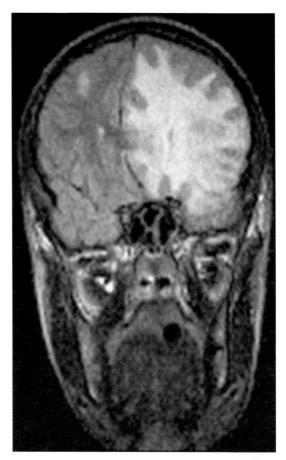

Figure 18.6 Large mass-like lesion with associated midline shift in 10-year-old with ADEM. The patient made a full recovery.

the UCSF pediatric MS cohort, MS and CIS patients who underwent a spinal cord MRI within 3 months from disease onset had extensive T2 bright cord lesions (more than 3 vertebral segments high) less commonly compared with ADEM patients (8.3% vs. 65%) [22]. If this is confirmed, the presence of extensive spinal cord lesions will be useful for diagnosing ADEM versus MS in children, and might need to be included in future diagnostic criteria.

ADEM variants

The classical MRI of ADEM is of disseminated asymmetrical white matter lesions. However, it has become clear that a number of different ADEM variants are common.

Tumefactive or "tumor-like" lesions

Solitary "tumor-like" lesions are seen occasionally in ADEM. In one study, 2/31 ADEM patients had a

A

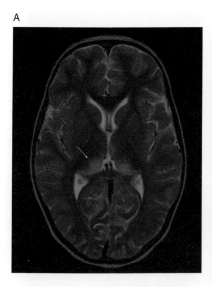

B

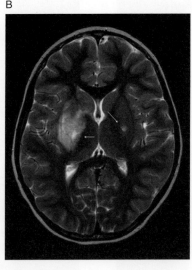

Figure 18.7 (A) A 2-year-old with ADEM shows bilateral thalamic MRI involvement. (B) A 5-year-old with ADEM shows a large hyperintense lesion of the left putamen and a smaller lesion affecting the right putamen.

tumor-like demyelinating lesion that required biopsy to confirm its inflammatory nature [3]. Solitary lesions such as this often have associated edema. Although described in both ADEM and MS, these mass-like lesions appear to be more common in ADEM [9]. Kepes described 31 patients with a focal tumor-like demyelinating lesion, of whom 24 had solitary lesions. The relapse rate and conversion to MS was low in this group suggesting solitary "tumor-like" lesions are more common in monophasic disease such as ADEM [14].

Bithalamic or bistriatal ADEM

As previously described, deep gray matter involvement is more common in ADEM than MS. In some patients, there is deep gray matter lesion involvement with relative sparing of the white matter. Bilateral basal ganglia (or striatal) involvement has been associated with a post-streptococcal variant of ADEM [23]. A bithalamic variant of ADEM is also well described, and Tenembaum et al. classified the bithalamic variant as one of four typical ADEM MRI patterns (Figure 18.7) [4]. This bithalamic form has been described as being unresponsive to steroids, yet responsive to plasmapheresis [7], suggesting that this variant may be immunologically distinct from more typical white matter variants. It is important to differentiate bithalamic ADEM from acute necrotizing encephalopathy, which has characteristic bithalamic and brainstem involvement (see differential diagnosis section) [24].

Acute hemorrhagic leukoencephalitis (AHLE)

This variant of ADEM classically runs a severe course and death is common if not treated. AHLE is considered to be caused by fulminant, inflammatory, and hemorrhagic demyelination. Steroids, IVIg, cyclophosphamide, and plasma exchange appear to improve outcome [21]. The radiological features are of secondary hemorrhage within the acute demyelinating lesions, best seen with inversion recovery sequences which can demonstrate blood [4,21]. AHLE appears to be rare, only 2/84 ADEM patients had hemorrhagic features compatible with AHLE [4].

Proposed new MRI diagnostic criteria for ADEM

Callen et al. have recently proposed MRI criteria to help differentiate ADEM from MS in children [10]. This was the first MRI diagnostic criteria created for this purpose. Previous MRI criteria were designed to specifically diagnose pediatric MS with no reference to ADEM (discussed elsewhere) [12]. Callen et al. proposed the following criteria for MS MRI versus ADEM MRI at the time of first demyelinating episode.

Criteria for predicting chronic relapsing demyelinating disease (MS). Any two of:

- ≥ 2 periventricular lesions, OR
- presence of black holes on T1 imaging, OR
- absence of diffuse bilateral lesion pattern (poorly demarcated).

Using ≥ 2 criteria, Callen found a sensitivity of 81% and specificity of 95% (discriminating MS from ADEM) [10]. Further cohorts are required to test the validity of these criteria. Other MS MRI criteria are discussed elsewhere in this book (Chapter 5). The MRI criteria to help demonstrate MS from ADEM proposed by Mikaeloff *et al.* and Callen *et al.* need to be tested in other cohorts to determine their validity. Definitions such as "diffuse bilateral lesions" have been criticized for being ambiguous. In order to improve reproducibility, a more precise definition of large lesion has been proposed – but still untested – that includes confluent T2 FLAIR lesions involving more than two adjacent gyri [18,25].

MRI outcome of ADEM lesions, and timing of repeat imaging

ADEM is a monophasic disease. New asymptomatic lesions seen on convalescent imaging more than 3 months after acute onset are incompatible with ADEM, and more suggestive of MS (or multiphasic disseminated encephalomyelitis, as discussed elsewhere) [6]. When considering the timing of re-imaging, most investigators agree that convalescent MRI too soon after a first event cannot define whether new lesions are part of the initial event, or suggestive of MS. Therefore, delaying repeat imaging until 6 months after the acute event can avoid this problem [1,3,5,26]. New lesions seen on repeat MRI after 6 months would be suggestive of MS. Convalescent and serial imaging in ADEM should not reveal any new lesions. Tenembaum *et al.* found no new lesions on serial MRI imaging of a large Argentinean ADEM cohort [4]. Although complete resolution of the ADEM lesions is reported in up to 50% [1,8], it is more common for there to be incomplete resolution of lesions (Figures 18.1 and 18.2) [1,5]. Residual gliosis and demyelination occurred in some ADEM patients [1,5,27]. The absence of new lesions after extended follow-up (5–10 years) in ADEM patients supports the theory that ADEM is a monophasic entity [27]. In view of the increasing emphasis on early treatment in MS, Tenembaum has recommended convalescent MRI at least twice over a period of 5 years after the ADEM event, to confirm the absence of new asymptomatic lesions [21]. It is recognized that the improvement in MRI lesions can lag behind the clinical improvements (personal observation).

Table 18.3 Differential diagnosis of radiological ADEM

Broad categories	Diseases (characteristic features)
Demyelinating	Clinically isolated syndrome of demyelination, Multiple sclerosis
Inflammatory/ infectious	Viral encephalitis (cortical lesions)
	VGKC or NMDA-R autoimmune encephalitis (limbic cortical encephalitis)
	Macrophage activation syndrome
	Cerebral vasculitis
	Systemic lupus erythematosus
	Anti-phospholipid syndrome
	Acute necrotizing encephalopathy (bithalamic)
	Langerhans histiocytosis (cerebellar white matter lesions)
	Fungal or bacterial abscesses (ring lesions)
	Tuberculomas
	Neurocysticosis (calcification)
	HIV encephalopathy
	Behçet syndrome
	Neurosarcoidosis
Structural	Tumor
	Metastatic malignancy
Vascular	Cerebral venous thrombosis
Metabolic/ genetic	Leukodystrophies
	Mitochondrial cytopathy
	Extrapontine myelinolysis
	Organic acidurias (basal ganglia)
	Infantile bilateral striatal necrosis (basal ganglia)

VGKC: voltage-gated potassium channel.
NMDA-R: NMDA- receptor.

Differential diagnosis of radiological ADEM

The differential diagnosis of ADEM is broad and requires a thorough clinical and investigation approach (see Chapter 17). Table 18.3 reviews the differential diagnosis of radiological ADEM.

Table 18.4 Summary of the differences between ADEM MRI and MS (trends only)

Lesion size	Larger lesions in ADEM compared to MS
Lesion number	Less lesions in ADEM compared to MS
Lesion margin	Poorly demarcated lesions in ADEM compared to MS
Lesion shape	"Dawson's fingers", PVPOL or well-defined ovoid lesions perpendicular to corpus callosum uncommon in ADEM compared to MS
Lesion T1 characteristic	Black holes less common in ADEM compared to MS
Lesion symmetry	Typically asymmetrical lesions in ADEM and MS
Lesion regional involvement	Periventricular white matter lesions less common in ADEM than MS Cortical and deep gray matter lesions more common in ADEM compared to MS
	Corpus callosum lesions less common in ADEM compared to MS
Spinal lesions	Large, edematous multi-segmental lesions more common in ADEM compared to MS
Lesion outcome	No new lesions in ADEM
	New asymptomatic lesions typical in MS

New techniques in ADEM

T2-weighted and FLAIR MR imaging are the best at defining demyelinating lesions. Newer MR techniques can be useful and informative. Magnetic resonance spectroscopy (MRS) is marginally useful, the most common finding being a reduced N-acetylaspartate (NAA):choline ratio [28–30]. The reduced NAA:choline ratio appears to be reversible, suggesting that this MRS finding is not always indicative of neuronal loss or damage [28]. Diffusion-weighted imaging (DWI) is primarily used to define vascular insults and stroke. However, diffusion restriction measured by apparent diffusion coefficient (ADC) is described in acute ADEM lesions. The ADC restriction (when present) appears to be potentially reversible [29,30].

Conclusions

In conclusion, there are certain characteristic features of ADEM as summarized in Table 18.4. These "trends" cannot definitely differentiate ADEM from MS, as there are no absolute specific features of ADEM. In addition, the variable nature of ADEM imaging supports the hypothesis that ADEM is a heterogenous syndrome with different immunopathological mechanisms, rather than one disease, and there may be some overlap with CIS/MS. Further detailed clinical, radiological, immunological and genetic studies will help clarify ADEM and associated disorders in the future.

References

1. Dale RC, de Sousa C, Chong WK, et al. Acute disseminated encephalomyelitis, multiphasic disseminated encephalomyelitis and multiple sclerosis in children. Brain 2000;123:2407–2422.

2. Murthy SN, Faden HS, Cohen ME, Bakshi R. Acute disseminated encephalomyelitis in children. Pediatrics 2002;110:e21.

3. Hynson JL, Kornberg AJ, Coleman LT, et al. Clinical and neuroradiologic features of acute disseminated encephalomyelitis in children. Neurology 2001; 56:1308–1312.

4. Tenembaum S, Chamoles N, Fejerman N. Acute disseminated encephalomyelitis: A long-term follow-up study of 84 pediatric patients. Neurology 2002; 59:1224–1231.

5. Kesselring J, Miller DH, Robb SA, et al. Acute disseminated encephalomyelitis. MRI findings and the distinction from multiple sclerosis. Brain 1990; 113:291–302.

6. Krupp LB, Banwell B, Tenembaum S. Consensus definitions proposed for pediatric multiple sclerosis and related disorders. Neurology 2007;68(Suppl 2):S7–12.

7. Khurana DS, Melvin JJ, Kothare SV, et al. Acute disseminated encephalomyelitis in children: Discordant neurologic and neuroimaging abnormalities and response to plasmapheresis. Pediatrics 2005; 116:431–436.

8. Atzori M, Battistella P, Perini P, et al. Clinical and diagnostic aspects of multiple sclerosis and acute monophasic encephalomyelitis in pediatric patients: A single centre prospective study. Mult Scler 2009;15:363–370.

9. Singh S, Prabhakar S, Korah IP, et al. Acute disseminated encephalomyelitis and multiple sclerosis: Magnetic resonance imaging differentiation. Australas Radiol 2000;44:404–411.

10. Callen DJ, Shroff MM, Branson HM, *et al.* Role of MRI in the differentiation of ADEM from MS in children. *Neurology* 2009;**72**:968–973.

11. Neuteboom RF, Boon M, Catsman Berrevoets CE, *et al.* Prognostic factors after a first attack of inflammatory CNS demyelination in children. *Neurology* 2008;**71**:967–973.

12. Mikaeloff Y, Adamsbaum C, Husson B, *et al.* MRI prognostic factors for relapse after acute CNS inflammatory demyelination in childhood. *Brain* 2004;**127**:1942–1947.

13. Ghassemi R, Antel SB, Narayanan S, *et al.* Lesion distribution in children with clinically isolated syndromes. *Ann Neurol* 2008;**63**:401–405.

14. Kepes JJ. Large focal tumor-like demyelinating lesions of the brain: Intermediate entity between multiple sclerosis and acute disseminated encephalomyelitis? A study of 31 patients. *Ann Neurol* 1993;**33**:18–27.

15. Mikaeloff Y, Caridade G, Husson B, *et al.* Acute disseminated encephalomyelitis cohort study: Prognostic factors for relapse. *Eur J Paediatr Neurol* 2007;**11**:90–95.

16. Alper G, Heyman R, Wang L. Multiple sclerosis and acute disseminated encephalomyelitis diagnosed in children after long-term follow-up: Comparison of presenting features. *Dev Med Child Neurol,* 2009;**51**:480–486.

17. Dale RC, Pillai SC. Early relapse risk after a first CNS inflammatory demyelination episode: Examining international consensus definitions. *Dev Med Child Neurol* 2007;**49**:887–893.

18. Chabas D, Pelletier D. Sorting through the pediatric MS spectrum with brain MRI. *Nat Rev Neurol* 2009;**5**:186–188.

19. Lim KE, Hsu YY, Hsu WC, Chan CY. Multiple complete ring-shaped enhanced MRI lesions in acute disseminated encephalomyelitis. *Clin Imaging* 2003;**27**:281–284.

20. Suppiej A, Vittorini R, Fontanin M, *et al.* Acute disseminated encephalomyelitis in children: Focus on relapsing patients. *Pediatr Neurol* 2008;**39**:12–17.

21. Tenembaum S, Chitnis T, Ness J, Hahn JS. Acute disseminated encephalomyelitis. *Neurology* 2007;**68**(Suppl 2):S23–36.

22. Mowry E. Long lesions ion initial spinal cord MRI predict a final diagnosis of acute disseminated encephalomyelitis versus multiple sclerosis in children. *Neurology* 2008;**70**(Suppl 1):A135.

23. Dale RC, Church AJ, Cardoso F, *et al.* Poststreptococcal acute disseminated encephalomyelitis with basal ganglia involvement and auto-reactive antibasal ganglia antibodies. *Ann Neurol* 2001;**50**:588–595.

24. Mizuguchi M, Yamanouchi H, Ichiyama T, Shiomi M. Acute encephalopathy associated with influenza and other viral infections. *Acta Neurol Scand Suppl* 2007;**186**:45–56.

25. Chabas D, Castillo-Trivino T, Mowry EM, *et al.* Vanishing MS T2-bright lesions before puberty: A distinct MRI phenotype? *Neurology* 2008;**71**:1090–1093.

26. Dale RC, Branson JA. Acute disseminated encephalomyelitis or multiple sclerosis: Can the initial presentation help in establishing a correct diagnosis? *Arch Dis Child* 2005;**90**:636–639.

27. O'Riordan JI, Gomez-Anson B, Moseley IF, Miller DH. Long-term MRI follow-up of patients with post infectious encephalomyelitis: Evidence for a monophasic disease. *J Neurol Sci* 1999;**167**:132–136.

28. Bizzi A, Ulug AM, Crawford TO, *et al.* Quantitative proton MR spectroscopic imaging in acute disseminated encephalomyelitis. *Am J Neuroradiol* 2001;**22**:1125–1130.

29. Balasubramanya KS, Kovoor JM, Jayakumar PN, *et al.* Diffusion-weighted imaging and proton MR spectroscopy in the characterization of acute disseminated encephalomyelitis. *Neuroradiology* 2007;**49**:177–183.

30. Kuker W, Ruff J, Gaertner S, *et al.* Modern MRI tools for the characterization of acute demyelinating lesions: Value of chemical shift and diffusion-weighted imaging. *Neuroradiology* 2004;**46**:421–426.

Chapter 19

Treatment and prognosis of acute disseminated encephalomyelitis

Amy T. Waldman and Marc Tardieu

Introduction

Acute disseminated encephalomyelitis (ADEM) is an inflammatory demyelinating disease of the central nervous system (CNS). Our understanding about the natural history of disease and its response to therapy is based on epidemiological studies of prospectively followed cohorts of patients as well as case series and case reports [1–3]. Although the prognosis is generally favorable, the acute phase can be severe and even life-threatening. As opposed to pediatric multiple sclerosis (MS), ADEM typically occurs as an isolated event and does not require long-term therapy. However, relapses do occur in some patients presenting a diagnostic challenge in differentiating recurrent or multiphasic disseminated encephalomyelitis from pediatric MS [4,5]. This chapter focuses on the treatment of ADEM in children. When possible, prognostic implications of the interventions will also be addressed.

Treatment of the acute phase of ADEM with high doses of corticosteroids

Adrenocorticotropic hormone (ACTH), given intramuscularly or by subcutaneous infusion, was one of the earliest therapies used to treat children and adults with demyelinating diseases, including ADEM [6]. Some patients responded rapidly to injections, prompting a large study to determine the efficacy of ACTH in adults with MS. Although it was perhaps better than placebo in reducing worsening during acute attacks, ACTH did not impact the outcome of patients with MS [7]. Nevertheless, the success of corticosteroids in treating acute attacks of demyelination led to its further use in patients with ADEM.

In 1980, Pasternak *et al.* reported seven pediatric cases with an "unusual, slowly progressive, parainfectious syndrome" treated with oral corticosteroids [8]. Five of the patients were treated with dexamethasone (0.5 mg/kg/day divided every 6 h, route not specified), and the other two children received oral prednisone (one received 25 mg daily and the other received 30 mg twice a day). All of the children improved with corticosteroids; one child was left with residual abnormalities (unsustained ankle clonus, bilateral Babinski signs, and emotional lability).

Early case series reported multiple regimens of corticosteroids for ADEM, including both oral and intravenous therapies, depending on the severity of neurologic impairment. The use of low-dose oral vs. high-dose intravenous corticosteroids in demyelinating diseases was studied in 1992 in the Optic Neuritis Treatment Trial [9]. Performed in adults, this study compared high-dose intravenous methylprednisolone, low-dose oral prednisone, and placebo for the treatment of acute optic neuritis (ON) (symptom onset within 8 days). This randomized, double-blind, placebo-controlled trial demonstrated that intravenous methylprednisolone followed by oral prednisone (see Table 19.1 for dosing regimens) hastened visual recovery compared to placebo over a two-year period (in a secondary objective of the trial). Oral prednisone had no benefit in a similar analysis. Moreover, the group treated with oral prednisone had an increased risk of recurrence of ON compared to placebo. As a result of this study, intravenous methylprednisolone followed by oral prednisone was recommended for acute ON.

The use of intravenous methylprednisolone to treat children with ADEM was later supported by a study of 84 children with ADEM conducted in Argentina [1]. Consecutive patients between 1988 and 2000 were enrolled (one patient from 1982 was

Demyelinating Disorders of the Central Nervous System in Childhood, ed. Dorothée Chabas and Emmanuelle L. Waubant. Published by Cambridge University Press. © Cambridge University Press 2011.

Table 19.1 Treatment regimens used in the Optic Neuritis Treatment Trial (adults aged 18–46 years) [9]

Group	Regimen
IV Methylprednisolone	Methylprednisolone 250 mg IV q6 for 3 days followed by Prednisone 1 mg/kg PO daily for 11 days*
Oral prednisone	Prednisone 1 mg/kg PO daily for 14 days*
Placebo	Same schedule as the oral prednisone group

Note:
* Rounded to the nearest 10 mg.

Table 19.2 Corticosteroid regimens used in the Argentina ADEM study [1]

Corticosteroid	Dose	No. patients (%)
Dexamethasone	1 mg/kg/day IV for 10 days*	43 (51%)
Methylprednisolone	30 mg/kg/day IV for children <30 kg for 3–5 days* 1 g/day IV for children >30 kg for 3–5 days*	21 (25%)
Prednisolone	2 mg/kg/day orally for 10 days*	10 (12%)
Deflazacort	3 mg/kg/day orally for 10 days*	6 (7%)
None	Not applicable	3 (4%)

Note:
* All patients received a 4–6 week taper.

also included) in the study in which the primary objective was to determine predictors of outcome. Eighty children (95%) received corticosteroids in this observational study. Children were not randomized; therefore, multiple treatment regimens were used (see Table 19.2). The authors performed a subanalysis to determine the efficacy of intravenous dexamethasone compared to intravenous methylprednisolone in 46 patients with severe disease, such as coma, ON, or spinal cord involvement. The clinical outcome was determined using Kurtzke's Expanded Disability Status Scale (EDSS) [10]. When the sub-groups receiving intravenous therapy were compared, the group receiving high-dose methylprednisolone had a more favorable outcome (median EDSS 1, range 0–3) compared with the dexamethasone group (median EDSS 3, range 0–6.5, $p = 0.029$). The authors concluded that high-dose intravenous methylprednisolone is the treatment of choice for children with ADEM with optic nerve or spinal cord involvement, impairment of consciousness, or large lesions with mass effect on neuroimaging.

The efficacy of high-dose methylprednisolone in demyelinating disease in children was further supported by a study evaluating transverse myelitis using a historical control group [11]. Patients with transverse myelopathy were given intravenous methylprednisolone. Four patients received 1 g/1.73 m², and one patient received 0.5 g/1.73 m² for 3–5 days followed by an oral prednisone taper (1 mg/kg/day) for a total treatment duration of 14 days. The treated group had a quicker recovery, including median time to independent walking (23 vs. 96.5 days, $p = 0.01$), percentage of patients recovering independent

walking by 4 weeks (100% vs. 20%, $p = 0.007$), percentage of patients making a full recovery at 3 months (60% vs. 0%, $p = 0.02$), and percentage of patients making a full recovery at 12 months (80% vs. 10%, $p = 0.01$). Other case series have also supported the beneficial effect of intravenous methylprednisolone for transverse myelopathy [12,13].

The optimal dose of methylprednisolone has not been established. Most physicians use 10–30 mg/kg/day (to a maximum of 1000 mg/day) of methylprednisolone by intravenous infusion for 3–5 days [13–16]. It should be emphasized that for young children (15–35 kg), the different modes of calculation (30 mg/kg, 500 mg/m², or 1 g/1.73 m²) lead to very different doses. Although intravenous methylprednisolone is accepted as the first-line therapy, the administration, dose, and duration of an oral taper of corticosteroids are debated. A favorable outcome has been reported after a three-day intravenous course without an oral taper in an adult [13]; however, a shorter duration of corticosteroids may impact the chance of recurrence (see the next section).

The precise therapeutic effects of corticosteroids are unknown. However, a number of mechanisms have been proposed including T-cell apoptosis [17], suppression of pro-inflammatory cytokines [18], disruption of leukocyte migration across the blood–brain barrier [19], and a shift from a Th1 to a Th2 response [20,21].

Corticosteroids are generally well-tolerated. Potential side effects include hyperglycemia, hypokalemia, insomnia, hypertension, and psychosis. Although rare, death due to gastrointestinal bleeding has been reported [22]. Gastric ulcer prophylaxis is generally recommended for patients receiving high-dose corticosteroids [23]. Avascular necrosis has occurred, even with less than 1 month of corticosteroid therapy, and this risk should be discussed with patients [24,25]. The impact of corticosteroids on bone health has been studied in adults. To prevent glucocorticoid-induced osteoporosis in adults taking >3 months of these medications, lifestyle modifications (cessation of smoking and alcohol use), supplements (calcium, vitamin D), and weight-bearing physical exercise are recommended [26]. Long-term glucocorticoid use (>6 months) has not shown a decrease in bone mineral density in children [27,28]; however, many children do not get recommended daily amounts of calcium. Vitamin D is also important for bone health. Moreover, vitamin D may play a role in susceptibility to MS [29], and its role in preventing or treating demyelinating diseases is under investigation. In summary, corticosteroids have many side effects, even with short-term use, and children may benefit from diet modification (low-salt, low-sugar), vitamin supplementation (calcium, vitamin D), gastrointestinal prophylaxis, and exercise during therapy to reduce the possibility of glucocorticoid-induced hypertension, diabetes, avascular necrosis, osteoporosis, gastric ulcers, and weight gain.

Corticosteroid treatment and the risk of subsequent relapses

Although ADEM is typically considered a monophasic disease, relapses have been demonstrated in several series. A relapse may be associated with corticosteroid withdrawal or may signify an alternative diagnosis, such as recurrent acute disseminated encephalomyelitis, multiphasic disseminated encephalomyelitis, or MS (see Prognosis, below) [4,30,31]. A relapse may occur within 4 weeks of tapering corticosteroids. In these children, the diagnosis is "steroid-dependent ADEM" [23]. Although no prospective, randomized trials have compared the corticosteroid dosing regimens, a few studies have questioned whether treatment with corticosteroids impacts the development of

relapsing disease. A prospective study was performed in France to determine the prognostic factors for relapse after ADEM in children [3]. This study included 132 patients with a mean follow-up of 5.4 ± 3.3 years. In this cohort, the use of intravenous methylprednisolone was not statistically significant between those patients who developed a relapse and those with monophasic disease.

Another study suggested that relapses may be associated with a shorter steroid taper after intravenous methylprednisolone (30 mg/kg/day for 5 days) [2]. Among children with ADEM who relapsed, the mean duration of oral prednisone was 3.17 weeks (range 0.5–8 weeks), whereas the children with monophasic disease received a mean 6.3 weeks (range 0.5–16 weeks) of oral prednisone. Anlar et al. also reported an association between a prolonged steroid taper and decreased risk of relapse [14]. However, both of these studies were observational and retrospective.

Other therapies for the acute phase of ADEM, especially in life-threatening situations

Several other therapeutic options have been proposed either in association with methylprednisolone or as a second-line treatment for life-threatening (such as acute hemorrhagic leukoencephalitis) or prolonged attacks (in which the acute phase lasts more than 10 days). While considering additional therapy, other diagnoses should be investigated as described in Chapter 18. In children with prolonged and resistant acute phases, the differential diagnosis should include macrophage activation syndromes, tumors, and mitochondrial respiratory chain disorders, since these conditions require alternative treatment.

Repetition of intravenous methylprednisolone

Children in the acute phase of disease that do not respond to the first course of methylprednisolone might improve with a repeat course. Some physicians advocate for an additional 3–5 days of intravenous therapy at the same dose given 10–14 days after the initial treatment. This is a pragmatic and clinical practical approach used in several centers; however, no formal investigation of its efficacy has been published.

Intravenous immunoglobulin

Intravenous immunoglobulins (IVIg) have been used successfully as an alternative therapy for autoimmune diseases including ADEM [32,33]. Possible mechanisms include cytokine inhibition, complement disruption, and autoantibody neutralization. The fragment crystalizable (Fc) region of human immunoglobulins binds to Fc receptors on lymphocytes and monocytes thereby suppressing cytokine production (including IL-1, IL-6, and tumor necrosis factor (TNF)) [34–37]. IVIg also contain auto-antibodies that bind to cytokines directly [34,38,39]. They have been shown to disrupt complement-mediated damage in animal models and other autoimmune diseases [40]. IVIg also contains anti-idiotypic antibodies against pathogenic autoantibodies [41].

Only case reports and case series exist using IVIg for children with ADEM [32,33]. In two studies, four patients with impairment in consciousness and meningeal signs in addition to various neurologic signs and symptoms were treated with IVIg (0.4 g/kg/d for five days) [32,33]. All had pleocytosis in the cerebral spinal fluid (CSF), and one patient had a mumps infection [33]. IVIg was initiated within two weeks of symptom onset in three of the four patients, who showed improvement within 24 h of initiating therapy. The fourth patient was initially thought to have meningitis and received IVIg over seven weeks after the onset of symptoms. Despite the delay in therapy, this patient also responded to IVIg and clinically improved before therapy was even completed [27]. No adverse reactions were reported in these patients; however, aseptic meningitis, headache, nausea, and vomiting have been reported in patients receiving IVIg for other indications [42].

Shahar et al. reported 16 patients with "severe acute encephalomyelitis" defined as patients with a progressive course characterized by (1) deterioration in consciousness, cranial nerve abnormalities, and bulbar signs (four patients), (2) weakness evolving to para- or quadriplegia, with or without a sensory level or bowel or bladder involvement (11 patients), or (3) progressive vision loss (one patient, who also had left-sided weakness) [43]. The four children with brainstem involvement all responded to intravenous methylprednisolone alone and recovered within eight days of initiating therapy. In addition, the child with ON and weakness also responded to intravenous methylprednisolone with complete recovery within two months. Of the 11 patients with spinal cord involvement, five improved with intravenous methylprednisolone alone. These patients walked independently after an average of 5.83 days (range 2–9 days), and completely recovered within two weeks. One patient with paraplegia was initially treated with oral prednisolone without any benefit. Two weeks later, he was treated with IVIg (1 g/kg/day for two days). Four days later, he was able to walk, and he completely recovered within 10 days. The remaining five patients with spinal cord involvement received both intravenous methylprednisolone and intravenous immunoglobulin. Two patients did not recover and remain paraplegic; two patients fully recovered within three months, and one patient has multiple handicaps (including cognitive, speech, and motor dysfunction). The authors advocate for combined therapy in cases of severe encephalomyelitis characterized by encephalomyeloradiculoneuropathy.

Other authors recommend sequential therapies in progressive patients. Pradhan et al. initially treated four patients with intravenous methylprednisolone (10–15 mg/kg/day for 3–5 days) [44]. Three of the four patients were obtunded and quadriplegic. The fourth patient had diffuse cerebral involvement, including the brainstem. Two patients required mechanical ventilation. None of the patients improved while receiving corticosteroids, and IVIg (0.4 g/kg/day for five days) was initiated the day following the last corticosteroid dose. All patients demonstrated significant improvement while receiving IVIg, and two patients recovered completely. Although the temporal course suggests that these patients responded to IVIg, it is possible that their improvement was a delayed response to corticosteroids [44].

In conclusion, IVIg might be of value in children for whom corticosteroid therapy is contraindicated or in those who do not respond to corticosteroids. The usual dose is 2 g/kg divided over 2–5 days.

Plasma exchange

Plasma exchange, commonly referred to as plasmapheresis, has been used to treat many neurologic diseases including Guillain–Barré syndrome [45]. Although the mechanism of action is unknown, plasma exchange may decrease circulating antibodies or remove immune complexes, cytokines, or humoral factors that play a role in the pathogenesis of the disease [45–47].

Two double-blind randomized clinical trials using plasma vs. sham exchange have been reported in

Table 19.3 Treatment regimens used in the plasma exchange studies

Study	Year	Drug	Plasma exchange
Weiner et al. [48]	1989	ACTH 40 U IM q12 h for 7 days 20 U IM q12 h for 4 days 20 U IM q24 h for 3 days *plus* Cyclophosphamide 2 mg/kg orally qAM or following PE for 12 weeks	Continuous flow PE 60 ml/kg using 3.5% albumin in normal saline solution containing Ca^{2+} 6.9 mEq/l, Mg^{2+} 2 mEq/l, K^+ 4 mEq/l performed 5 times in 14 days, with at least 48 h between treatments
Weinshenker et al.* [47]	1999	Intravenous methylprednisolone 7 mg/kg/day or equivalent	Continous flow PE 54 mg/kg (1.1 plasma volume) using 5% albumin[†] and crystalloids performed 7 times over 14 days

Notes:
* Cross-over design.
† One patient received hydroxyethyl starch as replacement.

adults with demyelinating diseases [47,48]. In 1989, Weiner et al. studied patients ($\geq$18 years) with clinically definite MS experiencing a relapse [48]. Plasma exchange or sham treatment was performed in addition to the administration of ACTH and oral cyclophosphamide (see Table 19.3). The authors concluded that plasma exchange accelerated recovery from acute attacks in patients with relapsing–remitting MS; however, this benefit was not sustained over the duration of the study (24 months).

Weinshenker et al. performed a randomized trial of plasma vs. sham exchange in patients with idiopathic inflammatory demyelinating diseases who did not respond to intravenous corticosteroids [47]. After seven treatments (plasma vs. sham exchange), each patient was evaluated by two blinded neurologists. Rating scales and criterion for success were predetermined, and z scores were calculated for the primary analysis. If the physicians agreed that the patient made at least moderate improvement, the patient did not undergo further therapy; others crossed over to the opposite treatment arm. Of the 22 patients who were randomized, half of them received plasma exchange first. The diagnoses in this group were as follows: MS (6), acute transverse myelitis (ATM) (2), Marburg's variant of MS (1), neuromyelitis optica (NMO) (1), and recurrent myelitis (1). The other half, including patients with MS (6), ATM (2), ADEM (1), NMO (1), and focal cerebral demyelination (1), was randomized to sham treatment first. There was a difference between active and sham treatment ($p = 0.011$ for neurologist A and $p = 0.032$ for neurologist

B, one-sided rank sum test). Although this study showed a positive effect, 11 of 19 patients (58%) did not respond to plasma exchange (six received active treatment first and five received sham treatment first).

To determine which patients are likely to benefit from plasma exchange, a broader retrospective study of adults receiving plasma exchange at the same institution was performed [49]. Various treatment protocols were used, and a median of seven exchanges were performed (range 2–20). Out of 59 patients, 10 had ADEM. Response to plasma exchange was shown in male patients ($p = 0.021$), patients with preserved reflexes ($p = 0.019$), and those receiving early treatment ($p = 0.009$).

The largest series of children with ADEM treated with plasmapheresis reported combination therapy in six of 13 patients [50]. These six children had fulminant disease with brainstem and/or spinal cord involvement resulting in respiratory failure requiring mechanical ventilation. They received intravenous methylprednisolone (30 mg/kg/day for five days followed by a two-week prednisone taper), IVIg (0.4 mg/kg over five days), and plasma exchange (one volume using 5% albumin as replacement every other day for five exchanges). All patients receiving plasma exchange showed significant improvement. The timing of the improvement correlated with plasma exchange; however, it is possible that the prior treatments contributed to the patients' recovery. These authors recommended initiating corticosteroids (5 days) as first-line therapy followed by observation (3–5 days). If no improvement is seen, they advocate for the use of IVIg

(5 days) followed again by observation (3–5 days). Finally, if there is no change or worsening of symptoms, they suggest using plasma exchange (5 courses every other day). Of note, plasma exchange performed within days of IVIg therapy removes IVIg.

Several case reports also support plasmapheresis in severe ADEM [51,52]. One patient with extensive brain and spinal cord involvement developed respiratory failure and coma despite IVIg (0.125 g/kg/day for three days) and oral prednisone (60 mg/day for 1 day) followed by intravenous methylprednisolone (1 g/day for three days) [52]. She was treated with plasma exchange (54 ml/kg using 5% albumin) within three weeks of symptom onset. She improved after the first exchange, and she received three exchanges over four days. After 3 months, she completely recovered; however, she developed complex partial seizures one year later. The seizures were easily controlled with an anti-epileptic medication.

Another child developed respiratory failure, seizures, coma, paresis, and multiple neurologic signs and symptoms with large tumor-like lesions in the white matter of the brain and spinal cord [51]. She failed to improve with intravenous methylprednisolone (300 mg for 4 days), oral dexamethasone (0.5 mg/kg/day for 1 month then tapered over an additional month), two courses of IVIg (0.4 g/kg/day for 5 days each), and interferon beta-1b (45 00 000 units subcutaneously for 40 days). Four months after symptom onset, she continued to decline, and she was treated with plasma exchange (1400 cc exchanged every other day for six courses). Within two weeks, she dramatically improved, and she had no further relapses over two and a half years.

According to published case reports and case series, plasma exchange is well tolerated in children with ADEM [50–52]. However, the procedure often requires the placement of a central line, and complications associated with indwelling catheters, such as sepsis, have been reported [48]. Other common side effects include anemia and symptomatic hypotension [47,49]. Other rare events reported in adults include endotoxic shock, heparin-associated thrombocytopenia, pulmonary embolus, and death [47,48]. Most deaths are believed to be due to the underlying disease rather than a complication of treatment; however, one adult died during sham treatment from a pulmonary embolus associated with heparin-associated thrombocytopenia [47].

In conclusion, plasma exchange is probably beneficial for life-threatening acute demyelination and for a prolonged acute phase not responding to corticosteroids. Five to eight exchanges performed every two days is the usual choice.

Supportive care

The location of the lesions can cause a variety of neurologic deficits requiring additional treatment, such as anti-epileptic drugs for children with seizures [53,54] and mechanical ventilation for brainstem or upper cervical cord involvement. Mannitol has been used for increased intracranial pressure [8,53]. Admission to the intensive care unit may be necessary for those with impending neurologic or respiratory failure [55]. Patients with spinal cord involvement may have a neurogenic bladder or spasticity [1,2,12,16,54]. Additional services, such as physical therapy, occupational therapy, or speech therapy, may be helpful in affected patients.

Prognosis

The prognosis for children with ADEM is generally favorable. Some children recover without intervention while others receive combinations of the therapies described above. A summary of pediatric ADEM series, including treatment and outcome, is listed in Table 19.4. The average number of patients making a complete recovery was 77% regardless of the intervention. The studies for which the recovery was not reported were excluded from this calculation.

While most children with ADEM recover from their neurologic deficits, behavior problems or cognitive deficits can occur [2,16,53,56]. In one series, 11% of children had cognitive impairment after the acute event, and 11% had behavior problems [2]. Neurocognitive testing was performed in a small study of six children with ADEM. All of the patients had deficits in at least one domain, even though parents of four of the children did not report any abnormalities [57]. Lower scores were seen in the following areas: attention, processing speed, memory, executive function, and behavior. There have been no studies published to date examining the influence of treatment on cognitive outcome. Another study reported a child with ADEM following a *Mycoplasma* infection who presented with psychiatric symptoms [58]; however, to our knowledge, isolated psychiatric symptoms in the absence of other abnormalities have not been described in children with ADEM.

A child who develops neurologic symptoms after ADEM should be investigated thoroughly. Relapses of ADEM can occur, and multiphasic ADEM or

Table 19.4 Summary of pediatric ADEM case series – treatment and outcome[1]

Study	Year	Number of patients	Treatment		Number of patients with complete recovery (%)	Number of deaths (%)	Number of patients with 1 or more clinical relapse[3] (%)
			Therapy	Number of patients receiving therapy[2] (%)			
Pasternak [8]	1980	7	CS	7 (100%)	7 (86%)	0	0
Murthy [63]	1999	21	None	0 (0%)	13 (62%)	0	0
Pradhan [44]	1999	4	IVMP+IVIg	4 (100%)	1 (25%)	0	0
Nishikawa [33]	1999	3	IVIg	3 (100%)	3 (100%)	0	0
Dale [2]	2000	35	IVMP	25 (71%)	20 (57%)	0	7 (20%)
Cohen [5]	2001	21	NR	NR	NR	0	8 (38%)
Hynson [16]	2001	31	IVMP Oral dex+IVMP IVMPx2 IVIg	21 (68%) 1 (3%) 2 (6%) 2 (6%)	25 (81%)	0	4 (13%)
Hung [53]	2001	52	CS	24 (46%)	37 (71%)	0	1 (2%)
Murthy [54]	2002	18	Oral CS IVMP IVMP+IVIg None	8 (44%) 1 (6%) 2 (11%) 7 (39%)	15 (83%)	0	1 (6%)[4]
Shahar [43]	2002	16	IVMP Oral Pred+IVIG IVMP+IVIg	10 (63%) 1 (6%) 5 (31%)	13 (81%)	0	0
Tenembaum [1]	2002	84	IV Dex IVMP Oral Pred Deflazacort None	43 (51%) 21 (25%) 10 (12%) 6 (7%) 4 (5%)	75 (89%)[5]	0	8 (10%)
Anlar [14]	2003	46	IVMP CS IVIg None	28 (70%) 12 (26%) 3 (7%) 2 (4%)	71%	0	13 (28%)
Brass [59]	2003	7	NR	NR	3 (75%)[6]	1 (14%)	0 (0%)[6]
Gupte [15]	2003	18	IVMP Oral Pred IVMP+IVIg IV Dex+oral pred None	7 (50%) 2 (11%) 1 (6%) 2 (11%) 6 (33%)	12 (67%)[7]	0	2 (11%)
Idrissova [56]	2003	90	NR	NR	42 (47%)[8]	0	11 (12%)
Leake [61]	2004	42	IVCS IVCS+IVIg	25 (60%) 8 (19%)	36 (86%)	2 (5%)[9]	4 (10%)
Khurana [50]	2005	13	IVMP IVIg+IVMP	5 (38%) 1 (8%)	3 (23%)	0	1 (8%)

Table 19.4 (cont.)

Study	Year	Number of patients	Treatment		Number of patients with complete recovery (%)	Number of deaths (%)	Number of patients with 1 or more clinical relapse[3] (%)
			Therapy	Number of patients receiving therapy[2] (%)			
			IVMP+IVIg+PE	6 (46%)			
			None	1 (8%)			
Mikaeloff [3]	2007	132	NR	NR	NR	0	24 (18%)[10]
Suppiej [31]	2008	24	IVMP	19 (79%)	17 (71%)[7]	0	3 (13%)
			IVIg	2 (8%)			
			IVMP+ IVIg	3 (13%)			

Abbreviations: CS = Corticosteroids (includes route or drug not specified or various treatments used), IVCS = Intravenous corticosteroid (methylprednisolone or dexamethasone), IVIg = Intravenous immunoglobulins, IVMP = Intravenous methylprednisolone, IVMPx2 (2 courses of IV methylprednisolone), NR = Not reported, Oral CS = Oral corticosteroids (prednisone or dexamethasone), Oral dex (oral dexamethasone), PE = Plasma Exchange
Notes:
[1] Excludes case reports
[2] Not all patients are accounted for in the publication
[3] Relapses must be more than 3 months after symptom onset and greater than 1 month from steroid taper [4]
[4] One additional patient developed new MRI lesions without clinical signs 18 months after the initial presentation
[5] Complete recovery or "abnormal signs without disability"
[6] Excludes three patients who were lost to follow-up
[7] One patient was lost to follow-up
[8] "Full normalization of neurologic state" occurred in 70% of patients with "other ADEM" ($n = 20$), 54% of patients with ADEM after varicella infection ($n = 26$), and 43% of patients after rubella infection ($n = 33$). No patients with multiphasic ADEM recovered completely.
[9] Deaths: 1 patient with ADEM, 1 with "chronic MS-related complications"
[10] Ten percent were lost to follow-up

recurrent ADEM should be considered, although the latter is rare (see Chapter 17). New symptoms occurring at least 1 month after the completion of treatment (including a steroid taper) is suspicious for MS; however, a child whose initial presentation is consistent with ADEM must have two events that do not fulfill these criteria before a diagnosis of MS can be confirmed [4]. Relapses are treated using the same therapies as the initial ADEM presentation.

Death is rare in children; however, it can occur in patients with acute hemorrhagic leukoencephalitis or fulminant disease (causing increased intracranial pressure and subsequent herniation) or as a complication of treatment [22,59–61].

Conclusions

The clinical presentation and time to recovery is quite variable in children with ADEM. Some recover quickly without intervention [16]; others suffer from a progressive course [43,44,50]. The outcome is generally favorable regardless of treatment. Most children recover from their neurologic deficits, although some children have residual abnormalities depending upon the location of the lesions [62,63].

Prospective randomized clinical trials using rigorous research methodology are needed to evaluate the various treatment regimens used in clinical practice. Ideally, a formal evaluation of any treatment of ADEM should distinguish several outcomes including:

- the length of the acute phase (evaluated, for example, by the length of the comatose phase or the length of the intensive care unit stay);
- the motor functional recovery (evaluated using a recognized scale at a given time after the attack; for example, using Kurtzke's Disability Status Scale [10] at 3 and 6 months);
- the cognitive recovery (also evaluated at pre-established times); and
- the occurrence of further relapses and, accordingly, the risk of MS.

Early treatment of ADEM should target the inflammatory response, especially in children with disability or life-threatening disease. In the future, a better understanding of the immunological differences between ADEM, recurrent ADEM, multiphasic ADEM, and the initial attack of MS will allow the use of more specific immunomodulation than the commonly proposed pulses of high doses of corticosteroids.

References

1. Tenembaum S, Chamoles N, Fejerman N. Acute disseminated encephalomyelitis: A long-term follow-up study of 84 pediatric patients. *Neurology* 2002;**59**:1224–1231.

2. Dale RC, de Sousa C, Chong WK, Cox TCS, Harding B, Neville BGR. Acute disseminated encephalomyelitis, multiphasic disseminated encephalomyelitis and multiple sclerosis in children. *Brain* 2000;**123**: 2407–2422.

3. Mikaeloff Y, Caridade G, Husson B, Suissa S, Tardieu M, on behalf of the Neuropediatric KIDSEP Study Group of the French Neuropediatric Society. Acute disseminated encephalomyelitis cohort study: Prognostic factors for relapse. *Eur J Paediatr Neurol* 2007;**11**:90–95.

4. Krupp LB, Banwell B, Tenembaum S. Consensus definitions proposed for pediatric multiple sclerosis and related disorders. *Neurology* 2007;**68**(Suppl 2): S7–S12.

5. Cohen I, Steiner-Birmanns B, Biram I, Abramsky O, Honigman S, Steiner I. Recurrence of acute disseminated encephalomyelitis at the previously affected brain site. *Arch Neurol* 2001;**58**:797–801.

6. Miller HG. Acute disseminated encephalomyelitis treated with ACTH. *BMJ* 1953;**1**(4803):177–182.

7. Rose AS, Kuzma JW, Kurtzke JF, Namerow NS, Sibley WA, Tourtellotte WW. Cooperative study in the evaluation of therapy in multiple sclerosis: ACTH vs placebo final report. *Neurology* 1970;**20**:1–59.

8. Pasternak JF, De Vivo DC, Prensky AL. Steroid-responsive encephalomyelitis in childhood. *Neurology* 1980;**30**:481.

9. Beck RW, Cleary PA, Anderson MM, *et al.* A randomized controlled trial of corticosteroids in the treatment of acute optic neuritis. *N Engl J Med* 1992;**326**:581–588.

10. Kurtzke JF. Rating neurologic impairment in multiple sclerosis: An expanded disability status scale (EDSS). *Neurology* 1983;**33**:1444–1452.

11. Sebire G, Hollenberg H, Meyer L, Huault G, Landrieu P, Tardieu M. High dose methylprednisolone in severe acute transverse myelopathy. *Arch Dis Child* 1997;**76**:167–168.

12. Lahat E, Pillar G, Ravid S, Barzilai A, Etzioni A, Shahar E. Rapid recovery from transverse myelopathy in children treated with methylprednisolone. *Pediatr Neurol* 1998;**19**:279–282.

13. Straub J, Chofflon M, Delavelle J. Early high-dose intravenous methylprednisolone in acute disseminated encephalomyelitis: A successful recovery. *Neurology* 1997;**49**:1145–1147.

14. Anlar B, Basaran C, Kose G, *et al.* Acute disseminated encephalomyelitis in children: Outcome and prognosis. *Neuropediatrics* 2003;**34**:194–199.

15. Gupte G, Stonehouse M, Wassmer E, Coad NAG, Whitehouse WP. Acute disseminated encephalomyelitis: A review of 18 cases in childhood. *J Paediatr Child Health* 2003;**39**:336–342.

16. Hynson JL, Kornberg AJ, Colemen LT, Shield L, Harvey AS, Kean MJ. Clinical and neuroradiologic features of acute disseminated encephalomyelitis in children. *Neurology* 2001;**56**:1308–1312.

17. Schmidt J, Gold R, Schonrock L, Zettl UK, Hartung HP, Toyka KV. T-cell apoptosis in situ in experimental autoimmune encephalomyelitis following methylprednisolone pulse therapy. *Brain* 2000;**123**:1431–1441.

18. Sebire G, Delfraissy JF, Demotes-Mainard Oteifeh A, Emilie D, Tardieu M. Interleukin-13 and interleukin-4 act as interleukin-6 inducers in human microglial cells. *Cytokine* 1996;**8**:636–641.

19. Tischner D, Reichardt HM. Glucocorticoids in the control of neuroinflammation. *Molec Cell Endocrinol* 2007;**275**:62–70.

20. Tait AS, Butts CL, Sternberg EM. The role of glucocorticoids and progestins in inflammatory, autoimmune, and infectious disease. *J Leuk Biol* 2008;**84**:924–931.

21. van der Brandt J, Luhder F, McPherson KG, *et al.* Enhanced glucocorticoid receptor signaling in T cells impacts thymocyte apoptosis and adaptive immune responses. *Am J Pathol* 2007;**170**:1041–1053.

22. Thomas GS, Hussain IH. Acute disseminated encephalomyelitis: A report of six cases. *Med J Malaysia* 2004;**59**:324–351.

23. Tenembaum S, Chitnis T, Ness J, Hahn JS, for the International Pediatric MS Study Group. Acute disseminated encephalomyelitis. *Neurology* 2007;**68**:23–36.

24. Richards RN. Side effects of short-term oral corticosteroids. *J Cut Med Surg* 2008;**12**: 77–81.

25. Richards RN. Short-term corticosteroids and avascular necrosis: Medical and legal realities. *Cutis* 2007;**80**:343–348.

26. American College of Rheumatology Ad Hoc Committee on Glucocorticoid-induced Osteoporosis. Recommendations for the prevention and treatment of glucocorticoid-induced osteoporosis. *Arthritis Rheum* 2001;**44**:1496–1503.

27. Leonard MB, Feldman HI, Shults J, Zemel BS, Foster BJ, Stallings VA. Long-term, high-dose glucocorticoids and bone mineral content in childhood glucocorticoid-sensitive nephrotic syndrome. *N Engl J Med* 2004;**351**:868–875.

28. Cohran VC, Griffiths M, Heubi JE. Bone mineral density in children exposed to chronic glucocorticoid therapy. *Clin Pediatr* 2008;**47**:469–475.

29. Munger KL, Levin LL, Hollis BW, *et al*. Serum 25-hydroxyvitamin D levels and risk of multiple sclerosis. *JAMA* 2006;**296**:2832–2838.

30. Hahn JS, Siegler DJ, Enzmann D. Intravenous gammaglobulin therapy in recurrent acute disseminated encephalomyelitis. *Neurology* 1996;**46**:1173–1174.

31. Suppiej A, Vittorini R, Fontanin M, *et al*. Acute disseminated encephalomyelitis in children: Focus on relapsing patients. *Pediatr Neurol* 2008;**39**:12–17.

32. Kleiman M, Brunquell P. Acute disseminated encephalomyelitis: Response to intravenous immunoglobulin? *J Child Neurol* 1995;**10**: 481–483.

33. Nishikawa M, Ichiyama T, Hayashi T, Ouchi K, Furukawa S. Intravenous immunoglobulin therapy in acute disseminated encephalomyelitis. *Pediatr Neurol* 1999;**21**:583–586.

34. Abe Y, Horiuchi A, Miyake M, Kimura S. Anti-cytokine nature of natural human immunoglobulin: One possible mechanism of the clinical effect of intravenous immunoglobulin therapy. *Immunol Rev* 1994;**139**:5–19.

35. Andersson U, Björk L, Skansén-Saphir U, Andersson J. Pooled human IgG modulates cytokine production in lymphocytes and monocytes. *Immunol Rev* 1994;**139**:21–42.

36. Kurlander RJ. Reversible and irreversible loss of Fc receptor function of human monocytes as a consequence of interaction with immunoglobulin G. *J Clin Invest* 1980;**66**:773–781.

37. Kurlander RJ, Hall J. Comparison of intravenous gamma globulin and a monoclonal anti-Fc receptor antibody as inhibitors of immune clearance in vivo in mice. *J Clin Invest* 1986;**77**:2010–2018.

38. Hansen MB, Svenson M, Diamant M, Bendtzen K. High-affinity IgG autoantibodies to IL-6 in sera of normal individuals are competitive inhibitors of IL-6 in vitro. *Cytokine* 1993;**5**:72–80.

39. Svenson M, Hansen MB, Bendtzen K. Binding of cytokines to pharmaceutically prepared human immunoglobulin. *J Clin Invest* 1993;**92**:2533–2539.

40. Basta M, Dalakas MC. High-dose intravenous immunoglobulin exerts its beneficial effect in patients with dermatomyositis by blocking endomysial deposition of activated complement fragments. *J Clin Invest* 1994;**94**:1729–1735.

41. Dietrich G, Kazatchkine MD. Normal immunoglobulin G (IgG) for therapeutic use (intravenous Ig) contain antiidiotypic specificities against an immunodominant, disease-associated cross-reactive idiotype of human anti-thyroglobulin autoantibodies. *J Clin Invest* 1990;**85**:620–625.

42. Obando I, Duran I, Martin-Rosa L, Maria J, Garcia-Martin FJ. Aseptic meningitis due to administration of intravenous immunoglobulin with an usually high number of leukocytes in cerebrospinal fluid. *Pediatr Emerg Care* 2002;**18**:429–432.

43. Shahar E, Andraus J, Savitzki D, Pilar G, Zeinik N. Outcome of severe encephalomyelitis in children: Effect of high-dose methylprednisolone and immunoglobulins. *J Child Neurol* 2002;**17**:810–814.

44. Pradhan S, Gupta R, Shashank S, Pandey N. Intravenous immunoglobulin therapy in acute disseminated encephalomyelitis. *J Neurol Sci* 1999;**165**:56–61.

45. Anonymous. Assessment of plasmapheresis: Report of the Therapeutics and Technology Assessment Subcommittee of the American Academy of Neurology. *Neurology* 1996;**47**:840–843.

46. Weinshenker BG. Therapeutic plasma exchange for acute inflammatory demyelinating syndromes of the central nervous system. *J Clin Apheresis* 1999;**14**:144–148.

47. Weinshenker BG, O'Brien PC, Petterson TM, *et al*. A randomized trial of plasma exchange in acute central nervous system inflammatory demyelinating disease. *Ann Neurol* 1999;**46**:878–886.

48. Weiner HL, Dau PC, Khatri BO, *et al*. Double-blind study of true vs. sham plasma exchange in patients treated with immunosuppression for acute attacks of multiple sclerosis. *Neurology* 1989;**39**:1143–1149.

49. Keegan M, Pineda AA, McClelland RL, Darby CH, Rodriguez M, Weinshenker BG. Plasma exchange for severe attacks of CNS demyelination: Predictors of response. *Neurology* 2002;**58**:143–146.

50. Khurana DS, Melvin JJ, Kothare SV, *et al*. Acute disseminated encephalomyelitis in children: Discordant neurologic and neuroimaging abnormalities and response to plasmapheresis. *Pediatrics* 2005;**116**:431–436.

51. Balestri P, Grosso S, Acquaviva A, Bernini M. Plasmapheresis in a child affected by acute disseminated encephalomyelitis. *Brain Dev* 2000;**22**:123–126.

52. Miyazawa R, Hikima A, Takano Y, Arakawa H, Tomomasa T, Morikawa A. Plasmapheresis in fulminant acute disseminated encephalomyelitis. *Brain Dev* 2001;**23**:424–426.

53. Hung KL, Liao HT, Tsai ML. The spectrum of postinfectious encephalomyelitis. *Brain Dev* 2001;**23**:42–45.

54. Murthy SNK, Faden HS, Cohen ME, Bakshi R. Acute disseminated encephalomyelitis in children. *Pediatrics* 2002;**110**:21–27.

55. Markus R, Brew BJ, Turner J, Pell M. Successful outcome with aggressive treatment of acute haemorrhagic leukoencephalitis. *J Neurol Neurosurg Psychiatry* 1997;**63**:551.

56. Idrissova ZR, Boldyreva MN, Dekonenko EP, *et al.* Acute disseminated encephalomyelitis in children: Clinical features and HLA-DR linkage. *Eur J Neurol* 2003;**10**:537–546.

57. Hahn CD, Miles BS, MacGregor DL, Blaser SI, Banwell BL, Hetherington CR. Neurocognitive outcome after acute disseminated encephalomyelitis. *PediatrNeurol* 2003;**29**:117–123.

58. Omata T, Arai H, Tanabe Y. Child with acute disseminated encephalomyelitis (ADEM) initially presenting with psychiatric symptoms. *[Japanese] No to Hattatsu [Brain and Development]* 2008;**40**:465–468.

59. Brass SD, Caramanos Z, Santos C, Dilenge ME, Lapierre Y, Rosenblatt B. Multiple sclerosis vs. acute disseminated encephalomyelitis in childhood. *PediatrNeurol* 2003;**29**:227–231.

60. Kuperan S, Ostrow P, Landi MK, Bakshi R. Acute hemorrhagic leukoencephalitis vs. ADEM: FLAIR MRI and neuropathology findings. *Neurology* 2003;**60**:721–722.

61. Leake JA, Albani S, Kao AS, *et al.* Acute disseminated encephalomyelitis in childhood: Epidemiologic, clinical, and laboratory features. *Pediatr Infect Dis J* 2004;**23**:756–764.

62. Kimura S, Nezu A, Ohtsuki N, Kobayashi T, Osaka H, Uehara S. Serial magnetic resonance imaging in children with postinfectious encephalitis. *Brain Dev* 1996;**18**:461–465.

63. Murthy JMK, Yangala R, Meena AK, Reddy J. Acute disseminated encephalomyelitis: Clinical and MRI study from south India. *J Neurol Sci* 1999;**165**:133–138.

Chapter

20

Pediatric optic neuritis

Amy T. Waldman and Laura J. Balcer

Introduction

Optic neuritis (ON) is an inflammatory disorder of the optic nerve. Associated with a variety of disorders, ON is most commonly considered a demyelinating disease, and it is often the initial manifestation of multiple sclerosis in children and adults. The incidence of pediatric ON as a first demyelinating event regardless of etiology in Canadian residents is 0.2 per 100 000 children (95% CI 0.16–0.3) [1]. The incidence of pediatric ON in the United States is unknown; however, the prevalence of pediatric multiple sclerosis in the USA is estimated at 1.4–2.5 per 100 000 [2].

Adults with ON have been thoroughly studied through the Optic Neuritis Treatment Trial (ONTT) [3–10]. The ONTT was a multicenter, randomized clinical trial designed to evaluate the efficacy and safety of corticosteroids (intravenous high dose and oral low dose) compared to placebo in adults with acute ON [4]. This trial showed a faster recovery in adults with ON receiving intravenous steroids; however, there were no differences in visual outcome [3]. In contrast, ON in children has been studied primarily through retrospective or small prospective studies at single academic centers, and there is a need for clinical trials in this age group. This chapter will review the presentation of children with ON and compare these children to the 457 adults enrolled across the 15 institutions who participated in the ONTT. Inclusion and exclusion criteria for the ONTT are listed in Table 20.1 for comparison [5]. Of note, 15% of adults enrolled in the ONTT had probable or definite MS at the time of entry into the study [10]. This chapter addresses the potential differences between adult- and pediatric-onset disease and reviews the diagnosis, treatment, and prognosis for ON in children.

Clinical features of pediatric optic neuritis

Optic neuritis in the pediatric age group is diagnosed by the same criteria used in adults, including sudden or sub-acute visual loss, central or cecocentral visual field defect, impairment of color vision, afferent pupillary defect, and ocular pain on eye movements.

The visual symptoms described by adults in the ONTT include scotoma (45%), blurry vision (40%), complete loss of vision (6%), other descriptions (6%), and intermittent blurring (1.3%) [5]. Children typically present with loss of vision (98–100%) [11,12]. Adults may also experience positive visual phenomena such as colors or flashing lights (30%) [5], a finding that has not been systematically reported in children. Ocular pain was present in 92% of adults in the ONTT: mild in 50%, moderate in 38%, and severe in 12% [5]. Eye pain has been reported in 37–77% of children presenting with ON [11–15]. Children often have a preceding illness in the month prior to the onset of visual symptoms [16–18].

Visual acuity is quite variable in children with ON. An affected eye may have a visual acuity of 20/20 or better while others have no light perception. While 64% of adults in the ONTT had visual acuities of 20/190 or better on their initial evaluation [3], the same percentage (64–69%) of children present with visual acuities of 20/200 or worse in retrospective studies [14,19]. Adults were enrolled into the ONTT within 8 days of symptom onset [4], whereas the time elapsed between initial symptoms and ophthalmologic exam is not available for retrospective studies. In addition, it is possible that children do not notice subtle impairments in their visual acuity, thus introducing bias in the direction of poorer vision for children compared to adults. Abnormalities of color vision are frequently

Demyelinating Disorders of the Central Nervous System in Childhood, ed. Dorothée Chabas and Emmanuelle L. Waubant. Published by Cambridge University Press. © Cambridge University Press 2011.

Table 20.1 Inclusion and exclusion criteria for the Optic Neuritis Treatment Trial [5]

Inclusion criteria

1. Presence of acute unilateral optic neuritis of unknown or demyelinating etiology

2. Visual symptoms $\leq$8 days

3. Age 18–46 years

4. Presence of a relative afferent pupillary defect and a visual field defect in the affected eye

Exclusion criteria

1. Treatment for optic neuritis already instituted

2. Previous diagnosis of optic neuritis in the fellow eye or diagnosis of multiple sclerosis for which the patient already received corticosteroids or ACTH

3. Diagnosis or evidence of any systemic condition, other than MS, which might cause optic neuritis, or for which corticosteroids would be contraindicated

4. Previous history consistent with optic neuritis or evidence of optic disc pallor in the currently affected eye

5. Ocular findings suggestive of a nondemyelinating cause for optic neuritis (such as macular exudates, vitreous cells more than trace, or iritis)

6. Pre-existing ocular abnormalities that might affect assessment of visual function

7. Reliability indices (fixation losses, false positives, or false negatives) on Humphrey field analyzer not exceeded in the eye with the best vision (almost always the fellow eye)

8. Painless visual loss associated with disc swelling and either (1) disc or peripapillary hemorrhage, or (2) altitudinal (or other nerve fiber bundle) type visual field defect

9. Myopia measuring >6 D (spherical equivalent) or hyperopia or astigmatism measuring 3 D in the affected eye

10. Narrow angle glaucoma induced by pupillary dilation

11. Intraocular pressure >30 mmHg in the affected eye currently or in the past, with or without treatment

12. Patient receiving medication that may produce retinal or optic nerve toxicity (e.g. ethambutol, plaquenil, phenothiazines)

13. Patient received systemic corticosteroid treatment or corticotrophin for any condition for any duration within the past 3 months or for >7 days within the past 6 months

14. Blood pressure >180 mmHg systolic or 110 mmHg diastolic; heart rate >120/min or presence of a pathologic arrhythmia

15. Blood glucose level >11.1 mmol/l in a patient who is not receiving medical treatment for diabetes (which would exclude the patient)

detected in adults using the Famsworth-Munsell 100-hue test or Ishihara color plates (94 and 88%, respectively) and children using Ishihara or Hardy Rand Rittler plates (86%) [5,14]. An afferent pupillary defect was required for inclusion in the ONTT (further defining unilateral or asymmetrical bilateral disease). An afferent pupillary defect was seen in 53% of children in one study [14], perhaps affected by the frequency of bilateral disease in children (as discussed elsewhere in this chapter).

Inflammation in ON may occur anywhere along the course of the optic nerve. When the inflammation occurs at the papilla, vascular changes or swelling around the optic nerve may be seen on funduscopic exam, and in this case, the term papillitis is used (Figure 20.1). In the ONTT, optic disc swelling and peripapillary hemorrhages were seen in 35% and 6% of adults, respectively [5]. While one pediatric study reported a similar percentage of optic disc swelling (40%) [11], most studies have found a higher

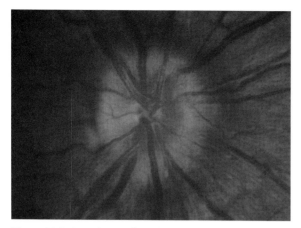

Figure 20.1 Optic disc swelling, also called papillitis, in an adult patient. (Courtesy of Dr. Nicholas J. Volpe, Department of Ophthalmology, University of Pennsylvania School of Medicine, Scheie Eye Institute, Philadephia.) [24,51].

incidence of disc swelling in children (67–69%) [14,19]. Peripapillary hemorrhages are present in 4–21% of children [19,20]. The inflammation in ON may occur in the retrobulbar portion of the nerve, perhaps extending to the optic chiasm. In the case of retrobulbar ON, optic disc swelling is not present clinically. With resolution of the inflammation, the optic disc appears pale; therefore, patients with optic atrophy in the affected eye were excluded from the ONTT as these patients were likely to have had a prior clinical or subclinical event. Pediatric studies have included patients who already had optic nerve atrophy (17–35%) [13,14].

The presence of a visual field defect in the affected eye was required for adults in the ONTT [4]. A central or cecocentral scotoma is often associated with ON in adults and children thus reflecting the central visual acuity loss that characterizes ON in both populations [5,12]. Moreover, many visual field deficits were detected in adults with acute ON in the ONTT, including altitudinal and hemianopic defects [5]. Similar abnormalities were seen in children with ON. Younger children may not be able to cooperate with formal testing [19].

The symptoms and examination findings described above are used to classify the presentation as unilateral or bilateral. However, not all authors have used the same definitions (Table 20.2). Bilateral ON is often further differentiated into bilateral simultaneous ON if both eyes are affected at the same time or within 1–2 weeks [12,13,18,19] or 1

month [22] of each other. If one eye is affected followed by the second eye, the child is diagnosed with bilateral sequential ON [13,18]. Some authors define bilateral sequential ON as both eyes being affected between 2 weeks and 3 months of each other [12,19]. Bilateral recurrent disease has been defined as one or both eyes affected more than once [22]. Adults with unilateral disease only were eligible for the ONTT; however, sub-clinical fellow eye abnormalities were detected, especially visual field abnormalities which were present in the fellow ("normal") eye in 69% of adults [23]. Bilateral disease in children may be defined by clinical symptoms, findings on examination, or radiographic abnormalities (MRI) [19].

Differential diagnosis and evaluation

Optic neuritis is part of a broader category of disorders, collectively referred to as the optic neuropathies, causing dysfunction of the optic nerve. Typically, these disorders present with deficits in visual acuity, color vision, or visual fields. The history and ophthalmologic examination are crucial in identifying the cause of optic nerve dysfunction. A comprehensive list of disorders of the optic nerve can be found in Table 20.3.

Congenital disc anomalies, such as optic disc drusen, optic pits, or optic disc colobomas, may cause decreased visual acuity or visual fields defects [24]. Kjer's dominant optic atrophy causes gradual vision loss in both eyes with variable acuities along with cecocentral scotomas, blue–yellow dyschromatopsia, and temporal pallor of the optic discs [25]. The onset usually occurs in the first decade of life. The family history is important in recognizing Kjer's dominant optic atrophy, although some family members may not recognize subtle deficits in visual acuity, color vision, or visual fields. Kjer's is caused by mutations of the *OPA1* gene located on chromosome 3 (3q28-q29) [26–29]. Leber's hereditary optic neuropathy (LHON) causes painless bilateral simultaneous or sequential vision loss during the second or third decade [30]. LHON also causes a centrocecal scotoma and color vision deficits. Classically, the funduscopic examination reveals tortuosity of the central retinal vessels, circumpapillary telangiectatic microangiopathy, or swelling and hyperemia of the nerve fiber layer [31]. Men are affected more than women. LHON is caused by mutations in mitochondrial DNA with

Table 20.2 Definitions of bilateral and recurrent optic neuritis

Kriss et al. (1988) [18], Lana-Peixoto and de Andrade (2001) [13]	Bilateral simultaneous optic neuritis	Involvement of both eyes at the same time or within a period of 2 weeks
	Bilateral sequential optic neuritis	Involvement of both eyes more than 2 weeks apart
Visudhiphan et al. (1995) [21]	Bilateral optic neuritis	Involvement of both eyes simultaneously or within 1 week
Lucchinetti et al. (1997) [12]	Bilateral simultaneous optic neuritis	Involvement of both eyes immediately or within a period of 2 weeks
	Bilateral sequential optic neuritis	Involvement of both eyes more than 2 weeks but less than 3 months apart
	Recurrent optic neuritis	A second episode of optic neuritis occurring in either eye more than 3 months after the initial event
Brady et al. (1999) [22]	Bilateral simultaneous optic neuritis	Involvement of both eyes within 1 month of each other
	Bilateral recurrent optic neuritis	One or both eyes affected more than once
Wilejto et al. (2006) [14], Alper and Wang (2009) [11]	Bilateral optic neuritis	Involvement of both eyes within 2 weeks of each other
Bonhomme et al. (2009) [19]	Bilateral simultaneous optic neuritis	Involvement of both eyes by clinical features, neuro-ophthalmologic examination, or radiographic features within a period of 2 weeks
	Bilateral sequential optic neuritis	Involvement of both eyes as above between 2 weeks and 3 months of each other
	Recurrent optic neuritis	Relapses of either unilateral or bilateral simultaneous optic neuritis separated by at least 3 months

maternal inheritance. Most patients (95%) have a point mutation in one of three genes (*MT-ND4, MT-ND6, MT-ND1*) encoding complex I subunits of the mitochondrial respiratory chain [32,33]. Genetic testing is commercially available.

Other causes of optic neuropathy include infectious, neoplastic, traumatic, and toxic/metabolic disorders as listed in Table 20.3 [16,19,24,34]. Papilledema is defined as disc swelling due to increased intracranial pressure. Causes of papilledema include pseudotumor cerebri (idiopathic intracranial hypertension), intracranial mass lesions, and sinus venous thrombosis. Papilledema can be differentiated from a swollen disc due to optic neuropathies by history and ophthalmologic examination. Papilledema may be accompanied by other signs of increased intracranial pressure such as headache, nausea and vomiting, and a sixth nerve palsy. Papilledema is typically bilateral whereas optic neuropathies may be unilateral.

Unilateral or bilateral asymmetrical disease of the optic nerve may result in an afferent pupillary defect. Early papilledema may cause a markedly swollen nerve with preservation of visual acuity [24]. Patients with papilledema often have an enlarged blind spot or peripheral field constriction compared with the central or cecocentral deficits seen in optic neuropathies.

Acute demyelinating ON may occur as a clinically isolated syndrome as in adults, or it may be concurrent with widespread demyelination as in acute disseminated encephalomyelitis [35]. According to the International Pediatric Multiple Sclerosis Study Group, acute disseminated encephalomyelitis is a multiphasic/polysymptomatic illness that includes encephalopathy [36]. ON may also be the presenting symptom of MS or neuromyelitis optica (NMO) [14,15,19,37–39] (see Chapters 8 and 23).

The approach to a patient with visual loss begins with a detailed history and careful neuro-ophthalmologic

Table 20.3 The differential diagnosis of optic neuropathy [24]

Congenital/hereditary	Congenital disc anomalies
	Hereditary optic neuropathy
	Kjer's dominant optic atrophy
	Leber's hereditary optic neuropathy
	Recessive optic atrophy
	Wolfram (DIDMOAD) syndrome
Infectious	*Bartonella henselae* bacillus (Cat scratch disease)
	Herpes infections
	Human immunodeficiency syndrome
	Lyme
	Mucocele
	Sinusitis
	Syphilis
	Toxoplasmosis
	Uveitis
Inflammatory/demyelinating	Acute disseminated encephalomyelitis (ADEM)
	Idiopathic optic neuritis
	Juvenile rheumatoid arthritis
	Multiphasic acute disseminated encephalomyelitis
	Multiple sclerosis
	Neuromyelitis optica (Devic's disease)
	Optic perineuritis
	Recurrent acute disseminated encephalomyelitis
	Sarcoidosis
	Sjögren
	Systemic lupus erythematosus
	Uveitis
Neoplastic	Carcinomatous meningitis
	Compressive optic neuropathy
	Pituitary adenomas
	Craniopharyngiomas
	Suprasellar meningioma
	Infiltrative optic neuropathy
	Lymphoma
	Leukemia
	Metastatic tumor
	Optic nerve tumors
	Optic nerve glioma
	Optic nerve sheath meningioma
	Radiation-induced optic neuropathy
Papilledema	Causes of increased intracranial pressure
	Idiopathic intracranial hypertension (pseudotumor cerebri)
	Intracranial mass lesions
	Meningitis
	Sinus venous thrombosis
Toxic/nutritional/metabolic	B12 deficiency
	Charcot Marie Tooth
	Friedreich's ataxia
	Neuronal lipid storage diseases
	Mucopolysaccharidoses
	Olivopontocerebellar atrophy
	Spinocerebellar degeneration (spinocerebellar ataxia)
Medication side effect	Amiodarone
	Cisplatin
	Digitalis
	Isoniazide
	Lead
	Methotrexate
	Organophosphates
	Tacrolimus
	Vincristine
Traumatic	Traumatic optic neuropathy
Vascular	Aneurysm (due to compression)
	Vasculitis

examination. A thorough neurologic examination may be warranted to assess for other signs of demyelination as seen in acute disseminated encephalomyelitis (ADEM), MS, and NMO. The presence of neurologic abnormalities excluding the ON was 36% in one study [14]. In adults with a typical history and classic features of ON, laboratory studies are not necessary [5]. The history and physical examination should be used to direct laboratory testing in atypical cases, such as Lyme titers in a patient with erythema chronicum migrans living in a Lyme-endemic area or a B12 level in patients with pernicious anemia [5].

All patients with ON should undergo neuroimaging (MRI of the brain and orbits with and without contrast) (Figure 20.2). While an MRI of the orbits may be useful to confirm the clinical findings and identify subclinical disease in the fellow eye, an MRI of the brain is often performed to identify T2/FLAIR abnormalities. Abnormalities of the brain excluding the optic nerves have been shown in 38–54% of children presenting with ON [14,19]. Imaging of the spinal cord should be included in patients presenting with widespread demyelination, such as extremity weakness or a sensory level, to assess for longitudinally extensive lesions as seen in NMO. MRI not only provides a useful tool in identifying the extent of the illness, but also has prognostic value as discussed elsewhere in this chapter.

Optic neuritis remains a clinical diagnosis. A lumbar puncture is not required for the diagnosis of isolated ON; however, it may provide supportive evidence in atypical cases. Cerebrospinal fluid analysis is recommended in children suspected of having MS [40]. A few retrospective studies have reported CSF findings in children with acute ON. A pleocytosis in the CSF has been found in up to 70% of children with ON (range 43–70%) [11,14,22]. Approximately 10% of patients have elevated protein in the CSF [11,14]. Among those children tested, oligoclonal bands were present in 11–17% of children [11,14].

Treatment of acute optic neuritis

The treatment of pediatric optic neuritis has not been evaluated through a clinical trial. Only descriptive and cohort studies have been performed in children, and most pediatric studies do not include specific treatment regimens such as the dose and length of therapy. One study reported the use of methylprednisolone 10–30 mg/kg/day (one patient received dexamethasone 8 mg/kg/day) but did not include length of therapy or the use of an oral taper [22].

Despite the lack of data in children, the use of corticosteroids has been thoroughly investigated in adults. In the ONTT, adults were randomized to one of three treatments (Table 20.4) [3]. When each treatment regimen was compared to placebo, patients receiving IV methylprednisolone perhaps recovered from deficits of contrast sensitivity, visual fields, and color vision faster than those in the oral group; however, there was no difference in visual acuity [3]. Moreover, at one year, there was no difference between the groups for any of these outcomes [41]. While early data suggested a decreased risk of developing MS at 2 years in patients receiving IV corticosteroids compared to oral, there was no difference in the risk of developing MS between the groups beyond 3 years [6–8].

In a volunteer survey of pediatric and adult neurologists who treat children with demyelinating diseases, 86% of respondents agreed that acute demyelinating events (not only ON) do not necessarily require treatment (personal communication). The clinical symptoms were the most important factor in the decision to treat an event. All of the respondents use intravenous corticosteroids as first-line therapy for acute ON in children. Weight-based dosing was primarily recommended, although dosing regimens (including the exact mg/kg and frequency) and length of therapy did not reach a consensus in the study. The use of an oral taper was also physician-dependent.

In summary, physicians may treat children with severe or bilateral vision loss less than 8 days in duration, with IV methylprednisolone (15–30 mg/kg/day, maximum of 1 g/day) for 3 days, followed by a 2-week oral taper (beginning with 1 mg/kg/day). While this regimen did not have long-term benefits in adults, it may shorten the duration of some deficits (contrast sensitivity, visual fields, color vision). Patients should be carefully followed for side effects from corticosteroids (see Chapter 8). A pediatric randomized clinical trial is needed in this population.

Prognosis after optic neuritis in childhood

Visual recovery is usually good in children with ON. Despite the poor visual acuity at presentation,

A

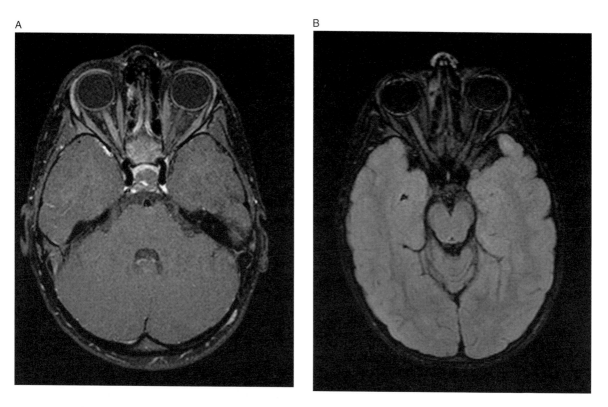

B

C

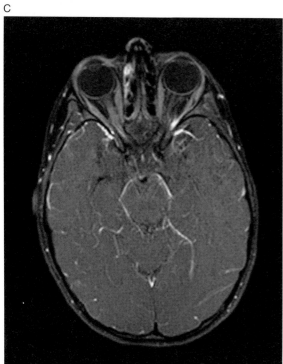

Figure 20.2 MRI of the orbits in a 5-year-old girl who presented with decreased visual acuity (20/200) and decreased color vision in the right eye. Further examination reviewed a right afferent pupillary defect and disc edema. Shown here are the T1-weighted (A), FLAIR (B), and post-contrast images (C) which demonstrate mild enlargement of the intraorbital and intracanalicular segments of the right optic nerve, associated with signal abnormality and enhancement.

Table 20.4 Treatment regimens used in the Optic Neuritis Treatment Trial [3]

Group	Days 1–3	Days 4–14	Days 15–18
IV	Methylprednisolone 250 mg IV every 6 h	Prednisone 1 mg/kg* by mouth daily	Day 15: Prednisone 20 mg
			Day 16: Prednisone 10 mg
			Day 17: None
			Day 18: Prednisone 10 mg
Oral	Prednisone 1 mg/kg* by mouth daily		Day 15: Prednisone 20 mg
			Day 16: Prednisone 10 mg
			Day 17: None
			Day 18: Prednisone 10 mg
Placebo	Placebo given on the same schedule as the oral group		

Note:
* Rounded to the nearest 10 mg

most children (83–96%) have acuities of 20/40 or better at the time of their last follow-up examination [14,19]. In the ONTT, 92% of adults reached 20/40 or better [42]. As for the long-term prognosis, ON can recur in children [16,19]. Moreover, it may be the presenting symptom of MS or NMO [14,19,35,37–39].

The relationship between ON and MS has been more thoroughly investigated in adults than in children. The risk of MS after unilateral ON has been defined in adults. The risk of developing MS within 15 years after unilateral ON is 50% [10]. Using Kaplan–Meier methods and including patients with both bilateral and unilateral disease, Lucchinetti et al. found that the risk of MS is lower in children than adults. The risk of MS was estimated to be 13% at 10 years, 19% by 20 years, 22% by 30 years, and 26% by 40 years [12]. However, retrospective studies have varied widely in determining the risk of developing MS in children after ON. This risk has been estimated from 17 to 36% over an average of 2–7 years [11,14,19]. Furthermore, there are conflicting studies regarding the risk of MS after unilateral compared to bilateral ON. A greater risk of MS after unilateral ON compared with bilateral simultaneous ON was reported by Morales and Riikonen [16,17], whereas bilateral ON was associated with the development of MS according to Wilejto [14]. Lucchinetti reported an increased risk of MS after bilateral sequential or recurrent ON [12].

The risk of developing MS after ON has been further defined in adults using brain MRI. The overall risk of developing MS is 50% at 15 years; however, in adults with a normal MRI at presentation, the risk was 25% at 15 years compared to 72% in those with one or more white matter lesions (measuring at least 3 mm) [10]. Although the risk of MS varies by study, data have also shown a decreased risk of developing MS in children with a normal MRI scan of the brain at presentation. During the follow-up phase of three separate retrospective studies, less than 10% of patients with ON and a normal MRI of the brain developed MS [11,14,19]. One study suggested that a normal MRI of the brain is also associated with a better visual recovery in children [22].

The ONTT has had a tremendous impact on the use of MS therapies (also called immunomodulators or disease-modifying therapies) in adults with ON and other clinically isolated syndromes. Using MRI to identify patients at high risk for MS, multiple adult studies have shown that the initiation of an immunomodulator (such as interferon-beta or glatiramer acetate) after a first clinical event (such as ON) decreases the conversion to clinically definite MS [43,44]. Furthermore, early treatment reduces disease activity as measured by clinical attacks and MRI (including T2 lesion volume and the presence of a new or gadolinium-enhancing lesion) [44–46]. Because of the benefits of early therapy, children with clinically isolated syndromes, such as ON, at high risk for MS may be offered an immunomodulator. One author uses the following criteria to initiate disease-modifying therapy: a child (>12 years of age) with a monosymptomatic presentation (such as ON), multiple white matter lesions on brain MRI, including periventricular perpendicular ovoid lesions, positive CSF for oligoclonal bands, and negative serum NMO IgG antibody [11].

Optical coherence tomography (OCT) is a high-resolution imaging technique that uses near infrared light to quantify the thickness of ocular structures, particularly the retinal nerve fiber layer (RNFL). The RNFL contains nonmyelinated ganglion cell axons. By measuring the average RNFL thickness around the optic disc, as well as the temporal, superior, nasal, and inferior retinal quadrants, OCT provides a method to quantify the axonal and neuronal loss in the anterior visual pathway. In adults, the RNFL thickness is significantly decreased in the eyes of patients with ON and MS. Furthermore, it is also decreased in the apparently unaffected eyes of patients with MS compared to controls [47]. In fact, at autopsy, almost all adults with MS have characteristic changes in the retina and optic nerve, regardless of whether they previously experienced acute ON [48,49]. Children with demyelinating disorders also have axonal loss as measured by OCT. Similar to the adult data, the RNFL thickness is decreased in children with demyelinating diseases (ADEM, transverse myelitis, MS), and it is further decreased in children with a history of ON [50]. While OCT may become a useful tool in the diagnosis and management of ON, OCT is mostly currently available for ON in the research setting.

Conclusion

Optic neuritis in children is diagnosed using the same clinical criteria as applied to adults including deficits in visual acuity, visual fields, and color vision, with or without pain on eye movements, an afferent pupillary defect, or disc swelling. There are some important differences between pediatric and adult ON, some of which may impact the rate and prevalence of MS development in children. Based mostly on case series or cohort studies, children have greater impairments in visual acuity and more often present with bilateral disease compared to adults. Despite these features, most children have excellent visual recovery. Similar to

adults, ON may be a clinically isolated syndrome or may occur in the setting of MS or NMO. MRI is useful in identifying patients at high risk for MS. A normal MRI of the brain at the onset of ON is prognostically favorable. Treatment is based on adult studies and includes short-term (IV corticosteroids followed by an oral taper) and long-term (immunomodulators) therapies, which may hasten some aspects of visual recovery and decrease the disease burden and risk of MS, respectively. Collaborative efforts among pediatric centers are needed to further explore the clinical presentation, treatment, and prognosis of pediatric ON.

References

1. Banwell B, Kennedy J, Sadovnick D, et al. Incidence of acquired demyelination of the CNS in Canadian children. Neurology 2009;72:232–239.

2. Gadoth N. Multiple sclerosis in children. Brain Dev 2003;25:229–232.

3. Beck RW, Cleary PA, Anderson MM, et al. A randomized controlled trial of corticosteroids in the treatment of acute optic neuritis. N Engl J Med 1992;326:581–588.

4. Cleary PA, Beck RW, Anderson MM, et al. Design, methods, and conduct of the Optic Neuritis Treatment Trial. Contr Clin Trials 1993;14:123–142.

5. Optic Neuritis Study Group. The clinical profile of optic neuritis: Experience of the Optic Neuritis Treatment Trial. Arch Ophthalmol 1991;109: 1673–1678.

6. Optic Neuritis Study Group. The 5-year risk of MS after optic neuritis: Experience of the Optic Neuritis Treatment Trial. Neurology 1997;79: 1404–1413.

7. Optic Neuritis Study Group. Visual function 5 years after optic neuritis: Experience of the Optic Neuritis Treatment Trial. Arch Ophthalmol 1997;115: 1545–1552.

8. Optic Neuritis Study Group. High- and low-risk profiles for the development of multiple sclerosis within 10 years after optic neuritis. Arch Ophthalmol 2003;121:944–949.

9. Optic Neuritis Study Group. Neurologic impairment 10 years after optic neuritis. Arch Neurol 2004;61:1386–1389.

10. Optic Neuritis Study Group. Multiple sclerosis risk after optic neuritis: Final Optic Neuritis Treatment Trial follow-up. Arch Neurol 2008;65: 727–732.

11. Alper G, Wang L. Demyelinating optic neuritis in children. J Child Neurol 2009;24:45–48.

12. Lucchinetti CF, Kiers L, O'Duffy A, *et al.* Risk factors for developing multiple sclerosis after childhood optic neuritis. *Neurology* 1997;**49**:1413–1418.

13. Lana-Peixoto MA, de Andrade GC. The clinical profile of childhood optic neuritis. *Arq Neuropsiquiatr* 2001;**59**:311–317.

14. Wilejto M, Shroff M, Buncic JR, *et al.* The clinical features, MRI findings, and outcome of optic neuritis in children. *Neurology* 2006;**67**:258–292.

15. Kennedy C, Carter S. Relation of optic neuritis to multiple sclerosis in children. *Pediatrics* 1961;**28**:377–387.

16. Morales DS, Siatkowski M, Howard CW, *et al.* Optic neuritis in children. *J Pediatr Ophthalmol Strabismus* 2000;**37**:254–259.

17. Riikonen R, Donner M, Erkkila H. Optic neuritis in children and its relationship to multiple sclerosis: A clinical study of 21 children. *Dev Med Child Neurol* 1988;**30**:349–359.

18. Kriss A, Francis DA, Cuendet F, *et al.* Recovery after optic neuritis in childhood. *J Neurol Neurosurg Psychiatry* 1988;**51**:1253–1258.

19. Bonhomme GR, Waldman AT, Balcer LJ, *et al.* Pediatric optic neuritis: Brain MRI abnormalities and risk of multiple sclerosis. *Neurology* 2009;**72**:881–885.

20. Parkin PJ, Hierons R, McDonald WI. Bilateral optic neuritis: A long-term follow-up. *Brain* 1984;**107**:951–964.

21. Visudhiphan P, Chiemchanya S, Santadusit S. Optic neuritis in children: Recurrence and subsequent development of multiple sclerosis. *Pediatr Neurol* 1995;**13**:293–295.

22. Brady KM, Brar AS, Lee AG, *et al.* Optic neuritis in children: Clinical features and visual outcome. *J AAPOS* 1999;**3**:98–103.

23. Keltner JL, Johnson CA, Spurr JO, *et al.* Baseline visual field profile of optic neuritis: The experience of the Optic Neuritis Treatment Trial. *Arch Ophthalmol* 1993;**111**:231–234.

24. Liu GT, Volpe NJ, Galetta SL. Visual loss: Optic neuropathies. In *Neuro-ophthalmology: Diagnosis and Management.* 2nd edn. London, UK: Saunders Elsevier; 2010:103–198.

25. Kjer P. Infantile optic neuropathy with dominant mode of inheritance: A clinical and genetic study of 19 Danish families. *Acta Ophthalmol* 1959;**37** (suppl 54):1–46.

26. Alexander C, Votruba M, Pesch UE, *et al.* OPA1, encoding a dynamin-related GTPase, is mutated in autosomal dominant optic atrophy linked to chromosome 3q28. *Nat Genet* 2000;**26**:211–215.

27. Delettre C, Lenaers G, Griffoin JM, *et al.* Nuclear gene OPA1, encoding a mitochondrial dynamin-related protein, is mutated in dominant optic atrophy. *Nat Genet* 2000;**26**:207–210.

28. Eiberg H, Kjer B, Kjer P, *et al.* Dominant optic atrophy (OPA1) mapped to chromosome 3q region, I. *Hum Mol Genet* 1994;**3**:977–980.

29. Kjer B, Eiberg H, Kjer P, *et al.* Dominant optic atrophy mapped to chromosome 3q region. II. Clinical and epidemiological aspects. *Acta Ophthalmol Scand* 1996;**74**:3–7.

30. Leber T. Ueber hereditaere und congenital angelegte sehnervenleiden. *Graefes Arch Clin Exp Ophthalmol* 1871;**17**:249–291.

31. Smith JL, Hoyt WF, Susac JO. Ocular fundus in acute Leber optic neuropathy. *Arch Ophthalmol* 1973;**90**:349–354.

32. Man PYW, Turnbull DM, Chinnery PF. Leber hereditary optic neuropathy. *J Med Genet* 2002;**39**:162–169.

33. Yu-Wai-Man P, Chinnery PF. Leber hereditary optic neuropathy. 2008. Available online at: http://www.ncbi.nlm.nih.gov/bookshelf/br.fcgi?book=gene&part=lhon. (Accessed 2 February 2010.)

34. Cassidy L, Taylor D. Pediatric optic neuritis. *J AAPOS* 1999;**3**:68–69.

35. Dale RC, de Soussa C, Chong WK, *et al.* Acute disseminated encephalomyelitis, multiphasic disseminated encephalomyelitis and multiple sclerosis in children. *Brain* 2000;**123**:2407–2422.

36. Krupp LB, Banwell B, Tenembaum S, for the International Pediatric MS Study Group. Consensus definitions proposed for pediatric multiple sclerosis and related disorders. *Neurology* 2007;**68**:7–12.

37. Boiko A, Vorobeychik G, Paty D, *et al.* Early onset multiple sclerosis: A longitudinal study. *Neurology* 2002;**59**:1006–1010.

38. Duquette P, Murray TJ, Pleines J, *et al.* Multiple sclerosis in childhood: Clinical profile in 125 patients. *J Pediatr* 1987;**111**:359–363.

39. Sindern E, Haas J, Stark E, *et al.* Early onset MS under the age of 16: clinical and paraclinical features. *Acta Neurol Scand* 1992;**86**:280–284.

40. Hahn S, Pohl D, Rensel M, Rao S, for the International Pediatric MS Study Group. Differential diagnosis and evaluation in pediatric multiple sclerosis. *Neurology* 2007;**68**:13–22.

41. Beck, RW, Cleary, PA, and the Optic Neuritis Study Group. Optic neuritis treatment trial: One-year follow-up results. *Arch Ophthalmol* 1993;**111**:773–775.

42. Optic Neuritis Study Group. Visual function 15 years after optic neuritis: A final follow-up report from the Optic Neuritis Treatment Trial. *Ophthalmology* 2008;**115**:1079–1082.

43. CHAMPIONS Study Group. IM interferon beta-1a delays definite MS 5 years after a first demyelinating event. *Neurology* 2006;**66**:678–684.

44. Comi G, Filippi M, Barkhof F, *et al*. Effect of early IFN treatment on conversion to definite MS. *Lancet* 2001;**357**:1576–1582.

45. Kappos L, Polman CH, Freedman MS, *et al*. Treatment with interferon beta-1b delays conversion to clinically definite and McDonald MS in patients with clinically isolated syndromes. *Neurology* 2006;**67**:1242–1249.

46. Comi G, Martinelli, V, Rodegher M. Effect of glatiramer acetate on conversion to clinically definite multiple sclerosis in patients with clinically isolated syndrome (PreCISe study): A randomized double-blind, placebo-controlled trial. *Lancet* 2009; **374**:1503–1511.

47. Fisher JB, Jacobs DA, Markowitz CE, *et al*. Relation of visual function to retinal nerve fiber layer thickness in multiple sclerosis. *Ophthalmology* 2009; **113**:324–332.

48. Ikuta F, Zimmerman HM. Distribution of plaques in seventy autopsy cases of multiple sclerosis in the United States. *Neurology* 1976;**26**:26–28.

49. Toussaint D, Perier O, Verstappen A, *et al*. Clinicopathological study of the visual pathways, eyes, and cerebral hemispheres in 32 cases of disseminated sclerosis. *J Clin Neuroophthalmol* 1983;**3**:211–222.

50. Yeh EA, Weinstock-Guttman B, Lincoff N, *et al*. Retinal nerve fiber layer thickness in inflammatory demyelinating diseases of childhood onset. *Mult Scler* 2009;**15**:802–810.

51. Balcer LJ. Optic neuritis. *N Engl J Med* 2006; **354**:1273–1280.

Recurrent isolated optic neuritis in the pediatric population

Bianca Weinstock-Guttman and Grant T. Liu

Introduction

Optic neuritis (ON) is an inflammatory disorder of the optic nerve characterized by loss or dimming of vision that typically progresses over several days, frequently preceded by ocular pain and followed usually by recovery over a period of weeks to months. In contrast to adults, children with ON often present with bilateral optic nerve involvement, profound visual loss, and prominent disc swelling [1]. Despite the severe visual loss during the acute events, the recovery rate is usually excellent (over 80% with complete recovery) [1–3].

The etiology of ON in childhood is most often post-infectious, a preceding viral infection being reported between 16 and 46% [5–7] The differential diagnosis of ON in the pediatric population should also include other causes of acute and sub-acute optic neuropathies such as systemic vasculitis (systemic lupus erythematosis, Sjögren's disease), granulomatous diseases (sarcoidosis), toxic, and metabolic causes, compressive or infiltrative lesions (meningioma, glioma), as well as mitochondrial and other genetic abnormalities, especially in cases of progressive visual loss or recurrent events [2,5–7]. A more detailed description of ON and its differential diagnosis can be found in Chapter 20.

Recurrent optic neuritis

A sub-group of patients following an initial episode of ON may experience recurrent events of ON (RON) without clinical evidence of a systemic disease or other areas of CNS involvement. This entity of RON was classified as MS in earlier studies [8,9]. During the last decades, along with the advance in neuroimaging and development of new biological markers as the NMO-IgG antibodies for neuromyelitis optica

(NMO), it became evident that while some patients convert to MS or NMO, the clinical presentation and often the prognosis differs from patients with isolated ON. Recurrent ON is less well characterized in the published pediatric ON series. The cohorts are usually small and the reports focus primarily on the risk ascertainment of conversion to MS, or more recently to NMO [2,10]. As previously mentioned, the recovery of ON, is usually very good in the pediatric series that often includes a few RON cases.

The incidence of RON in the adult population is low. Using the central record system of the Mayo Clinic, Pirko and colleagues identified 72 patients with RON (5.7%) out of 1274 patients with a first episode of ON seen at Mayo between 1994 and 2000. All patients had normal brain and spinal cord MRI scans at the time of their first and second ON events. The risk of conversion to MS or NMO within the 5-year reported follow-up was 12 and 14.4%, respectively. The "non-converters", i.e. those who remained RON (two-thirds of this group), presented with a more severe disease (worse visual loss, seen from the first event), similar to that seen in NMO patients. However, at the time of the aforementioned publication, the NMO diagnosis was made according to the initial Wingerchuck criteria (i.e. before the availability of NMO-IgG testing). Thus, the diagnosis required having optic nerve and longitudinal extensive spinal cord involvement/transverse myelitis (LETM).

The chronic recurrent inflammatory optic neuritis (CRION) recently described in an adult population by Kidd *et al.* refers to an even more limited and particular type of recurrent ON [11]. The clinical characteristics differ somewhat from the classical demyelinating optic neuropathy with respect to the severity of visual loss (65% of patients have a reduced

Demyelinating Disorders of the Central Nervous System in Childhood, ed. Dorothée Chabas and Emmanuelle L. Waubant. Published by Cambridge University Press. © Cambridge University Press 2011.

acuity in the worse affected eye of 20/200 or lower) and pain, its persistence after onset of the visual loss, and the relapsing and steroid-dependent nature of the disease. The prevalence of this entity in the pediatric population is much lower, usually being reported as isolated cases within the ON pediatric series. Nevertheless, RON in general requires an accurate, timely diagnosis in the pediatric as well as in the adult group, as the therapeutic intervention is different than for the typical isolated ON (see later in the therapy section).

Recurrent ON in the pediatric population

Discrepancies across pediatric ON reports may occur more frequently than in the adult ON series. This may be mostly related to the smaller sample size and shorter follow-up in the pediatric group, notwithstanding the lack of standardized definitions across studies. For example, simultaneous bilateral vs. sequential ON cutoff period varies between 2 and 4 weeks; recurrent disease varies between 1 and 3 months. Finally, a referral bias may also contribute to these differences [3,10,12] (see Chapters 20 and 23).

In the pediatric Mayo Clinic series, Lucchinetti and colleagues identified 79 pediatric patients (less than 16 years of age) who presented with an initial isolated ON. Only 3% of these cases presented with recurrent ON. Using life-table analysis, 13% of the ON patients progressed to clinically or laboratory-supported definite MS by 10 years of follow-up, and 19% by 20 years. Gender, age, fundus findings, visual acuity, or family history of either ON or MS were not associated with the development of MS. However, the presence of bilateral sequential or RON increased the risk of developing MS ($p = 0.002$; hazard ratio = 5.09; 95% CI 1.84–14.06) [10]. This latter finding was not reproduced in the most recent studies, and therefore these data should be interpreted with caution, especially since no brain MRI data were available [2–4].

In the series reported by Kriss and colleagues that included 39 children (age range 3–15 (mean 8.6 years)) who presented with an initial ON, and were followed for a mean of 8.8 years (range 3 months to 29 years), six patients (15%) developed MS [4]. Four patients (10%), two with an initial unilateral ON and two with an initial bilateral ON, had one or more recurrent attacks of isolated ON. Only one of these patients developed further evidence of MS,

suggesting a lower risk for MS in this RON cohort. Referral bias as pediatric neurology outpatient setting vs. MS clinics can partially explain the contradictory results.

Another recent Turkish pediatric ON series evaluated the records of 31 children (aged 4–15 years) who were followed for a mean of 2.2 years (range 6 months to 15 years), 8/31 (25%) of whom ultimately received a diagnosis of MS. An increased risk of developing MS was associated with presence of unilateral ON and female gender [2]. Seven patients (22.5%) of the cohort developed RON before a final diagnosis was established; two developed MS, two NMO, one Sjögren's disease, and two patients remained RON during a three-year follow-up period. The recovery in the RON sub-group was reported as partial or poor in 3/7 patients (43%), while only 2/24 (8%) within the isolated ON group had a poor or incomplete recovery – both cases actually being later diagnosed with an underlying mitochondrial dysfunction and ischemic ON, respectively.

A Canadian study reported on 36 children (female/male ratio 1.6; ages 2.2–17.8 years (mean 12.2 years) with unilateral ON in 58% and bilateral ON in 42% of the patients, 69% of whom had a severe visual deficit (visual acuity (VA) <20/200). However, full or almost full (>20/40) recovery occurred in 83% (39/47 affected eyes). Seven patients (19%) had recurrent ON events in addition to other CNS events and were later diagnosed with MS [3].

A more recent study reviewing data available from Children's Hospital of Philadelphia (CHOP) identified 29 children with an initial idiopathic ON, of whom 38% had white matter T2-bright foci on their brain MRI [1]. Nine patients (31%) had relapses of ON during the study period and five had more than one relapse. The pattern and location of the recurrent episodes showed no specific pattern. For example, three patients who initially presented with bilateral ON had subsequent unilateral relapses. In contrast, the remaining six patients presented with unilateral optic neuritis, half of whom ultimately met criteria for bilateral sequential ON and the other half for RON. Of the nine patients with RON, two developed MS. The relative risk of developing MS among patients with RON was 4.0 ($p = 0.25$). It is unclear whether this will be confirmed in larger cohorts. Patients with bilateral simultaneous or sequential ON did not have a greater risk of MS compared to patients presenting with unilateral disease ($p = 0.53$).

The recovery rate was also, in general, very good, as reported in the previous pediatric ON series. Although at initial presentation 89% of affected eyes (40 out of 45 eyes) exhibited impaired visual acuities, quantified by Snellen, or the H-O-T-V, or Lea charts for pre-schoolers, worse than 20/25, at the time of last follow-up examination (median of 36 months) 96% of affected eyes (47 of 49 eyes, including four initially normal eyes affected by ON during the study period) had visual acuities that were 20/40 or better. In contrast, at the time of last follow-up, 3/9 (33%) within the RON group had a VA of 20/40 or worse, while only 1/19 (5%) of the isolated ON cases was left with a VA of 20/40, suggesting that RON is associated with a more severe and cumulative destructive process to the optic nerve [1]. The worst outcome (VA 20/200) was seen in the patient with three recurrent events.

As part of a prospective natural history study at the Pediatric MS Center of the Jacobs Neurological Institute, Buffalo, NY, one of the centers of the US Pediatric MS Network, we studied consecutive children under 18 years of age who had at least one documented clinical episode of an acquired demyelinating event. Within 3 years (2006–2008), 17 of 75 patients had ON as their first demyelinating event (mean follow-up of 25.2 months from event onset, range 3 months to 10 years) (Weinstock-Guttman, personal communication; partly reported in [13]). Within this time frame, seven of the 17 (41%) patients with an initial ON developed MS and six remained isolated ON. Eight of 17 (47%) had recurrent ON events. Four of these eight patients with RON (50%) developed MS after the second ON, all of whom had abnormal brain MRI at presentation. While none of the four patients with RON who did not convert to MS developed NMO or had positive NMO-IgG antibodies, two fulfilled the diagnosis of CRION characterized by recurrent severe ON (VA ≤20/40) and clear steroid dependence without evidence of a systemic autoimmune disease. None of these patients (RON and CRION) had an abnormal brain MRI. The initial presentation was bilateral in four of the seven (57%) cases that converted to MS. Within the isolated ON, three presented with bilateral and three with unilateral ON, while in the RON group three of four (75%) presented with bilateral ON. Most of the subsequent episodes were unilateral. Although at presentation the majority of patients presented with a VA worse than 20/50 (13/17; 76%), the recovery was very good (VA of 20/30 or better) in 13 of 17 (76%)

patients. Only four patients remained with a VA of 20/50 or worse; three (75%) were RON and one converted to MS. Our findings are very similar to the children from the CHOP report, suggesting a worse visual prognosis in the RON group.

Recurrent ON and NMO-IgG antibodies

The discovery of NMO-IgG serum autoantibody that binds to the CNS-dominant water channel, aquaporin-4 with its well-defined high sensitivity (73%) and specificity (92%) for NMO, opened a new era and brought hope for the future identification of potential new biomarkers within the heterogeneous class of inflammatory demyelinating diseases of the CNS [14–16]. For instance, recent studies identified a 20–25% seroprevalence of NMO-IgG among adult patients presenting with isolated RON without myelopathy [17,18]. The visual disability recorded for patients in both of these publications was worse than previously reported for patients with ON. The initial ON episode was more severe in NMO-IgG seropositive patients ($p = 0.05$) and VA in the affected eye was worse than 20/200 at the nadir in all seropositive patients compared to 64.7% in seronegative patients ($p = 0.05$) [17]. Similarly, the mean final visual status score was worse in the seropositive compared to seronegative group (10.22±9.0 vs. 6.38±1.0, $p = 0.02$). The number of RON patients who converted to NMO was higher in the NMO antibody-positive group (3/6, 50%) than in the NMO antibody-negative group (2/18, 11.1%) ($p > 0.05$). The MRI of the optic nerve in NMO patients is usually associated with nerve swelling and gadolinium enhancement, often followed by optic nerve atrophy. As seen in Figures 21.1A, B, the recurring events can affect each eye separately within an interval of a few months.

In a recent international collaborative study, Banwell and colleges studied the clinical, radiologic, and serum NMO-IgG status in 87 children: 41 with relapsing–remitting multiple sclerosis (RRMS), 17 with NMO, and the rest with a first isolated demyelinating syndrome [19]. Ten of the 87 children (11%) were seropositive for the NMO-IgG, of whom eight were within the 17 NMO cases (47%). This series also included 13 patients with ON (8 with isolated and five with recurrent ON). Only one of the five children with RON had positive NMO-IgG (20%), similar to the 20–25% frequency reported for adult patients with RON [17], supporting the concept that this disorder has a similar

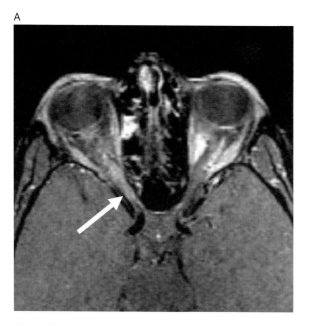
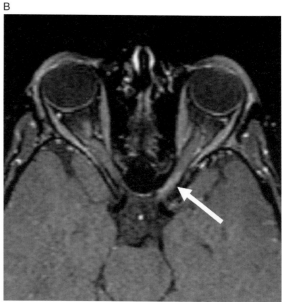

Figure 21.1 Recurrent optic neuritis in a child with NMO-Ab. (A) Optic neuritis in the right eye, February 2007. Axial gadolinium-enhanced brain MRI demonstrating right optic nerve swelling with enhancement (arrow). (B) Optic neuritis in the left eye, June 2007. Axial gadolinium-enhanced brain MRI demonstrating left optic nerve enhancement (arrow) and resolution of the right optic nerve enhancement.

pathogenesis in childhood and adulthood. No seropositive cases were identified among the 41 patients with RRMS (14% of whom developed longitudinal extensive myelitis at some point in their clinical course). The presence, although rare, of NMO-IgG in the RON group especially when associated with severe irreversible damage emphasizes the importance of testing for NMO-IgG in this group of patients.

Most of the pediatric RON cases are not associated with the presence of oligoclonal bands (OCB). The reported cases with available CSF data usually displayed an increased white blood cell count and sometimes increased total proteins [4,10]. CSF evaluation in most of the reported pediatric RON series was less informative in predicting the conversion to MS, especially at the time of the initial presentation. A few of the cases that were followed and converted to MS did later develop OCB, although this was not seen at the time of their first event. This might, in part, be related to age at disease onset as reported by the US Pediatric MS Network [20].

Optical coherence tomography in RON

Objective evidence of damage to the visual pathways in MS may also be found using optical coherence tomography (OCT) [21–23]. OCT is a new technology that uses infrared light to produce cross-sectional images of the retina, with high-resolution images of the retinal nerve fiber layer (RNFL, which contains only non-myelinated axons) and macula [21] (see more on the OCT and ON in Chapter 20).

In the adult RON series, Matiello and collegues used OCT in an attempt to discriminate between the different types of ON. Interestingly, the only difference they found was a greater RNFL reduction observed in NMO antibody-positive compared with negative patients, although not statistically different probably due to the small sample size [17]. The more substantial loss of RNFL in NMO antibody-positive patients is in line with a more severe axonal damage already suspected from the worse visual outcome in NMO patients.

In a recent study, our group evaluated 38 consecutive pediatric patients (74 eyes) diagnosed with a demyelinating inflammatory process with OCT [13]. All patients were evaluated during stable disease usually 1 month or more following an acute attack of ON. The demographic and clinical characteristics of our control and patient populations are summarized in Table 21.1. Children with comorbid ocular conditions

Table 21.1 Clinical and demographic characteristics of the cohort

Characteristic	All patients	MS	ADEM/TM	ON	CRION
N	38	17	12	7	2
Females:Males (% Female)	23:15 (61%)	11:6 (65%)	4:8 (33%)	6:1 (86%)	2 (100%)
Age, years	13.3±3.9	14.3±3.0	10.6±5.0	14.9±1.7	14.7±1.2
Age of onset, years	10.1±4.4	11.6±3.6	7.0±4.9	12.7±2.1	8.0±1.4
Number with history of ON	19 (50%)	7 (41%)	3 (25%)	7 (100%)	2 (100%)
Number with recurrent disease	23 (61%)	17 (100%)	2 (20%)	1 (14%)	2 (100%)
EDSS*	1.0±1.0	1.5±1.0	1.25±2.0	1.0±1.0	2.0

Note:
* Data are mean ± SD, except for EDSS, which is expressed as median ± inter-quartile range.

Table 21.2 Visual acuity (VA) and low-contrast letter acuity (LCLA) parameters of the cohort

Group	VA LogMAR		LCLA LogMAR	
	Unaffected	Affected	Unaffected	Affected
Healthy controls	−0.06±0.06 [13]	–	0.44±0.15 [13]	–
ON	0.1 [10]	0.23±0.21 [11]	0.80 [10]	0.80±0.14 [11]
MS	0.018±0.11 [8]	0.17±0.23 [3]	0.63±0.21 [9]	0.50±0.22 [28]
ADEM/TM	0.18±0.27 [9]	–	0.46±0.097 [7]	–
CRION	–	0.5±0.12 [28]	–	0.95±0.07 [1]

Note:
* Average of both eyes for patients unaffected by optic neuritis.
Data are mean ± SD (number of eyes).

not related to MS, significant refractive errors (±5 diopters) and previously known history of retinal pathology (i.e. diabetic retinopathy) as ascertained by a detailed history and examination were excluded. Three of 38 patients had RON and two additional patients had an initial ADEM with ON followed by recurrent episodes of demyelination without recurrent encephalopathy.

All children underwent a complete ophthalmologic evaluation including pupillary and fundus examination, assessment of best-corrected visual acuity (using Snellen charts). All patients and controls had additional visual testing using Low Contrast Letter Acuity (LCLA) charts, OCT, and pattern reversed visual evoked potentials (PRVEP) testing shown previously to be useful in monitoring visual function and outcomes in the adult population [24,25]. Visual acuity, as measured using Snellen and LCLA 2.5%

charts (converted to LogMAR scores, where lower scores represent better VA), was affected in this cohort (see Table 21.2). LCLA 2.5% testing in affected eyes was worse than controls in all the disease groups, being worse in the CRION group (Table 21.2).

Average retinal nerve fiber layer thickness (RNFLT) of affected eyes in all children with a clinical history of ON was lower (77±18 μm) compared to the healthy controls (107±12 μm) ($n = 30$) and the other neurological disorder controls (108±5 μm) ($n = 10$) (Figure 21.2). In children with MS, average RNFLT±SD was 99±14 μm in unaffected ($n = 24$) vs. 83±12 μm in ON-affected eyes ($n = 10$). The lowest RNFLT was found in the CRION group (50±2 μm) and the ADEM/TM group (67±17 μm). The average RNFLT of the three RON cases (2 CRION+1 RON) was 59.8±SD 16.4 μm. The ADEM/TM group consisted of ADEM patients with ON (the TM also had

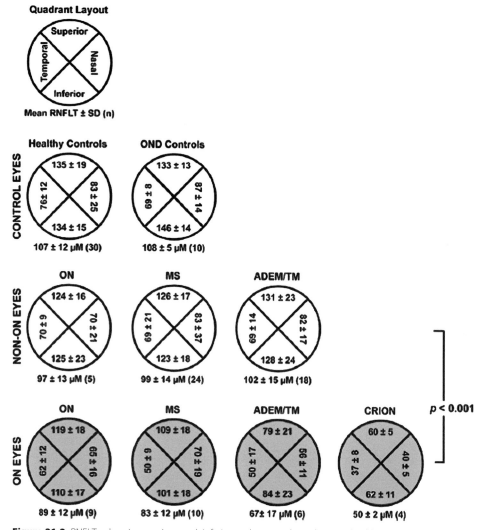

Figure 21.2 RNFLT values in superior, nasal, inferior, and temporal quadrants in healthy controls, OND controls, ON, MS, ADEM/TM, and CRION. Mean RNFLT±SD is shown below each circle. RNFLT values of unaffected eyes are in white and affected eyes in gray bars.

extensive brain lesions but did not have encephalopathy at presentation so did not fulfill the new ADEM criteria) [26]. Differences between the groups were statistically significant ($p<0.001$) (see Figure 21.2).

Although based on a small number, the CRION group appeared to differ from the other groups. The quadrant-wise averages for affected and unaffected eyes are summarized in Figure 21.2. As demonstrated in this figure, different patterns of decrease in RNFLT can be found in ON vs. MS vs. ADEM/TM and CRION. Macula volume was 7.1±0.57 μm in normal controls and 7.1±0.54 μm in OND controls. It was markedly lower in the affected eyes of children with ADEM/TM (6.2±0.19) and CRION (6.0±0.52 μm),

suggesting a more widespread and destructive disease process in CRION and ADEM affecting the retinal ganglion cells which are known to be primarily located in the macula. Average RNFLT decreased with increasing number of episodes of ON (Figure 21.3), suggesting that minor changes secondary to a single insult to the optic nerve may be picked up using serial OCTs.

The tissue loss in CRION/RON and ADEM in our small cohort appear more widespread as it affects all the quadrants in contrast to the preferential temporal quadrant involvement seen in MS. This distinct pattern suggests a different underlying pathobiology. These findings need to be confirmed on larger

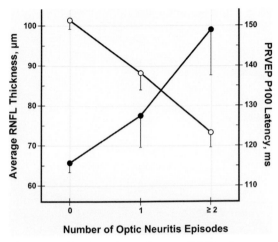

Figure 21.3 The dependence of average RNFLT and pattern reversed evoked potentials (PRVEP) on the number of optic neuritis episodes. The error bars are standard errors of the mean.

cohorts. OCT may serve as a diagnostic tool and surrogate marker for axonal loss/preservation in this population.

Therapy for RON

The therapeutic prerequisite for RON entails a double target: therapy for the acute events as well as the consideration for preventive or disease-modifying therapy (DMT). Isolated episodes of ON in the pediatric population are usually treated with steroids, although this is still controversial, similar to the adult population (see Chapter 20). Considering the relatively benign nature of pulse steroid therapy, most clinicians recommend it for ON in children, despite the fact that no clear benefit on final visual outcome has been established through randomized placebo-controlled adult clinical trials [2,12,27] (see Chapters 9 and 20 for more details on the treatment of ON).

In Kidd's adult series of CRION the treatment recommended is different from the isolated ON therapy and the outcome without treatment is likely very poor [11]. The standard treatment regimen used for MS relapses (see Chapter 9) may not be adequate for this condition; prolonged oral steroid taper may be necessary, with careful monitoring by the clinician for evidence of relapse [11].

The need for preventive therapy for RON remains controversial. As previously shown a certain percentage of RON cases may ultimately be diagnosed with MS or NMO. For these cases, the appropriate therapy should be considered (see Chapters 10 and 23). No specific recommendations are established for the other cases of RON, although most of the reports suggest to use immunosuppressive therapy (i.e. azathioprine, mycophenolate mofetil, cyclophosphamide) [2,11,18]. Anecdotal cases including our group's experience suggest a beneficial effect for IVIg therapy in the recovery from the acute events and a trend to decreased severity and partial benefit in preventing recurrent events. This needs to be confirmed on larger series. From the Buffalo author's practice the four RON cases (presenting with more than two recurrences) were initially treated with pulsed IV glucocorticosteroids but had incomplete or limited recovery (VA of 20/50 or worse 2 weeks after treatment). Two patients required longer oral steroid taper (more than 4 weeks) because of worsening symptoms after steroid discontinuation and were diagnosed with CRION. All patients were given an additional 2 g of IVIg, followed by monthly IVIg 0.4 g/kg for 6 months. Three of the four CRION patients stabilized and improved during IVIg therapy, not requiring further steroid or other preventive therapy (mean follow-up of 18 months). However, the other CRION patient required continuous immunosuppression consisting of low-dose oral steroids and mycophenolate mofetil 1000 mg bid. No specific conclusions or recommendations can be determined from these small case series in the absence of controlled trials.

Conclusions and future directions

RON remains a challenging diagnosis, in part due to its rarity within the large group of acquired demyelinating diseases of the CNS affecting the adult and pediatric populations. The risk of conversion to MS or NMO from RON is relatively low (approximately 20%), being primarily influenced by the presence of brain MRI lesions or of NMO-IgG antibodies, respectively. Although pediatric, like adult, RON is associated with a more severe and cumulative destructive process to the optic nerve often identified from the initial bout, the consideration of initiating preventive therapy and the timing and type of therapy remain controversial. Therefore, prospective data on larger cohorts using more sensitive surrogate outcome measures (i.e. NMO-IgG and OCT) will be helpful in better characterizing this entity as well as providing a more appropriate, scientific therapeutic approach.

References

1. Bonhomme GR, Waldman AT, Balcer LJ, *et al*. Pediatric optic neuritis: Brain MRI abnormalities and risk of multiple sclerosis. *Neurology* 2009;**72**:881–885.

2. Cakmakli G, Kurne A, Guven A, *et al*. Childhood optic neuritis: The pediatric neurologist's perspective. *Eur J Paediatr Neurol* 2009;**13**:452–457.

3. Wilejto M, Shroff M, Buncic JR, Kennedy J, Goia C, Banwell B. The clinical features, MRI findings, and outcome of optic neuritis in children. *Neurology* 2006;**67**:258–262.

4. Kriss A, Francis DA, Cuendet F, *et al*. Recovery after optic neuritis in childhood. *J Neurol Neurosurg Psychiatry* 1988;**51**:1253–1258.

5. Chen YH, Wang AG, Lin YC, Yen MY. Optic neuritis as the first manifestation of rheumatoid arthritis. *J Neuroophthalmol* 2008;**28**:237–238.

6. Eggenberger ER. Inflammatory optic neuropathies. *Ophthalmol Clin North Am* 2001;**14**:73–82.

7. Brady KM, Brar AS, Lee AG, Coats DK, Paysse EA, Steinkuller PG. Optic neuritis in children: Clinical features and visual outcome. *J AAPOS* 1999;**3**:98–103.

8. Kahana E, Alter M, Feldman S. Optic neuritis in relation to multiple sclerosis. *J Neurol* 1976;**213**:87–95.

9. Alter M, Good J, Okihiro M. Optic neuritis in Orientals and Caucasians. *Neurology* 1973;**23**:631–639.

10. Lucchinetti CF, Kiers L, O'Duffy A, *et al*. Risk factors for developing multiple sclerosis after childhood optic neuritis. *Neurology* 1997;**49**:1413–1418.

11. Kidd D, Burton B, Plant GT, Graham EM. Chronic relapsing inflammatory optic neuropathy (CRION). *Brain* 2003;**126**:276–284.

12. Boomer JA, Siatkowski RM. Optic neuritis in adults and children. *Semin Ophthalmol* 2003;**18**:174–180.

13. Yeh EA, Weinstock-Guttman B, Lincoff N, *et al*. Retinal nerve fiber thickness in inflammatory demyelinating diseases of childhood onset. *Mult Scler* 2009;**15**:802–810. Epub 2009 May 22.

14. Cree B. Neuromyelitis optica: Diagnosis, pathogenesis, and treatment. *Curr Neurol Neurosci Rep* 2008;**8**:427–433.

15. Lennon VA, Wingerchuk DM, Kryzer TJ, *et al*. A serum autoantibody marker of neuromyelitis optica: Distinction from multiple sclerosis. *Lancet* 2004;**364**:2106–2112.

16. Loma IP, Asato MR, Filipink RA, Alper G. Neuromyelitis optica in a young child with positive serum autoantibody. *Pediatr Neurol* 2008;**39**:209–212.

17. Matiello M, Lennon VA, Jacob A, *et al*. NMO-IgG predicts the outcome of recurrent optic neuritis. *Neurology* 2008;**70**:2197–2200.

18. de Seze J, Arndt C, Jeanjean L, *et al*. Relapsing inflammatory optic neuritis: Is it neuromyelitis optica? *Neurology* 2008;**70**:2075–2076.

19. Banwell B, Tenembaum S, Lennon VA, *et al*. Neuromyelitis optica-IgG in childhood inflammatory demyelinating CNS disorders. *Neurology* 2008;**70**: 344–352.

20. Chabas D, Ness J, Belman A, Yeh EA, Kuntz N, Gorman MP. Younger children with MS have a distinct CSF inflammatory profile at disease onset. *Neurology* 2010;**74**:399–405.

21. Frohman EM, Fujimoto JG, Frohman TC, Calabresi PA, Cutter G, Balcer LJ. Optical coherence tomography: A window into the mechanisms of multiple sclerosis. *Nat Clin Pract Neurol* 2008;**4**:664–675.

22. Trip SA, Schlottmann PG, Jones SJ, *et al*. Optic nerve atrophy and retinal nerve fibre layer thinning following optic neuritis: Evidence that axonal loss is a substrate of MRI-detected atrophy. *Neuroimage* 2006;**31**:286–293.

23. Costello F, Hodge W, Pan YI, Metz L, Kardon RH. Retinal nerve fiber layer and future risk of multiple sclerosis. *Can J Neurol Sci* 2008;**35**:482–487.

24. Balcer LJ, Baier ML, Cohen JA, *et al*. Contrast letter acuity as a visual component for the Multiple Sclerosis Functional Composite. *Neurology* 2003;**61**:1367–1373.

25. Balcer LJ, Baier ML, Pelak VS, *et al*. New low-contrast vision charts: Reliability and test characteristics in patients with multiple sclerosis. *Mult Scler* 2000;**6**:163–171.

26. Krupp LB, Banwell B, Tenembaum S. Consensus definitions proposed for pediatric multiple sclerosis and related disorders. *Neurology* 2007;**68**:S7–12.

27. Beck RW, Gal RL. Treatment of acute optic neuritis: A summary of findings from the optic neuritis treatment trial. *Arch Ophthalmol* 2008;**126**:994–995.

28. Arndt C, Labauge P, Speeg-Schatz C, *et al*. [Recurrent inflammatory optic neuropathy]. *J Fr Ophthalmol* 2008;**31**:363–367.

22

What is acute transverse myelitis in children?

Frank S. Pidcock and Guillaume Sébire

Acute transverse myelitis (ATM) is a potentially devastating immune-mediated disorder of the spinal cord that affects all ages. The onset is often unaccompanied by any identifiable cause, and although the results of immediate treatment may be effective in moderating the damage, long-term sequelae in children are common. Because of its rarity, the causes, optimal treatment, and outcomes for ATM in children are poorly known.

Epidemiology of ATM

Typical ATM is a monofocal and monophasic inflammatory disorder targeting primarily the spinal cord, resulting in motor, sensory, and autonomic dysfunction. Approximately 1400 new cases are diagnosed in the United States each year (1–8 per million inhabitants per year), resulting in a prevalence of around 34 000 people with residual disabilities related to ATM [1,2]. Only about 20% of these patients are diagnosed with ATM before the age of 18 years [3]. Similarly, the recent population-based Canadian Paediatric Surveillance Program evaluated the incidence of ATM at 0.2 per 100 000 children [4]. In this study, incidence did not differ according to season, the female:male ratio was 0.81:1, and occurrence was similar whether ATM started before or after the age of 10 years [4].

When classified as a sub-group of acute disseminated encephalomyelitis (ADEM), ATM accounted for 30% of the topographic spectrum of central nervous system (CNS) involvements [5]. If only a single episode of ATM in childhood was considered, the prevalence was 10 times lower than for pediatric multiple sclerosis (MS). However, the generally poorer outcome reported in children with ATM as compared to supraspinal ADEM raises the question of distinct etiopathological mechanisms [5].

The comparison of epidemiologic factors relevant to pediatric ATM and other pediatric neuroimmunologic disorders such as MS, ADEM, and neuromyelitis optica (NMO) is particularly challenging, given the rarity of these conditions and the clinical overlap [6,7].

Definitions of ATM

The most straightforward definition of ATM is a monophasic and localized demyelinating process of sudden onset limited to one site in the spinal cord. About 75–90% of transverse myelitis (TM) cases fit this profile [8]. In a minority of cases, a repeat CNS attack follows, and the possibility of a recurrent demyelinating myelopathy, such as relapsing TM, MS, or NMO, needs to be considered.

For the past 30 years, typical diagnostic criteria for ATM used in clinical practice have been: (1) absence of past history of neurological disease, (2) acute onset of bilateral spinal cord dysfunction, and (3) absence of trauma, compression, vascular disruption, or toxins identified [9,10].

In 2002, new diagnostic criteria were proposed by a consortium of expert adult neurologists in order to define more homogeneous pathophysiological subgroups of ATM for research purposes [11]. These criteria are more exclusive than inclusive, given the large spectrum of potential differential diagnoses. The positive diagnostic criteria include the development of a bilateral myelopathy over a period of four hours to 21 days, and some evidence of spinal cord inflammation as demonstrated by cerebrospinal fluid (CSF) analysis (pleiocytosis, elevated IgG index) or spinal cord MRI (gadolinium enhancement), at disease onset or up to seven days later. The exclusion criteria include: (1) evidence of extra-axial spinal cord

Demyelinating Disorders of the Central Nervous System in Childhood, ed. Dorotheé Chabas and Emmanuelle L. Waubant. Published by Cambridge University Press. © Cambridge University Press 2011.

compression (by MRI or myelography); (2) past history of spine irradiation in the last 10 years; (3) abnormal flow voids suggestive of vascular malformation (by MRI); (4) serological or clinical evidence of connective tissue disease (mostly sarcoidosis, Sjögren, Behçet, systemic lupus erythematosus [SLE]) or infectious diseases (syphilis, Lyme, HIV, HTLV-1, *Mycoplasma* pneumonia, *Campylobacter jejuni*, HSV-1, HSV-2, VZV, CMV, EBV, HHV6, enterovirus, hepatitis viruses); (5) evidence of MS by brain MRI; (6) past history of clinically evident optic neuritis (ON) (suggestive of NMO).

Overlap of ATM with MS and related diseases

These ATM diagnostic criteria have not been validated in children. In addition, the diagnosis of ATM is particularly challenging at onset, because of the potential overlap with MS. Indeed, some children with an initial diagnosis of ATM may end up developing MS, sometimes after a long period of time. A French multicenter cohort study reported that among 168 children with a final diagnosis of MS according to Poser criteria, 13 (8%) initially presented with ATM while, among 42 children presenting with ATM, only 29 (69%) remained relapse-free after a mean follow-up of 2.9 ± 3 years [12]. These data may underestimate the proportion of conversion from ATM to MS, given the limited length of follow-up. In fact, regardless of the symptoms at onset, it was recently reported that the median time from onset to secondary progression was 28 years, and the median age at conversion was 41 years, in a French cohort of 394 patients with pediatric MS onset (≤ 16 years) [13].

The risk of developing MS is greater after an incomplete than after a complete ATM. Incomplete ATM patients present with asymmetric neurological deficit, including partially spared motor, sensory, or sphincter functions [14]. In incomplete ATM the spinal cord MRI lesion spreads over one or two vertebral segments, while a more extensive spinal cord segment is usually involved in patients with complete TM. As a matter of fact, the term "clinically isolated syndrome" (CIS) has been applied to individuals with incomplete, but not complete, TM. A cranial MRI is also useful in evaluating the risk of developing MS. The presence of two or more brain lesions suggestive of MS is associated with a risk of

88% for developing MS within 20 years [14]. The decision to treat high-risk patients with disease-modifying agents before the second attack is highly controversial [15,16].

Although the risk for developing MS is low following complete TM, recurrence of myelitis or development of NMO is possible. Predictive serologic markers include anti-Sjögren's syndrome antibody (SS-A) and NMO-IgG [17]. The presence of NMO-IgG predicted the recurrence of a demyelinating myelopathy in all cases of adults who presented with TM, whereas SS-A did not [18]. Whether this also applies to children is unknown.

Clinically, ATM overlaps with ADEM [5]. Indeed, patients with ADEM involving spinal cord foci of inflammation can present with clinical manifestations similar to ATM, and ATM can occur in association with subclinical supramedullary inflammatory foci detected by MRI [19–21]. Thus, the distinction between the two entities may be particularly challenging in the clinical setting.

Immunopathogenesis

The etiology and underlying mechanisms of ATM remain largely unknown. A post-infectious inflammatory process has been strongly suspected, based on the association with a preceding viral infection or vaccination and the increased CSF cell count (see Table 22.1 and the following section on the clinical presentation of ATM). Also, anatomical studies showed focal or multi-focal infiltration of the spinal cord by immune cells. The myelin sheath appears to be the main target of the process, based on the clinical appearance of symptoms (reflecting the involvement of long myelinated spinal cord tracts). This has been confirmed by anatomical studies showing areas of demyelination within the spinal cord [22,23]. However, no specific triggering factor has been identified in 10–45% of cases [1,2,9,10,24–27].

Pathophysiologically, the mechanism(s) leading to either diffuse, multi-focal, heterogeneous CNS injury as seen in ADEM or focal spinal cord damage associated with complete ATM may share similarities. However, even in the most extended forms, normal and abnormal patches of tissue co-exist. Such a heterogeneous distribution may be driven by stochastic hits of a transient immune/inflammatory process, heterogeneous CNS antigen expression, selective areas of blood–brain barrier disruptions, or

Table 22.1 Historical, clinical, and paraclinical features of ATM according to the main series of the literature

	Pidcock et al., 2007 [6]	Sébire et al., 2003 [26]	Paine et al., 1968 [13]	Dunne et al., 1986 [15]
Methods				
Collection period	2000–04	1965–95	1929–52	1966–83
Cohort (n)	47	24	25	21
Retrospective	+	+	+	+
Multicenter/tertiary	−/+	+/+	−/+	−/+
Demographic features				
Sex ratio (M/F)	1.04	0.85	0.5	0.9
Mean age (range, years)	8 (0–17)	7 (0–19)	8 (0.5–15)	10 (0.6–14)
Age at onset <3 years (%)	38	13	8	10
Prior infection (%)	47	58	60	100
Mean time infection to onset (days)	11	5	10	NA
Initial period				
Pain (any site) (%)	75	83	90	70
Back pain (%)	NA	75	55	40
Neck stiffness (%)	NA	45	60	NA
Fever (%)	NA	60	60	NA
Plateau				
Mean duration (days)	NA	7	NA	6
Complete paraplegia (%)	42	65	NA	65
Upper limb motor deficit (%)	NA	40	40	50
Sensory level				
Cervical (%)	25	12	11	20
Upper thoracic (%)		35	30	45
Lower thoracic (%)	53	50	30	30
Lumbar/sacral (%)	8	0	26	5
Sphincter dysfunction (%)	82	95	95	85
Paraclinical investigations				
CSF findings (%)	71	62	60	91
Spinal cord MRI findings (%)	94	66	ND	ND
Outcome				
Complete recovery (%)	NA	40	35	40
Death (n)	2	1	1	0
Chronic bladder dysfunction (%)	50	33	38	29
Multiple sclerosis (%)	Excluded	0	4	0

Table 22.1 (cont.)

	Pidcock et al., 2007 [6]	Sébire et al., 2003 [26]	Paine et al., 1968 [13]	Dunne et al., 1986 [15]
Predictors of favorable prognosis				
Lower sensory level	+	NT	NT	NT
Lack of complete paraplegia	NT	+	NT	+
Lack of rapid deterioration (<24 h)	–	+	NT	+
Lack of T1 hypointensity	+	NT	NT	NT

NT: not tested; NA: not available

differential neuroinflammatory responses depending on genetic or epigenetic spatiotemporal factors (see Chapters 15 and 17 for more details on the pathobiology of MS and ADEM).

Alternatively, ATM can be viewed as a distinct entity unrelated to ADEM. Supporting this hypothesis are the observations that ATM has a different neuroanatomic distribution than ADEM and that the prognosis of ATM and ADEM are different (50–70% of ATM versus 10–20% of ADEM patients do not reach full recovery: see Table 22.1) [8,19–21, 28,29].

It was recently shown that NMO, previously considered an anatomical variant of ADEM, is associated with a distinct immune process involving a specific auto-antibody directed against aquaporin-4. However, this antibody has not been detected in acute demyelination solely restricted to the optic nerve or to the spinal cord [30,31], suggesting that ATM is an entity distinct from NMO.

Animal models of immune/inflammatory demyelination provide evidence that a wide range of distinct immune pathways, belonging to either innate or adaptive immune responses, is needed to mimic human CNS demyelinating disorders. Using such models, the ability of a self or non-self antigen-driven adaptive immune response, implicating various subsets of CD4+ T cells, CD8+ T cells, or B cells, to trigger immune/inflammatory demyelination was demonstrated [32]. Other models showed that components of the innate immune response (monocytes/macrophages, or some pro-inflammatory cytokine pathway, e.g. TNF-α) were also able to induce such diseases on their own [33,34]. However, among these numerous models, none consistently and reproducibly induced a disease limited to the spinal cord, as in ATM. Of course, classical animal models, such as

experimental autoimmune encephalomyelitis (EAE), Theiler's virus encephalitis, or encephalomyelitis induced by pathogen-associated molecular patterns, may present with spinal cord involvement, sometimes predominantly, but most often as part of a more disseminated process. In fact, most observations from animal models failed to identify any specific immunopathological mechanism that might differentially affect the spinal cord rather than other neuroanatomical locations. Only Kaplin et al. reported that interleukin-6 (IL-6) levels were dramatically increased in the CSF of six patients with idiopathic ATM compared with other CNS diseases (hydrocephalus, aseptic meningitis, spinal cord infarct, and spinal cord tumors; $n = 2$ per group) [35]. The authors showed that subarachnoid injection of high-dose IL-6 induced spinal cord injuries predominantly affecting oligodendrocytes and axons, mimicking ATM. IL-6 seemed to act solely in the spinal cord, sparing the brain, via activation of the microglial JAK/STAT pathway and subsequent increase of iNOS and polyADP-ribose polymerase (PARP) activities. The selective spinal involvement was thought to be related to spatially distinct soluble IL-6R responses that were weaker in the spinal cord compared to the brain. Inter-individual genetic differences involving the IL-6 response, combined with exogenous factors such as infections, might account for the rare individual susceptibility to ATM in humans [35,36].

Clinical presentation of ATM
Preceding illness or immunization: a controversial notion

A preceding illness including non-specific symptoms such as fever, nausea, and muscle pain, occurring within three weeks before onset, was reported in 47% of patients in a large case series of ATM in childhood [24]. Overall, a preceding infection was observed in 47–100% of patients, 5–11 days prior to ATM onset (Table 22.1). A confirmed immunization or allergy shot within 30 days before onset was documented in approximately 30% of cases [24]. A preceding trauma, usually involving a twisting or falling injury to the back, was noted in 13% of patients, eight days on average before symptom onset [24]. The connection between these preceding events and ATM remains questionable and requires further investigation.

Clinical features

ATM presents with sudden onset of rapidly progressive weakness that most often involves the lower extremities but may include the arms as well. There may also be alterations in sensation, sphincter dysfunction, and respiratory insufficiency. History, clinical, and paraclinical features are summarized in Table 22.1 [9,19,24,28].

Flaccidity is initially present in most cases, with development of spasticity occurring by the second week of illness. Rapidly progressive neurological deterioration occurs between four and 21 days after the onset of symptoms, with more than 80% of patients reaching their clinical nadir within 10 days [3]. Most children with ATM are unable to ambulate at this stage of the illness.

Sensory loss or numbness has been reported in over 90% of children with ATM. The sensory level was cervical in 25%, thoracic in 53%, lumbar in 5%, sacral in 3%, and unclear in 14% of cases in a large case series [24]. Positive sensory complaints during the acute phase of illness (e.g. burning, tingling, or electric shock sensations) were present alone or in combination with numbness in 33 of 38 patients [24].

Bladder dysfunction is common during the acute phase of illness and persists in many children; 82% required urinary catheterization acutely and 50% at follow-up [24]. Information about concomitant bowel dysfunction was not specified, but it may reasonably be assumed that sphincter dysfunction applied to bowel movements as well. Fifty-four percent of pediatric patients with TM reported modified or complete dependence on others for management of sphincter control issues [24].

Abnormal CSF findings were reported in 60–80% of children with ATM [5,13,15,26]. An elevation in CSF white blood cells of 136 $\pm$ 67 cells/ml (range 6–950) was reported in 50% of cases, and CSF protein was elevated in 48% of cases with a mean value of 173 $\pm$ 75 g/dl (range 45–1120) in a large case series [24]. Oligoclonal bands (OCB) and elevated IgG index were present in less than 5% of the CSF specimens evaluated in this cohort [24].

Although depression is increasingly recognized as occurring with greater than anticipated frequency in adults with TM, very little is known about this in children.

Death is uncommon in ATM affecting children. A pediatric mortality risk of 4% was derived from five pediatric TM case series [24]. Death is typically caused by respiratory dysfunction in complete cervical ATM.

MRI presentation of ATM

Few studies have described the MRI aspects of ATM in childhood [19,24,37]. Abnormal findings were reported in four out of six children with ATM who underwent spinal cord MRI in a case series published in 2003 [19]. One child had multiple lesions in the cervical region and conus medullaris and three had a single lesion in the thoracic segment of the spinal cord. Edema of the spinal cord was visible on T1-weighted sequences in only half of the children with abnormal MRI. On T2-weighted sequences, all lesions exhibited high signal intensity and extended along two or more vertebral segments. In three children with abnormal initial MRI, the T2-bright lesions were associated with nodular, diffuse, or peripheral post-gadolinium enhancement on T1 sequences [19]. Of note, two children had a normal spinal cord MRI.

In 2007, a report on ATM in childhood reported abnormal MRI findings in 34 out of 36 children (95%) with lesions spreading over an average of six spinal cord segments, suggesting that MRI techniques have become increasingly sensitive for diagnosing ATM [24]. T1 gadolinium enhancement was reported in 74% of available cases. A hypointense lesion on T1 imaging was observed in 38% of cases. The presence of T1 hypointense lesions independently correlated with worse ambulation outcome on follow-up [24].

Asymmetric spinal cord lesions of small size, with well-defined borders, were linked with CIS/MS in childhood. Conversely, large MRI lesions with poorly defined borders were associated with monophasic ATM and ADEM, without any significant difference between the two entities [12].

A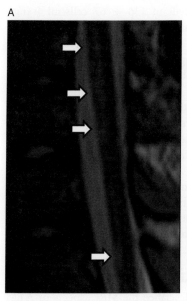

B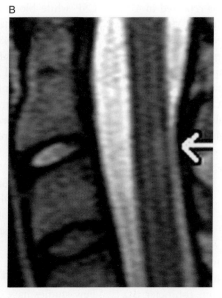

Figure 22.1 Typical spinal cord MRI presentation of ATM versus MS. (A) Sagittal section of T2-weighted MRI scan of the spinal cord performed in a 15-year-old boy presenting with ATM. Disease was characterized by acute paraplegia, sphincter dysfunction, T1 sensory level. Multiple fuzzy areas of hyperintensity irregularly extending from C5 to T1 were observed (arrows). T1-weighted images with or without gadolinium injection (not shown) were unremarkable. Three hours after initial symptoms the patient received high-dose intravenous methylprednisolone. At his six-month follow-up visit he presented a nearly full clinical recovery, and the repeat MRI scan was normal. (B) Sagittal section of T2-weighted MRI scan of the spinal cord in a 14-year-old girl presenting with a third attack of MS including proprioceptive ataxia and unilateral hemiparesthesia, sparing the face and upper cervical region. A single small, well-limited area of T2 hypersignal was seen (arrow), typical of an MS spinal cord lesion.

NMO has been associated in adulthood with longitudinally extensive transverse myelitis as seen on spinal cord MRI. However, this extended aspect of spinal cord lesions seems to be less predictive of NMO in childhood [30].

Figures 22.1 and 22.2 show MRI scans of pediatric ATM.

Outcome and prognosis

The clinical outcome for children with ATM is not well known, because of the rarity of the condition and the paucity of reliable information. Follow-up information about function in children who had TM is limited to only a few case series collected from single centers over a prolonged period of time (4–25 years after onset) [9,19,24,28,29].

A case series of ATM in childhood reported functional outcomes in a group of 33 individuals using the FIM and WeeFIM tools for measuring performance of daily skills at an average follow-up of eight years (95% CI 4.5–11.9 years) following the onset of disease [24,38]. The majority of patients were independent in self-care (73%), transfers (64%), communication (93%), and social cognition (93%). Regarding bowel and bladder sphincter control, 46% achieved independence. Locomotion, defined as the ability to walk or use a manual wheelchair for at least 150 feet, was eventually achieved by 67%. Some assistance in performing daily skills was reported in 30% for sphincter control and locomotion, 18% for transfers, and 12% for self-care. Complete dependence on an assistant was reported in 24% for sphincter control, 18% for performing transfers, 15% for self-care activities, and 3% for locomotion.

It is difficult to accurately determine the frequency of complete recovery from childhood-onset ATM, given the selection bias inherent in reported series from academic referral centers that treat the more severely affected cases. Another difficulty arises from the non-specific description of functional outcomes, leading to vague classifications of performance such as "minimal" or "mild" deficits. A case series published in 2003 reported full recovery in 31%, minimal sequelae in 25%, and mild to severe sequelae in 44% of 24 children [19]. It is estimated that approximately 33–50% of children with ATM have full recovery or minimal deficits, with the remainder experiencing lingering difficulties with bladder or bowel control

A

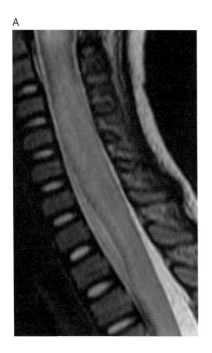

B

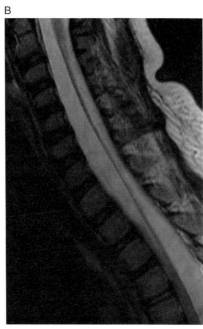

Figure 22.2 (A) Initial sagittal section of T2-weighted MRI scan of the cervical spinal cord of a one-year-old girl presenting with acute quadriplegia, severe sphincter dysfunctions, and bilateral multimodal anesthesia at a cervical level, showing a heterogeneous and diffuse hypersignal with a slight spinal cord swelling. (B) One year later, the clinical symptoms remained unchanged; repeat MRI showed a severe atrophic aspect of the spinal cord.

or mobility. Age of onset under three years was associated with a worse outcome [24]. Clinical factors associated with a better functional outcome include a shorter interval to diagnosis, absence of complete paraplegia, and lower sensory levels by neurologic examination [19].

Functional improvement typically occurs within six months from onset in most cases and continues at a slower rate for at least two years (personal experience). The influence of intensive therapies during this time on the speed and extent of recovery remains unknown and requires further investigation.

Diagnostic evaluation and differential diagnosis of sudden spinal cord dysfunction

ATM is a diagnosis made by exclusion. The sudden onset of rapidly progressive weakness involving the lower and sometimes upper limbs opens a wide range of differential diagnoses, some of which require specific and urgent therapeutic interventions.

Extraspinal differential diagnosis

The initial phase of Guillain–Barré syndrome (GBS) may be confused with ATM because of the similar presentation of muscle weakness, loss of reflexes, painful sensory and meningeal signs. The initial physical examination may not be helpful in determining a diagnosis, especially in young children, due to the accompanying severe pain. Helpful findings on examination that support the diagnosis of ATM include a spinal pattern of sensory deficits (i.e. not limited to myelinated fibers, often asymmetrical (except in complete ATM), and sensory level), a babinski sign, the lack of supramedullary symptoms, and the presence of significant sphincter dysfunction. Nearly all patients with GBS present with early cranial nerve dysfunction.

Ultimately, nerve conduction studies can provide useful diagnostic evidence. They are normal in ATM and typically abnormal in GBS, showing signs such as conduction blocks within the first days of illness [39]. Other acute peripheral pathologies, such as infectious meningoradiculitis (e.g. Lyme disease, cat scratch disease), and metabolic polyradiculoneuropathy (porphyria) can be distinguished from ATM based on a thorough history, clinical evaluation, and paraclinical investigations including CSF analysis. MRI studies are useful for identifying bacterial epiduritis and extraspinal intrameningeal pathologies such as hematoma or bacterial empyema.

Intraspinal conditions other than ATM

Various diseases lead to the sudden onset of a spinal cord syndrome in childhood: direct infections (e.g.

HIV-1, HTLV-1, *Bartonella henselae*, and parasites such as schistosomiasis), trauma, toxins (e.g. methotrexate), radiation, autoimmune diseases (mainly SLE), ischemic or hemorrhagic etiologies (e.g. arteriovenous malformation or cavernoma), tumors, and sudden worsening of occult malformations (e.g. tethered cord, neurenteric cyst) [40,41]. Spinal cord infarction is uncommon in children free of cardiovascular disease or other predisposing factors. Some of these conditions require specific and urgent treatment. Thus, spinal cord MRI should be performed urgently to rule out a compression that might require immediate neurosurgical treatment.

ATM vs. ADEM vs. CIS and MS

ATM can be the first manifestation of MS. However, the rate of conversion to MS after a first episode of demyelination seems to be lower if this initial manifestation is a myelitis (hazard ratio = 0.23; 95% CI 0.1–0.56) as compared to other CNS locations [12]. On initial MR imaging, brain lesions perpendicular to the long axis of the corpus callosum, CNS lesions purely focal and well defined (clear-cut borders), and a total of more than nine lesions were linked with subsequent occurrence of a second attack. Conversely, large MRI lesions with poorly defined borders and a "lesion load" > 50% were associated with a monophasic disease.

There is no specific biomarker that differentiates monophasic ATM from the first manifestation of MS at the time of initial presentation. However, the presence of CSF OCB increases the likelihood of a first episode of MS [42–45] (see Chapters 4 and 15). The overlap between ATM and MS is discussed above, including the predictive value of complete versus partial ATM.

ATM vs. NMO

Pediatric NMO seems to present some of the same distinctive features as previously described in adulthood [30], i.e. the association of recurrent manifestations of TM and ON. About 50% of children with NMO were serum NMO-IgG positive, including nearly all of the patients with a relapsing course. However, in contrast to adults, the typical MRI aspect of longitudinally extensive transverse myelitis seems to be less predictive of NMO in childhood [30] (see also Chapter 23). The overlap between ATM and NMO is discussed above.

ATM work-up

Whole (cervical to lumbar) T1- and T2-weighted spinal cord MRI including sagittal sections should be performed, with and without gadolinium injection. Additionally, T1- and T2-weighted axial sections at the level(s) determined by the clinical symptoms or by anomalies suspected on sagittal images provide important complementary information to further define the topography of the lesion (complete or not, symmetrical or not, vascular territory). Brain MRI, including the same sequences, is recommended to rule out mimicking diseases such as MS, ADEM, or NMO.

Once a compressive cause for acute myelopathy is ruled out by MRI, a lumbar puncture should be performed for CSF analysis including cell count and differential, total protein and glucose titers. IgG isofocalization should be performed on matched CSF and serum samples to look for a CSF-restricted IgG oligoclonal profile (OCBs), and the IgG index should be measured.

Serum antibody titration might be oriented by the recent medical history, such as exposure to an identifiable infectious disease (e.g. community outbreak of a specific infectious agent) or recent vaccination. Alternatively, a systematic infectious workup (cultures, serum antibodies titration performed twice at three-week intervals) could be performed based on the main infectious agents that have been linked with ATM (HSV-1, VZV, EBV, CMV, HHV-6, influenzae, enteroviruses, hepatitis A, B, or C). Particular attention should be paid to treatable infectious diseases requiring a specific antibiotic treatment such as *Mycoplasma* pneumonia, *Bartonella henselae* (even in the absence of cat scratch), and *Borrelia burgdorferi* (Lyme disease) [11,46–51].

The SLE markers (such as anti-nuclear antibodies, anti-double stranded DNA antibody, SS-A/Ro, SS-B/La, anti-cardiolipin antibody, lupus anticoagulant, and complement level) should be checked in the absence of any other obvious cause of ATM.

Ophthalmological examination is important to further characterize any sign either mentioned by the patient or detected by the neurological examination. If positive, it may suggest demyelinating disease other than ATM. Visual evoked potentials (VEPs) in the absence of any clinical sign do not seem to be useful and may even be misleading because of possible artifacts, which are particularly frequent in younger patients.

Acute interventions and medical treatments

At initial presentation, even before MRI is performed, some routine first-line therapeutic measures, which are mandatory in acute spinal cord injuries from undetermined origin, should be considered until spinal cord compression is ruled out. In particular, spinal cord immobilization should be considered, especially when a spine injury is suspected. If the patient reports significant back or neck pain, or is unable to describe the first symptoms and accompanying circumstances, at least a cervical collar should be used. The presence of a potential respiratory failure should be immediately evaluated, and treated with nasal oxygen or assisted ventilation depending on the severity. Continuous monitoring should be initiated, given the risk of worsening symptoms. Aspiration of gastric content should be prevented. Bladder catheterization should be performed in patients with significant urinary retention. Appropriate analgesic medication should be administered for management of dysesthetic pain, as needed.

Once imaging- and CSF-based assessments have led to the diagnosis of ATM, pharmacological treatments should be discussed. The likely immune-mediated mechanism of ATM, the high risk of residual disabilities, and the lack of evidence-based effective treatment has prompted investigators to evaluate the effect of intravenous methylprednisolone (IVMP) in severe childhood ATM. Using comparison between treated and untreated historical control groups, or observational studies, investigators showed that treatment with IVMP may be highly effective in children with ATM, in shortening the length of the disease and in improving outcome without any significant adverse effects [19,52–54]. In the largest therapeutic trial comparing 12 severe cases of ATM with at least complete flaccid paralysis of the lower limbs treated with IVMP (mean delay between onset and treatment: eight days) versus 17 untreated ATM cases, it was found that the proportion of patients who walked independently after one month was 66% in the IVMP group and 17% in the control group. At one year, 64% of treated patients had achieved a complete motor recovery, compared with 23% in the control group, and 75% of the patients in the treated group had normal sphincter function versus 17% in the control group. Full recovery within one year was seen in 54% of patients in the treated group versus 11% in the control group. Among patients who recovered walking, the median time to independent walking was 21 days in the treated group and 120 days in the control group [53]. Thus, even in the absence of randomized controlled trials, IVMP is now accepted as the standard first-line treatment of ATM. A usual therapeutic protocol is methylprednisolone at a dosage of 1 g/1.73 m^2/day every day for five consecutive days followed by an oral taper with prednisone (1 mg/kg/day for 14 days) then rapid withdrawal over four days [52–54]. The delay between initial symptoms and the beginning of the treatment might be important in terms of prognosis. By contrast, a low dose of oral or intravenous steroid did not seem to influence the outcome [5,9,27,28].

The experience with other immunomodulatory approaches, such as intravenous immunoglobulins (IVIg) or plasma exchanges, has been poorly documented, but these are used empirically as second-line treatments, in some centers, in the absence of a quick response to steroids.

Rehabilitation

Intervention during the acute phase of illness may be necessary to prevent the inactivity-related problems of skin breakdown and soft tissue contraction. Family education regarding the goals of physical and occupational therapy should be initiated at this time to develop a strategic plan for addressing the challenges to independence following return to the community. Assessment and application of appropriately fitting splints designed to passively maintain an optimal position for limbs that cannot be actively moved is an important part of the management of ATM.

Rehabilitation during the recovery phase from ATM, which may take up to two years, shares similarities with patients recovering from spinal cord injury. This includes the management of spasticity and weakness, bladder and bowel dysfunction, pain or dysesthesias, fatigue, and fragile bones.

Spasticity in children with ATM can be a disabling and painful long-term complication. The primary therapeutic goal is to maintain sufficient movement around large joints in the arms and legs to support functional skills such as walking, feeding, and dressing. To the extent that active movement is present or evolves, the physical or occupational therapist engages the patient in a series of repetitive graded activities to stimulate optimal return of movement. These activities are usually coupled with a stretching program that is provided actively by the therapists and families on a daily basis and passively through the use of custom-fitted orthoses worn according to a daily schedule. These splints are commonly used at the ankles, wrists, or elbows. A carefully monitored program for strengthening appropriate muscles may also be provided by the therapists. Additional measures to control painful spasms and reduce muscle tightness include antispasticity medications (e.g. diazepam, baclofen, dantrolene), medicinal botulinum toxin injections, and serial casting. These are adjunctive measures designed to enhance the effects of the primary interventions, which are daily repetitive and consistent exercise and stretching. Long-term rehabilitative care also includes effective compensatory strategies, anticipatory guidance with respect to adolescence and independent living, and holistic approaches to pain relief.

Effective management of bowel and bladder incontinence is an important component of long-term care. Elements of a successful bowel and bladder program include a high-fiber diet, adequate and timely fluid intake, medications to regulate bowel evacuations, and clean intermittent urinary catheterization. Regular evaluations by medical specialists for urodynamic studies and adjustment of the bowel program are recommended to prevent potentially serious complications.

In addition to the chronic medical problems there are ongoing psychosocial issues, which may be quite daunting. Issues include the ordering and maintenance of appropriate equipment, re-entry into the school and community, and coping with the psychological effects of this condition on the patients and their families. Emotional support to both child and family is an integral part of long-term care. Monitoring for sad affect or angry outbursts, which may be the early childhood depression equivalent, is appropriate as well as referral to mental health services as needed.

In summary, many children with ATM will require rehabilitative care to prevent secondary complications, to improve functional skills, and to optimize community reintegration. Involvement with family support groups and advocacy organizations such as the Transverse Myelitis Association (www.myelitis.org) will help individuals connect with other families facing similar challenges and professionals with expertise in addressing their issues.

Conclusions

Our current ATM knowledge is still limited at several levels from pathophysiology to treatment. Understanding ATM may be affected by referral bias (enrollment of cases from tertiary acute care centers) and the retrospective approach present in all of the case series reported in the literature. Thus, population-based prospective studies, such as the one recently launched in Canada and other countries, will be of crucial importance to enhance our understanding of childhood-onset ATM and its relationship to other neuroimmmunologic entities including MS, ADEM, and NMO [55].

References

1. Berman M, Feldman S, Alter M, *et al.* Acute transverse myelitis: Incidence and etiologic considerations. *Neurology* 1981;**31**:966–971.

2. Jeffery DR, Mandler RN, Davis LE. Transverse myelitis. Retrospective analysis of 33 cases, with differentiation of cases associated with multiple sclerosis and parainfectious events. *Arch Neurol* 1993;**50**:532–535.

3. Kerr DA, Krishnan C, Pidcock F. Acute transverse myelitis. In *Treatment of Pediatric Neurologic Disorders*, ed. HS Singer, EH Kossoff, AL Hartman, TO Crawford. Boca Raton, FL: Taylor and Francis; 2005:445–451.

4. Banwell B, Kennedy J, Sadovnick D, *et al.* Incidence of acquired demyelination of the CNS in Canadian children. *Neurology* 2009;**72**:232–239.

5. Dale RC, de Sousa C, Chong WK, Cox TC, Harding B, Neville BG. Acute disseminated encephalomyelitis, multiphasic disseminated encephalomyelitis and multiple sclerosis. *Brain* 2000;**123**:2407–2422.

6. Murthy SNK, Faden HS, Cohen ME, Bakshi R. Acute disseminated encephalomyelitis in Children. *Pediatrics* 2002;**110**:e1–e7.

7. Lotze TE, Northrop JL, Hutton GJ, Ross B, SChiffman JS. Spectrum of pediatric neuromyelitis optica. *Pediatrics* 2008;**122**:e1039–e1047.

8. Krishnan C, Kaplin AI, Pardo CA, Kerr DA, Keswani SC. Demyelinating disorders: Update on transverse myelitis. *Curr Neurol Neurosci Rep* 2006;**6**:236–243.

9. Paine RS, Byers RK. Transverse myelopathy in childhood. *AMA Am J Dis Child* 1968;**85**:151–163.

10. Ropper AH, Poskanzer DC. The prognosis of acute and subacute transverse myelopathy based on early signs and symptoms. *Ann Neurol* 1978;**4**:51–59.

11. Transverse Myelitis Consortium Working Group. Proposed diagnostic criteria and nosology of acute transverse myelitis. *Neurology* 2002;**59**:499–505.

12. Mikaeloff Y, Suissa S, Vallée L, *et al.* First episode of acute CNS inflammatory demyelination in childhood: Prognostic factors for multiple sclerosis and disability. *J Pediatr* 2004;**144**:246–252.

13. Renoux C, Vukusic S, Mikaeloff Y, *et al.* Natural history of multiple sclerosis with childhood onset. *N Engl J Med* 2007;**356**:2603–213.

14. Jacob A, Weinshenker BG. An approach to the diagnosis of acute transverse myelitis. *Semin Neurol* 2008;**28**:105–120.

15. Frohman EM, Havrdova E, Lublin F, *et al.* Most patients with multiple sclerosis or a clinically isolated demyelinating syndrome should be treated at the time of diagnosis. *Arch Neurol* 2006;**63**:614–619.

16. Pittock SJ, WEinshenker BG, Noseworthy JH, *et al.* Not every patient with multiple sclerosis should be treated at time of diagnosis. *Arch Neurol* 2006;**63**:611–614.

17. Hummers LK, Krishnan C, Casciola-Rosen L, *et al.* Recurrent transverse myelitis associates with anti-Ro (SSA) autoantibodies. *Neurology* 2004;**62**:147–149.

18. Weinshenker BG, Wingerchuk DM, Kryzer TJ, *et al.* Neuromyelitis optica IgG predicts relapse after longitudinally extensive transverse myelitis. *Ann Neurol* 2006;**59**:566–569.

19. Defresne P, Hollenberg H, Husson B, *et al.* Acute transverse myelitis in children: Clinical course and prognostic factors. *J Child Neurol* 2003;**18**:401–406.

20. Hynson JL, Kornberg AJ, Coleman LT, Shield L, Harvey AS, Kean MJ. Clinical and neuroradiologic features of acute disseminated encephalomyelitis in children. *Neurology* 2001;**56**:1308–1312.

21. Tenembaum S, Chitnis T, Ness J. Hahn JS, International Pediatric MS Study Group. Acute disseminated encephalomyelitis. *Neurology* 2007;**68**:S23–36.

22. Greenfield JO, Turner JWA. Acute and subacute necrotic myelitis. *Brain* 1939;**62**:227–252.

23. Hoffman HL. Acute necrotic myelopathy. *Brain* 1955;**78**:377–391.

24. Pidcock FS, Krishnan C, Crawford TO, Salorio CF, Trovato M, Kerr DA. Acute transverse myelitis in childhood: Center-based analysis of 47 cases. *Neurology* 2007;**68**:1474–1480.

25. Altrocchi PH. Acute transverse myelopathy. *Arch Neurol* 1963;**9**:21–29.

26. Christensen PB, Wermuth L, Hinge HH, *et al.* Clinical course and long-term prognosis of acute transverse myelopathy. *Acta Neurol Scand* 1990;**81**:431–435.

27. Lipton HL, Teasdall RD. Acute transverse myelopathy in adults. A follow-up study. *Arch Neurol* 1973;**28**:252–257.

28. Dunne K, Hopkins IJ, Shield LK. Acute transverse myelopathy in childhood. *Dev Med Child Neurol* 1986;**28**:198–204.

29. Knebusch M, Strassburg HM, Reiners K. Acute transverse myelitis in childhood: Nine cases and review of the literature. *Dev Med Child Neurol* 1998;**40**:631–639.

30. Banwell B, Tenembaum S, Lennon VA, *et al.* Neuromyelitis optica-IgG in childhood inflammatory demyelinating CNS disorders. *Neurology* 2008;**70**:344–352.

31. Lennon VA, Wingerchuk DM, Kryzer TJ, *et al.* A serum autoantibody marker of neuromyelitis optica: Distinction from multiple sclerosis. *Lancet* 2004;**364**:2106–2112.

32. Baxter AG. The origin and application of experimental autoimmune encephalitis. *Nat Rev Immunol* 2007;**7**:904–912.

33. Nguyen MD, Julien JP, Rivest S. Innate immunity: The missing link in neuroprotection and neurodegeneration? *Nat Rev Neurosci* 2002;**3**:216–227.

34. Furtado GC, Pina B, Tacke F, *et al.* A novel model of demyelinating encephalomyelitis induced by monocytes and dendritic cells. *J Immunol* 2006;**177**:6871–6879.

35. Kaplin AI, Deshpande DM, Scott E, *et al.* IL-6 induces regionally selective spinal cord injury in patients with the neuroinflammatory disorder transverse myelitis. *J Clin Invest* 2005;**115**:2731–2741.

36. Graber JJ, Allie SR, Mullen KM, *et al.* Interleukin-17 in transverse myelitis and multiple sclerosis. *J Neuroimmunol* 2008;**196**:124–132.

37. Andronikou S, Albuquerque-Jonathan G, Wilmhurst J, Hewlett R. MRI findings in acute idiopathic transverse myelopathy in children. *Pediatr Radiol* 2003;**33**:624–629.

38. Uniform Data System for Medical Rehabilitation. *The WeeFIM System clinical guide*, version 5.01. Buffalo, NY: UDSMR, 2000.

39. Delanoe C, Sébire G, Landrieu P, Huault G, Metral S. Acute inflammatory demyelinating polyradiculopathy in children: Clinical and electrodiagnostic studies. *Ann Neurol* 1998;**44**:350–356.

40. Kadhim H, Proano PG, Saint Martin C, *et al.* Spinal neurenteric cyst presenting in infancy with chronic fever and acute myelopathy. *Neurology* 2000;**23**:2011–2015.

41. Avcin T, Benseler SM, Tyrrel PN, Cucnik S, Silverman ED. A followup study of antiphospholipid antibodies and associated neuropsychiatric manifestations in 137

children with systemic lupus erythematosus. *Arthritis Rheum* 2008;**15**:206–213.

42. Callen DJ, Shroff MM, Branson HM, *et al.* Role of MRI in differentiation of ADEM from MS in children. *Neurology* 2009;**72**:968–973.

43. Banwell B, Ghezzi A, Bar-Or A, Mikaeloff Y, Tardieu M. Multiple sclerosis in children: Clinical diagnosis, therapeutic strategies, and future direction. *Lancet Neurol* 2007; **6**:887–902.

44. Chabas D, Strober J, Waubant E. Pediatric multiple sclerosis. *Curr Neurol Neurosci Rep* 2008;**8**:434–441.

45. Mikaeloff Y, Adamsbaum C, Husson B, *et al.* MRI prognostic factors for relapse after acute CNS inflammatory demyelination in childhood. *Brain* 2004;**127**:1942–1947.

46. Baar I, Jacobs BC, Govers N, Jorens PG, Parizel PM, Cras P. *Campylobacter jejuni*-induced acute transverse myelitis. *Spinal Cord* 2007;**45**:690–694.

47. de Silva SM, Mark AS, Gilden DH, *et al.* Zoster myelitis: Improvement with antiviral therapy in two cases. *Neurology* 1996;**47**:929–931.

48. Galanakis E, Bikouvarakis S, Mamoulakis D, Karampekios S, Sbyrakis S. Transverse myelitis associated with herpes simplex virus infection. *J Child Neurol* 2001;**16**:866–867.

49. Van Baalen A, Muhle H, Straube T, Jansen O, Stephani U. Nonparalytic poliomyelitis in Lyme borreliosis. *Arch Dis Child* 2006;**91**:660.

50. Baylor P, Garoufi A, Karpathios T, Lutz J, Mogelof J, Moseley D. Transverse myelitis in 2 patients with *Bartonella henselae* infection (cat scratch disease). *Clin Infect Dis* 2007;**15**:42–45.

51. Hmaimess G, Kadhim H, Saint Martin C, Abu Serieh B, Mousny M, Sébire G. Cat scratch disease presenting as meningomyeloradiculopathy. *Arch Dis Child* 2004;**89**:691–692.

52. Sébire G, Hollenberg H, Meyer L, Huault G, Landrieu P, Tardieu M. High dose methylprednisolone in severe acute transverse myelopathy. *Arch Dis Child* 1997;**76**:167–168.

53. Defresne P, Meyer L, Tardieu M, *et al.* Efficacy of high dose steroid therapy in children with severe acute transverse myelitis. *J Neurol Neurosurg Psychiatry* 2001;**71**:272–274.

54. Lahat E, Pillar G, Ravid S, Barzilai A, Etzioni A, Shahar E. Rapid recovery from transverse myelopathy in children treated with methylprednisolone. *Pediatr Neurol* 1998;**19**:279–282.

55. Banwell B. The long (-itudinally extensive) and the short of it: Transverse myelitis in children. *Neurology* 2007;**68**:1447–1449.

Chapter

23

Neuromyelitis optica in children

Andrew McKeon and Timothy Lotze

Neuromyelitis optica (NMO; also known historically as Devic disease) is a rare inflammatory, demyelinating disease of the central nervous system (CNS) that has a predilection for the optic nerves and spinal cord [1]. Disease attacks are usually severe, often resulting in blindness and paraplegia [1]. Although the median age of onset of NMO is 39 years [2], cases have been observed across all age groups, including children and the elderly [3–6]. Clinical, serological, immunological, and pathological data which have emerged in the past 15 years has indicated that NMO is a disease distinct from multiple sclerosis (MS). In particular, the discovery of a disease-specific IgG antibody biomarker, NMO-IgG [7], has revolutionized the classification of demyelinating disorders of childhood [3–5]. Recent studies of NMO in children have provided new insights into idiopathic demyelinating CNS disorders in that age group. While radiological brain abnormalities are common in adults with NMO, symptomatic disease is rare [1,8]. In children, symptomatic brain attacks are distinctly common, occurring in nearly half [4]. In light of these novel clinical findings and the emergence of aquaporin-4 (AQP4; the most abundant water channel in the CNS [9]) as the target autoantigen of NMO-IgG [10], a new previously unrecognized entity has emerged of an astrocytic AQP4 autoimmune channelopathy of the CNS [11].

In this chapter, we review the growing clinical and scientific literature regarding NMO and AQP4 autoimmunity, with the emphasis on recent studies in children.

Aquaporin-4: the target autoantigen in NMO

Most of the clinical, immunological, and pathological insights into NMO in recent years has emanated from

the identification of the disease-specific NMO-IgG antibody and its antigenic target, AQP4 [10]. AQP4 is a homotetrameric protein highly expressed in the polarized plasma membrane of astrocytic end-feet associated with CNS microvessels, ventricular ependyma and interneuronal synaptic junctions [9,10]. AQP4 regulates bidirectional flux of water between brain and spinal fluid, accompanying potassium ion fluxes. Similar to the paradigm of the muscle acetylcholine receptor autoantibody in myasthenia gravis [12], an antibody to a CNS cell membrane protein may be pathogenic in NMO. Clinical, pathologic, and immunologic observations described later in this chapter support a pathogenic role for an AQP4-specific autoantibody in NMO.

The historical perspective

NMO was first recognized as a clinical and pathological entity in the latter half of the nineteenth century. Clifford Allbutt inferred from five cases of myelitis seen that "changes at the back of the eye do not infrequently follow spinal disease" [13]. In 1894, Devic and Gault summarized their reported cases of the newly coined syndrome of "neuromyelitis optica" [14,15]. Their case descriptions included patients with monophasic and relapsing courses. In the first half of the twentieth century, several authors further described cases of severe myelitis occurring simultaneously or in close temporal association with optic neuritis, which was often severe and bilateral, as summarized by McKee and McNaughton [16]. Historically, some authors considered NMO a form of MS, while others considered NMO a distinct and chronic relapsing disease, and this debate has continued in recent times [17,18]. Contrary to many early descriptions of NMO as a monophasic illness, Beck described

Demyelinating Disorders of the Central Nervous System in Childhood, ed. Dorothée Chabas and Emmanuelle L. Waubant. Published by Cambridge University Press. © Cambridge University Press 2011.

in 1927 a case of severe recurrent NMO in a 15-year-old girl. Of particular note, the first presentation was compatible with an encephalitic illness [19]:

> On April 3rd 1926, thirteen months before admission to the National Hospital, the patient was taken suddenly ill with headache, vomiting, malaise and some drowsiness . . . she recovered entirely and for a period of five or six weeks, felt very well, until at the beginning of June, she awoke one morning to find that the vision of the left eye was hazy and indistinct. [19]

The patient subsequently had a relapsing NMO course, with attacks of both optic neuritis (ON) and transverse myelitis (TM). Post-mortem examination demonstrated evidence of bilateral optic neuritides and a longitudinally extensive myelopathic process. Despite this and other early descriptions, there has been a perception that NMO was, for the most part, a monophasic and mild disease when it occurred in childhood. In 1996, Jeffery *et al.* published a large case series, describing a benign course for NMO in nine pediatric patients; over five years of follow-up no recurrence or residual neurological deficit was observed in any patient [20]. However, with the development of accepted diagnostic criteria in 1999 (revised in 2006), and a serological disease antibody biomarker, pediatric NMO patients have more recently been described to have a relapsing and severe clinical course, with rapid accrual of attack-related disability [4,5].

Current diagnostic criteria

In 2007, the International Pediatric Multiple Sclerosis Study Group published consensus definitions for pediatric multiple sclerosis and related disorders to include NMO for children under 18 years. Utilizing the recent availability of the disease biomarker, NMO-IgG, the group suggested the following criteria for the diagnosis of NMO in children: (1) optic neuritis and transverse myelitis required as major criteria; and (2) either longitudinally extensive transverse myelitis (LETM) with MRI demonstrating involvement of three or more spinal segments *or* NMO IgG seropositivity [21]. Importantly, this definition did not incorporate brain imaging findings. Wingerchuk *et al.* proposed revised diagnostic criteria for adult NMO in 2006 utilizing likelihood ratios to develop several diagnostic models including the incorporation of NMO IgG as well as spinal cord and brain MRI findings [22]. The authors proposed revised NMO diagnostic criteria that removed the restriction on

CNS involvement beyond the optic nerves and spinal cord, since it was observed that brain lesions (although usually absent or non-specific in adults) did not preclude the diagnosis of NMO. Further work has demonstrated that symptomatic brain lesions are, in fact, common in children with NMO [4,5] (see the section on Clinical Presentation). Future revisions of the pediatric NMO criteria might need to include brain imaging abnormalities in the pediatric NMO population to better assure an accurate diagnosis in this age group.

Demographic features

Female sex predominates in a ratio of about 9:1 in children with NMO [4,5]. Female sex also predominates in pediatric MS, but with a smaller ratio of 3:1 [23,24]. There is a higher proportion of African-American children with NMO (34–44%) compared to other racial groups [4,5]. In North America, Caucasians, Latin American white non-Caucasian, and Asians make up the remainder of the racial groups [4,5]. However, this information is based on relatively small case series, and more systematic population-based studies of NMO disease prevalence and seroprevalence of the NMO-IgG antibody are needed to determine demographic information more definitively. One population-based study of MS and NMO in Martinique has been reported. NMO accounted for 17.3% of a French-Afro Caribbean cohort of demyelinating diseases on that island, with no cases of NMO found among French Caucasian patients [25].

The median age of disease onset in NMO patients is 39 years (and 29 years for MS) [1,26]. To date, children (under age 18) make up a minority (5%) of NMO-IgG seropositive patients, with median age of disease onset of 12–14 years [4,5], although a child presenting with a first NMO attack under the age of two years has also been reported [27].

Clinical presentation

Optic neuritis occurs at disease onset in 53% of pediatric patients, 15% of whom have bilateral ON [4]. Twenty-two percent of patients present with TM, which is often longitudinally extensive, with a contiguous lesion extending more than three vertebral segments (Figure 23.1) [4]. Simultaneous ON and TM is the presenting symptoms in 9% [4]. Symptomatic brain involvement (including encephalopathy and seizures) is more common in pediatric

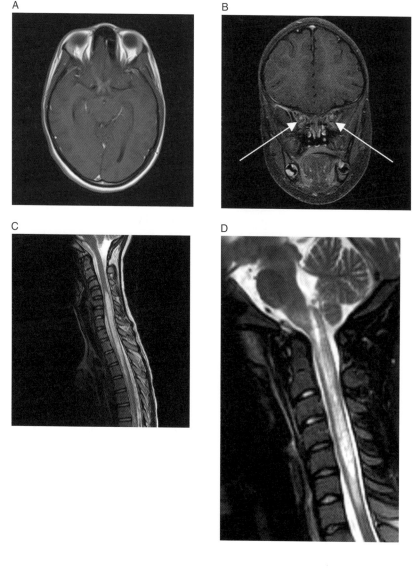

Figure 23.1 MRI abnormalities in three children with NMO showing characteristic sites of clinical involvement. (A) Bilateral optic nerve and optic chiasmal enhancement on a T1 post-contrast axial MRI of head in a 12-year-old girl with optic neuritis. (B) Bilateral optic nerve enhancement (arrows) on T1 post-contrast coronal MRI of head in a 2-year-old girl with optic neuritis. (C) An 11-year-old girl with a transverse myelitis, sagittal MRI of cord demonstrates an 11-vertebral segment long T2 signal abnormality. (D) The longitudinally extensive spinal T2 signal abnormality in this 17-year-old girl with intractable vomiting extends to the dorsal medulla, where the vomiting center of the area postrema is located. Copyrighted and modified with permission, Lippincott, Williams and Wilkins, 2008.

NMO patients compared to adults, occurring in 16–22% of patients [4,5]. Prodromal symptoms may also occur including fever, flu-like symptoms, nausea, vomiting, and meningismus. Patients may also present with site-restricted forms of the disease that include recurrent optic neuritis (RON) and recurrent TM in association with NMO-IgG seropositivity. The term NMO spectrum disorders (NMOSD) is often used to describe patients with restricted forms of NMO.

Brain involvement in NMO

Traditionally, NMO was considered to require absence of clinical disease outside the optic nerve or spinal cord, although clinically silent brain lesions were recognized as common in NMO [8,28]. Diagnostic criteria published in 1999 proposed negative brain MRI at onset as a supportive (but not required) criterion to differentiate NMO from MS [1]. Further study of patients with NMO, particularly following the discovery of the NMO-IgG antibody in 2004, revealed that patients with a well-established diagnosis of NMO may develop either asymptomatic or symptomatic brain lesions. Pittock *et al.* described the MRI brain findings in 36 NMO patients (as defined by the 1999 criteria) seen at Mayo Clinic, including a small number of children [8]. Brain MRI lesions were common, detected in 60% of patients studied. Most lesions were non-specific, but six patients (10%) had MS-like lesions, usually asymptomatic. Another five (8%), predominantly children, had diencephalic, brainstem or cerebral lesions, atypical for MS [8]. A further study by Pittock et al. revealed that diencephalic and periventricular MRI abnormalities found in these NMO patients correspond to sites of high AQP4 expression [29]. Misu et al. reported medullary and medullospinal T2 hyperintense MRI lesions involving the periventricular region, the area postrema and nucleus of tractus solitarius in six of eight patients with intractable hiccup and nausea in the setting of relapsing NMO [30]. With these findings in mind, the original criteria were revised in 2006 to include patients with brain MRI lesions atypical for MS and NMO-IgG seropositivity as a supportive criterion [22].

Unlike in adults, symptomatic brain disease is common in children with NMO (see Figures 23.1–23.3). McKeon et al. found symptoms referable to brain or brainstem lesions in 45% of NMO-IgG seropositive pediatric patients, occurring as the presenting syndrome in 16% [4]. Syndromes include intractable hiccoughs and vomiting, ataxia, ophthalmoparesis, and respiratory failure. Encephalopathy and seizures have also been described by McKeon and Lotze [4,5]. Some children presenting with a polysymptomatic encephalopathy and brain MRI lesions (including large hemispheric and thalamic lesions) were initially thought to have acute disseminated encephalomyelitis (ADEM) based upon current diagnostic criteria [4]. However, subsequent relapses and NMO-IgG seropositivity led to the diagnosis of NMO. The hypothalamic–pituitary axis is sometimes affected clinically and radiologically in NMO. Vernant et al. reported eight patients (all women) with relapsing NMO and endocrinopathies, most commonly amenorrhea and galactorrhea [31]. In children, reported disorders include the syndrome of inappropriate anti-diuretic hormone secretion (SIADH) and menstrual irregularities, with normalization of the menstrual cycle during remission while on immunosuppressive treatment [5]. Catamenial exacerbation of symptoms has also been noted in one patient, with an improved clinical course seen with introduction of an oral contraceptive agent [5]. Raised intracranial pressure has been reported in two children with NMO [4,32], one of whom had evidence of an obstructive hydrocephalus that improved with CSF shunting [4]. Recurrent hypersomnia and reduced hypocretin levels have been

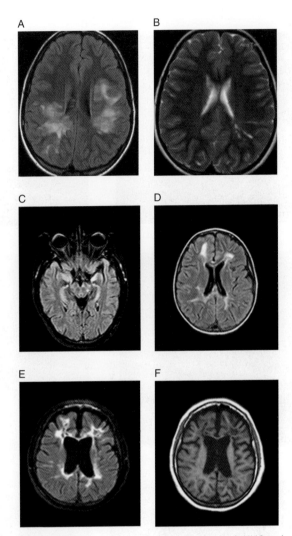

Figure 23.2 MRI abnormalities in four children with NMO and hemispheric involvement: typical of the spectrum of CNS AQP4 autoimmunity. (A) A 12-year-old girl with delirium and coma has confluent, hemispheric T2 signal abnormalities. (B) An 8-year-old girl with encephalopathy has radial T2 signal abnormality extending from the occipital horn of the left lateral ventricle through parietal subcortical white matter. (C) A 15-year-old boy with seizures and encephalopathy has T2 signal abnormality in the left mesial temporal region. (D–F) An 8-year-old girl presenting with encephalopathy and seizures has radial T2 white matter abnormalities extending from the lateral ventricles into frontal and parietal white matter (D). At age 16, follow-up MRI demonstrates persisting T2 signal abnormalities (E) and evidence of cerebral atrophy on T1 sequence (F). Copyrighted and modified with permission, Lippincott, Williams and Wilkins, 2008.

reported in an NMO-IgG seropositive Japanese patient with radiological evidence of hypothalamic disease and transverse myelitis [33].

Although attacks of ON and LETM predominate in NMO, brain symptomatology is common, and

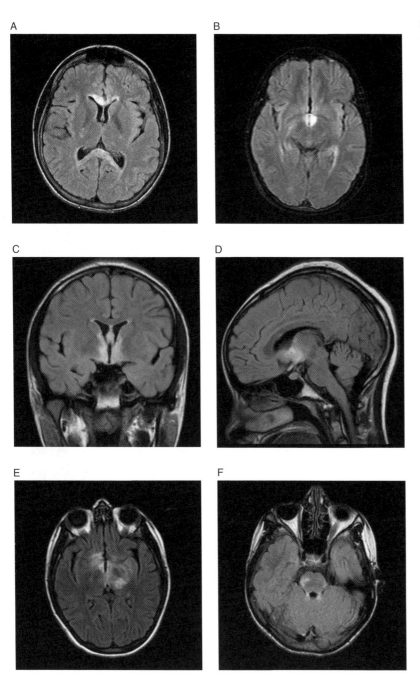

Figure 23.3 MRI abnormalities in five children with NMO showing the spectrum of periventricular abnormalities in the cerebral hemispheres, diencephalon, and brainstem, regions known to have high levels of AQP4 expression. (A) A 17-year-old girl with confluent T2 signal abnormality of the genu of the corpus callosum. (B) A 15-year-old patient with syndrome of inappropriate ADH secretion and menstrual irregularities has a hypothalamic T2 signal abnormality. (C, D) Hypothalamic and peri-third-ventricular diencephalic FLAIR abnormalities seen on coronal (C) and sagittal (D) MRI of head of a 12-year-old girl who presented with optic neuritis. (E) A 15-year-old boy with left thalamic and right hypothalamic FLAIR abnormalities. (F) The same patient as in (A) also has peri-fourth-ventricular FLAIR abnormalities in the superior cerebellar peduncles and in the right pons. Copyrighted and modified with permission, Lippincott, Williams and Wilkins, 2008.

therefore a broader concept of "CNS aquaporin-4 autoimmunity" in children has evolved [4].

Cerebrospinal fluid findings

McKeon *et al.* described that the most common CSF finding in NMO is a lymphocytic or neutrophil predominant leukocytosis (55%) and elevated protein (74%) [4]. Unlike in MS, where oligoclonal bands are almost always present and persist, in NMO oligoclonal bands are infrequently seen. Bergamaschi *et al.* reported 27% of adult patients with NMO had oligoclonal bands, and that they always disappeared with repeated testing, unlike in MS patients

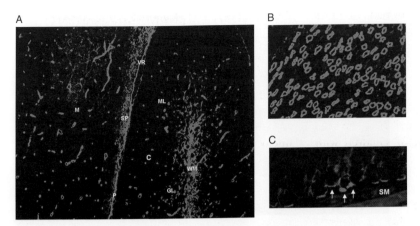

Figure 23.4 Immunofluorescence pattern of NMO-IgG in mouse CNS (A), kidney (B), and stomach (C). (A) Linearly stained pia (P), subpia (SP), and a Virchow–Robin (VR) space divide a section of mouse midbrain (M) on the left and cerebellum (C) on the right. Capillaries in the white and gray matter of the midbrain and cerebellum are stained, and are most prominent in central cerebellar white matter (WM) and in the granular (G) and molecular (ML) layers. The subpial region is stained in a mesh-like pattern. (B) Kidney: a subset of distal urine-collecting tubules in the renal medulla are stained. (C) Mucosa: the basolateral membranes of epithelial cells deep in the gastric mucosa are stained (arrows). SM = smooth muscle (unstained). Images provided courtesy of Dr. Vanda A. Lennon, Neuroimmunology Laboratory, Mayo Clinic, Rochester, MN. (See plate section for color version).

were oligoclonal bands persisted [34]. McKeon *et al.* found that only 6% of NMO-IgG seropositive children had CSF oligoclonal bands [4]; adult patients seldom have oligoclonal bands detected also [1]. Nakashima *et al.* reported that the total IgG concentration was elevated in the CSF of patients with NMO and MS, but that the percentage of IgG1 and the IgG1 index was elevated in the CSF of MS patients only [35].

Differential diagnosis

In children, the differential diagnosis for relapsing NMO is broader than it is for adults, making a definitive clinical diagnosis more challenging. Unlike in adults, LETM (a contiguous lesion more than three vertebral segments in length) is common among children with CNS inflammatory demyelinating disorders other than NMO. Banwell and colleagues demonstrated a high incidence of longitudinally extensive cord lesions in children with monophasic TM (83%), ADEM (100%), and relapsing–remitting MS (14%), among 87 children studied [3]. Thus, the presence of a longitudinally extensive lesion seems to be less predictive of NMO in children, and unlike in adults, seronegative monophasic NMO cases are common [3].

Symptomatic brain lesions may further complicate the diagnosis of NMO in children. In fact, several

reported pediatric NMO-IgG seropositive children had clinical symptoms at onset consistent with contemporary diagnostic criteria for ADEM (a polysymptomatic encephalopathy with focal or multifocal white matter-predominant brain lesions) [4,5,36]. However, unlike MS and ADEM, relapsing NMO is characterized by recurrent attacks of predominantly optic nerve and spinal cord disease, with rapid accrual of disability [4]. The presence of NMO-IgG in children with CNS inflammatory, demyelinating disorders predicts a relapsing NMO course and thus mandates initiation of long-term immunosuppressive therapies [4].

Antibody testing in NMO

The availability since 2004 of indirect immunofluorescence (IF) testing for the AQP4-specific autoantibody NMO-IgG has revolutionized the classification of idiopathic, inflammatory, demyelinating CNS disorders, allowing the distinction of NMOSD from MS [7,10]. In that original description of NMO-IgG, the antibody was 73% sensitive and 91% specific for clinically defined NMO [7]. Data from groups in Spain [37], the UK [38], Turkey [39], and France [40] have confirmed the high specificity of this antibody. NMO-IgG has a specific immunofluorescence pattern, binding selectively to the abluminal face of microvessels, pia, subpia and Virchow–Robin sheaths (Figure 23.4)

[7]. This deposition parallels the immune complex deposition in the spinal cord lesions of NMO [41]. NMO-IgG also binds to a subset of distal medullary collecting ducts in kidney, and basolateral membranes of gastric parietal epithelial cells, although the clinical significance is unclear [10]. These NMO-IgG immunoreactivity enriched sites were the clue that AQP4 was the autoantigen in NMO. Banwell *et al.* reported NMO-IgG seroprevalence among 87 children with demyelinating CNS disorders; 11% of all children were seropositive, and 47% of NMO patients were seropositive [3]. Eight of 17 pediatric NMO cases in that series had a monophasic course, and the seroprevalence of NMO-IgG was much higher in relapsing NMO (78% for relapsing versus 12.5% for monophasic disease) [3].

Immunoprecipitation (IP) assays employing recombinant human AQP4 have also been described [10]. Some recent reports suggest that antigen-specific IP and cell-binding assays for NMO-IgG (sometimes referred to as AQP4-IgG in this context) are more sensitive for NMOSD than IF [42,43]. Waters *et al.* reported that among 36 NMOSD patients tested, a green fluorescent protein (GFP) linked AQP4 IP assay [10] (76% sensitivity) was superior to their own IF assay (58% sensitivity) [43]. The authors also found specificity rates for NMO of 96% for NMO-IgG and 100% for the IP assay. Among 835 consecutive patients tested in Mayo Clinic neurology clinics (2004–2007), McKeon and colleagues demonstrated a sensitivity of 58% for NMO-IgG as tested by IF, but a sensitivity of only 33% for the IP assay [44]. Specificities were 99% for both assays in that study [44].

A cell-based assay where seropositivity is determined by loss of expression of AQP4 by a transfected human cell line after exposure to patient serum has also been studied. Both Waters *et al.* and Takahashi *et al.* found a sensitivity of 80% among a total of 35 patients tested for this technique [42,43], which may be limited when applied to the high throughput demands of a large clinical laboratory service. A novel AQP4-specific ELISA has shown early promise and appears to be as sensitive and specific as the NMO-IgG IF [45]. Combined assay testing may improve sensitivity. Seronegative cases may be explained by sub-optimal assay sensitivity, or perhaps some patients have an autoimmune disease with an antibody marker against a different neural target that remains to be identified.

Co-existing autoimmune disorders and autoantibodies in NMO

Co-existing autoimmune disorders are infrequently seen in multiple sclerosis, and do not occur with any higher frequency than in the general population [46]. In NMO, co-existing autoimmune disorders and co-existing markers of autoimmunity are distinctly common [47]. These disorders include systemic lupus erythematosus (SLE), Sjögren's syndrome, autoimmune thyroid disease, celiac disease, rheumatoid arthritis, the anti-phospholipid syndrome, and myasthenia gravis [47,48]. McKeon *et al.* demonstrated co-existing autoimmunity in 42% of NMO-IgG seropositive children, including SLE, Sjögren's syndrome, juvenile rheumatoid arthritis, and Grave's disease [4]. Lotze *et al.* demonstrated that a family history of autoimmunity is common among children with NMO; two-thirds of patients studied had a family history of an autoimmune disease in a first- or second-degree relative [5]. By contrast, among Canadian children with all acquired demyelinating syndromes, the incidence of autoimmune diseases reported among family members was low: thyroid disease, 4%; type 1 diabetes, 4% and SLE, 2% [49].

Non-organ-specific and organ-specific autoantibodies are also common among children and adults with NMO. McKeon *et al.* reported co-existing autoantibodies in 76% of NMO-IgG seropositive children, which included anti-nuclear antibody in 64%, antibodies to extractable nuclear antigen (ENA) in 17%, thyroid antibodies in 13%, and a variety of neural-specific antibodies in 19%, most commonly GAD65 antibody [4]. Other antibodies detected had specificities for neural cation channels (calcium channels [P/Q and N-type] and voltage-gated potassium channel) or for ganglionic acetylcholine receptors [4]. McKeon *et al.* systematically evaluated the frequency of neurological disorders and muscle and neural autoantibodies in 177 patients with NMO and in 250 control subjects (173 healthy; 77 MS patients) [47]. An excess of myasthenia gravis (MG, 2%), and muscle-type acetylcholine receptor antibody (11%) was detected among NMO patients [47]. The presence of neural or muscle autoantibodies was more common in NMO patients (34%) than in MS patients or healthy controls (8%) [47].

Disease course and outcome

Ninety percent of adult and pediatric patients with NMO have a relapsing course principally characterized by attacks of ON and LETM [1,4]. NMO-IgG seropositivity correlates with risk for relapsing disease. A prospective study by Weinshenker and colleagues demonstrated that 56% of NMO-IgG seropositive patients presenting with a first episode of transverse myelitis had a further attack of ON or TM within 12 months, whereas none of 14 seronegative patients with the same clinical presentation relapsed during that time frame [50]. McKeon et al. found in their series that 93% of NMO-IgG seropositive patients had a second attack within the median duration of follow-up (12 months) [4]. Wingerchuk et al. found that relapses occurred within 12 months in 60% of NMO patients, and that truly monophasic cases were rare and occurred principally in NMO-IgG seronegative patients [1,3]. Banwell et al. found that eight of 17 pediatric patients with a clinical diagnosis of NMO had a monophasic course (47%), all but one of whom were NMO-IgG seronegative (12%) [3]; the duration of follow-up was short in the monophasic group (1.1 years vs. 4.95 years for relapsing NMO). The detection of NMO-IgG seropositivity is important since it predicts a relapsing course as well as being a diagnostic biomarker.

It should be borne in mind that while some patients have an apparent monophasic course, other patients will have relapses separated by several years [1]. For the most part, patients with relapsing NMO will present with either ON or TM, and then fulfill diagnostic criteria for NMO only at a later attack, usually months or sometimes years later. Wingerchuk et al. reported an interval of one year or more between the index and second attack in just four of 31 cases with a relapsing course fulfilling strict diagnostic criteria for NMO [1]. Patients with a truly monophasic course generally develop simultaneous or almost simultaneous bilateral optic neuritis and transverse myelitis [1].

Most attacks of NMO are sub-acute with disability accrued over days and weeks. Unlike many MS relapses, recovery from NMO attacks is often incomplete. The development of chronic disability in NMO is attack-related, and a secondary progressive course is rare [51]. Prospective studies of outcome in NMO are lacking. Retrospective studies have shown that many children with NMO have a poor prognosis, with rapid development of attack-related disability. After a median follow-up of 12 months, residual visual impairment after attack resolution was documented in 54% of NMO-IgG seropositive children (27% had binocular blindness) and 44% had residual motor weakness [4]. Patients with RON who are NMO-IgG seropositive also have a worse visual outcome than those with RON who are seronegative [52].

Outcomes for NMO in childhood may be worse than for pediatric MS. Median EDSS scores for children with NMO were 3–4 after a median of one year of follow-up [4,5] in two small retrospective studies. In contrast, a prospective study of patients with childhood-onset MS recently demonstrated a median EDSS of 4.0 after 20 years of the disease [53].

The overall five-year survival rate for adults with NMO is 68%, with deaths occurring due to neurogenic respiratory failure in the setting of NMO-related rhombic encephalitis [1,54]. In a retrospective Brazilian study of 60 patients (59% were of African ancestry) mortality rates were noted to be higher among patients of Afro-Brazilians (accounting for 12 of 14 deaths) than among other racial groups [55].

To date, no reliable serological predictors of attack outcome or attack recurrence have emerged. Takahashi et al. found a positive correlation between titer of NMO-IgG antibody and severity of visual outcome, size of MRI-measured length of TM lesion, and size of cerebral lesions [56]. Waters et al. did not confirm a correlation between NMO-IgG antibody titers and length of spinal cord lesions [38]. Jarius and colleagues reported that NMO-IgG antibody levels increased in the months prior to an attack in a retrospective series of eight patients [57]. However, this finding was variable, as in three of these patients, the antibody titers decreased immediately prior to an attack, and in other instances no attack occurred in the setting of rising antibody levels [57].

The impact of NMO on cognitive function of patients has likely been underestimated until recent times. Even in the setting of clinical attacks restricted to optic nerve and spinal cord, and normal brain MRI, the brain may be abnormal in patients with NMO. Abnormalities in normal-appearing gray matter of NMO patients may be seen with magnetic transfer and diffusion tensor MRI techniques [58,59]. Blanc et al. reported that cognitive performance was significantly lower in patients with NMO than in healthy controls matched for age, sex, and educational level [60]. The degree of overall cognitive impairment

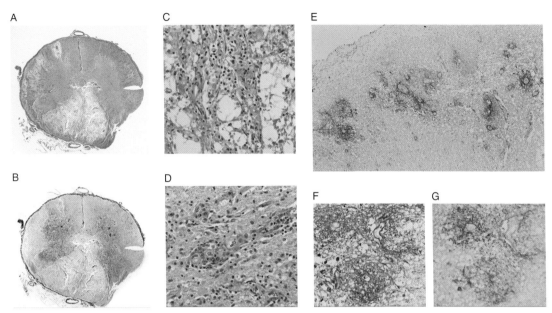

Figure 23.5 Pathological and immunopathological findings in NMO. (A) Extensive demyelination of the gray matter and white matter at the level of the thoracic cord (Luxol fast blue–Periodic acid Schiff stain for myelin; 10×). (B) Extensive axonal injury, necrosis, and associated cavitation (Bielschowsky silver impregnation; 10×). (C, D) The inflammatory infiltrate contains perivascular and parenchymal eosinophils and granulocytes (100×). (E) Prominent vasculocentric complement activation, in a characteristic rosette and rim pattern surrounding thickened blood vessels (immunocytochemistry for C9neo antigen [red]; 200×). (F) Higher magnification (1000×) of rosette pattern of immunoglobulin deposition (immunocytochemistry for IgG). (G) Rosette pattern of C9neo antigen in a similar distribution around the same vessels as in (F). Copyrighted and modified with permission from Elsevier, 2007. (See plate section for color version).

was similar in patients with NMO and in patients with MS in that report. The most common abnormalities seen in NMO patients were in the domains of long-term memory, information processing speed, executive dysfunction, and language dysfunction [60]. Long-term cognitive sequelae have also been reported in NMO-IgG seropositive children after resolution of acute encephalopathic attacks [4,5].

Immunopathology

In NMO, demyelination and necrosis affect the gray and white matter of optic nerves and spinal cord (Figure 23.5) [41]. Blood vessels are thickened and have a hyalinized (pink, glassy) appearance [41,61,62]. Eosinophils and neutrophils (as well as lymphocytes) are commonly observed in the inflammatory infiltrate of an active NMO lesion [41]. The pathogenic role of AQP4 IgG is supported by pathological studies of active NMO lesions demonstrating activation of terminal complement cascade components and immunoglobulin, deposited in a vasculocentric pattern, corresponding to the normal expression of AQP4 in the end-feet of astrocytes [41]. Unlike in

MS lesions (where AQP4 expression is upregulated), AQP4 staining is absent in NMO lesions (Figure 23.6) [63]. In MS, immune complexes may also be deposited along myelin sheaths, but not in a vasculocentric pattern [64]. NMO brain lesions have been shown to have identical pathological features to optico-spinal lesions [25,65].

Pathogenesis

The immunizing event in NMO is usually unknown. There have been case reports of patients developing NMO in the course of documented infections to include HIV [66], and varicella zoster [67–69]. NMO-IgG and clinical NMO have also been observed in a paraneoplastic context. Pittock *et al.* reported 31 patients who had NMO-IgG identified incidentally on paraneoplastic immunofluorescence, eight of whom had a neoplasm (breast, 3; lung, 2; thymus, 1; uterine cervical, 1; lymphoma, 1) [70]. Two patients in that study with NMO-IgG seropositivity had carcinoma in the absence of an NMO spectrum disorder [70]. Genetic factors may also have a role to play (although

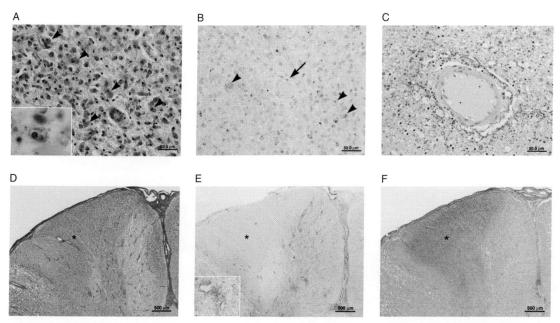

Figure 23.6 AQP4 immunoreactivity in MS (acute pattern II; A–C) and NMO (D–F) lesions. (A) In MS, numerous macrophages containing myelin debris are dispersed throughout the active lesion (arrowheads and inset). (B) C9neo antigen is present within macrophages (arrowheads), but absent around blood vessels (arrow). (C) Higher magnification reveals AQP4 immunoreactivity is prominent in a rosette pattern surrounding a penetrating blood vessel in the lesion. (D) In NMO, there is extensive demyelination involving both gray and white matter, *indicates preserved myelin in the periplaque white matter (PPWM). (E) C9neo is deposited in a vasculocentric rim and rosette pattern (inset) within the active lesions, but not in the PPWM. (F) The lesions lack AQP4, which is retained in the PPWM (*) and gray matter. (A,D), Luxol fast blue–Periodic Acid Schiff stain for myelin; (B,E), C9neo immunohistochemistry; (C,F), AQP4 immunohistochemistry. Copyrighted and modified with permission from Oxford University Press, 2007. (See plate section for color version).

reports of familial NMO are rare). Hereditary cases have been reported in two sets of sisters [71,72], a mother and daughter pair (the mother was NMO-IgG seropositive, the daughter had co-existing myasthenia gravis) [73], and identical twins [74].

The inciting factor in NMO is currently thought to be the AQP4-specific NMO-IgG from the peripheral immunoglobulin pool. AQP4 is highly expressed in astrocytic end-feet, which form a component of the blood–brain barrier (BBB) by binding to the basal lamina of endothelium [9]. AQP4 is conspicuously absent from myelin and oligodendrocytes. NMO-IgG produced by peripheral plasma cells is thought to traverse the BBB (through endothelial endocytosis, or at areas of relative BBB permeability or injury), and thus have access to the extracellular domains of AQP4-enriched astrocytic end-feet [2]. It is unlikely that pathologic NMO-IgG producing plasma cells are principally located and undergoing clonal expansion in the CNS since oligoclonal bands are at least three times less common in NMO than in MS [34]. Through crosslinking of bivalent IgG on the extracellular domain of AQP4, NMO-IgG can cause

endocytosis and targeting of the antigen to the endolysosomal pathway (antigenic modulation) [11,75]. The glutamate transporter critical for reuptake of cytotoxic glutamate (EAAT2) is coupled to AQP4, and is also degraded in the process of modulation, thus contributing to astrocytic and neuronal cytotoxicity [75]. A glutamate receptor antibody has been reported in one Japanese patient with NMO-IgG and TM [76]. NMO-IgG also induces activation of the complement cascade [11,75]. This contributes to loss of AQP4 from astrocytic end-feet, adversely altering osmotic regulation, BBB function, granulocyte recruitment, and maintenance of neural microenvironment [11,75,77]. Increased permeability of the BBB leads to a massive infiltration of leukocytes, including polymorphonuclear cells (eosinophils and neutrophils). Interleukins 8 and 17 likely play a role in inducing neutrophil infiltration. Ishizu *et al.* reported upregulation of interleukins 5, 8 and 17 in CSF supernatants of Japanese patients with opticospinal MS [78]. Complement-mediated cell injury and inflammatory cellular influx causes neuronal injury, demyelination, and necrosis.

Gene expression profiles of NMO brain lesions have revealed upregulation of molecules associated with immune regulation including interferon gamma-inducible protein 30, CD163 and osteopontin [79]. These molecules are likely regulated by nuclear factor-kappa B (NF-κB) and B-lymphocyte-induce maturation protein-1 (Blimp-1) [79]. Elevated matrix metalloproteinase-9 levels are found in the CSF of patients with MS but not in the CSF of NMO patients [80].

Treatment

Currently, treatment for NMO is based upon small case series, most of which describe adult populations. There have been no large randomized clinical trials in NMO. However, there is general consensus on current effective therapies for NMO. Treatment must include effective therapies for acute attacks as well as the use of chronic immunosuppressive treatments to help prevent further attacks and related disability. There are long-term safety concerns regarding the use of immunosuppressant medications in children, and close monitoring is required, even after the discontinuation of these agents. Chapter 11 provides further detailed discussion of these risks (Figure 23.7).

Corticosteroids are the typical initial treatment for patients with acute attacks associated with significant neurological disability. Methylprednisolone is most commonly used at a dosing of 30 mg/kg/day (maximum of 1 g) for five days. Patients with severe neurological deficits failing to respond within seven days may benefit from plasma exchange (PLEX) 1:1 plasma volumes every other day for five days [81,82]. Some institutions use higher volumes of exchange in circumstances of severe attack-related disability. A single dose of cyclophosphamide (750–1000 mg/m^2) may offer further benefit in combination with PLEX for patients with complete paralysis secondary to TM or for patients with comorbid autoimmune disease [83]. Other treatment options described for acute treatment have included IVIg 2 g/kg divided over five days [4,5].

Long-term treatment with immunosuppressive therapies is indicated for relapsing forms of NMO or in those patients found to have NMO-IgG seropositivity at the time of their initial attack. Chronic daily low-dose corticosteroids have been described to prevent relapses in previous small case series. Watanabe *et al.* analyzed relapse frequency in a group of nine

patients, comparing the relapse rate before and after initiation of corticosteroid monotherapy. They found a significant decrease in the annualized relapse rate after initiation of corticosteroid treatment compared to the rate before corticosteroid use (median 0.49 vs. 1.48, respectively) [84]. They additionally noted an increased relapse frequency when corticosteroid dosing was less than 10 mg/day. Mandler *et al.* prospectively followed seven NMO patients receiving treatment with daily corticosteroids and azathioprine for 18 months [85]. Each of these patients also received high-dose intravenous methylprednisolone for five days at the start of the study. None of the patients had relapses during the follow-up period, and there was a significant decrease in EDSS scores from a mean of 9 at baseline to a mean of 3 at 18 months ($p<0.005$). Based upon these studies as well as other case series, corticosteroids in combination with either azathioprine or mycophenolate mofetil are recommended as initial treatment for NMO [4,5]. Typically, prednisone is initiated at a dosing of 1 mg/kg/day. Azathioprine (2–3 mg/kg/day) or mycophenolate mofetil (15 mg/kg twice daily) is initiated three weeks later. Blood counts and liver function tests should be performed weekly for the first month and then monthly for at least the next three months with these agents. Pending response and tolerability to these medications, attempts can be made at the end of the first month of prednisone therapy for tapering by 5–10 mg every month until reaching a daily dosing of 10 mg. Patients should be monitored for complications of long-term steroid treatment to include cataracts, excessive weight gain, gastric irritation, and osteoporosis. The side effects of azathioprine and mycophenolate mofetil are reviewed in Chapter 11.

Patients failing to respond to corticosteroids in combination with either azathioprine or mycophenolate mofetil or who are having intolerable side effects should be considered for other alternate immunosuppressive treatments. Rituximab is a genetically engineered, chimeric, murine/human monoclonal antibody directed against the CD20 antigen found on the surface of normal B cells. It was initially developed as a treatment for non-Hodgkin's lymphoma and rheumatoid arthritis, and its use in NMO is off-label. However, given the suspected involvement of NMO-IgG in NMO, targeted therapy to reduce the B cell population might offer benefit in these patients. Cree *et al.* initially described benefits of rituximab treatment in an open-label study of eight

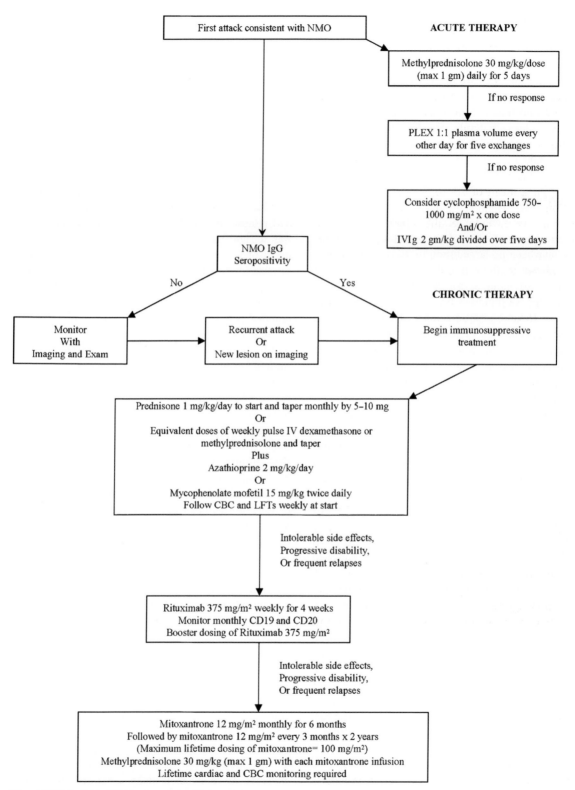

Figure 23.7 Pediatric NMO treatment algorithm.

adult patients over an average of one year follow-up [86]. In this study, patients received rituximab dosed at 375 mg/m^2, administered once per week for 4 weeks. B-cell counts were followed bimonthly. When B-cell counts became detectable, patients were given the option to be retreated with rituximab, consisting of two IV infusions of 1000 mg administered 2 weeks apart. Six of the patients were relapse-free with a reduction in annual relapse rate from a mean of 2.6 to 0 ($p = 0.0078$). Disability as measured by the EDSS was also reduced through the 12-month time course, going from a mean of 7.5 to 5.5 ($p = 0.013$). B-cell depletion was sustained for 6–12 months, allowing some patients to only require yearly retreatment. Jacob *et al.* recently described a retrospective cohort of 25 NMO patients (including two children) who were treated with rituximab and followed for a median of 19 months [87]. Patients received either 375 mg/m^2, administered once per week for four weeks or 1000 mg infused twice, with a two-week interval between the infusions. Median time for re-treatment was eight months. They found a similar significant reduction in annualized relapse rate before and after treatment (median annualized relapse rate of 1.7 vs. 0, respectively; $p<0.001$). The EDSS scores stabilized in nine patients and improved in 11. EDSS scores worsened in five patients. Complications of treatment included an increased number of infections, including one death from septicemia, and infusion-related reactions. Notably, in both of these studies and others, not all patients responded to rituximab, suggesting that an alternate or additional pathophysiologic mechanism may be occurring in these individuals. The off-label use of rituximab in NMO should be considered in patients with disease refractory to other agents. Alternatively, rituximab may be considered as first-line therapy for individuals with a more aggressive disease course to include fixed disability or a history of multiple relapses at the time of their initial presentation. Rituximab may be initiated at a dosing of 375 mg/m^2 weekly for four weeks. Currently, most institutions using rituximab treatment for NMO simplify this regimen to 1000 mg given on days 1 and 15. CD19 and CD20 levels are monitored every three months to assure adequate depletion of B cells. CD19 is used as an additional surrogate treatment marker, as rituximab will compete with CD20 antibodies used in flow cytometry, possibly resulting in false negative results for up to six months following treatment. A booster dosing of rituximab 375 mg/m^2 or 500–1000 mg once or twice two weeks apart is given yearly or when CD19 or CD20 counts begin to rise (see Chapter 11). Quantitative serum immunoglobulins should also be monitored on a routine basis to assure that the patient does not develop hypogammaglobulinemia. While this has not been reported in the literature, interval treatment with IVIg could be considered if this situation were to occur. While rituximab is generally well tolerated, it can have significant side effects, including infusion reactions, transient leukopenia or thrombocytopenia, and increased risk for infection. These are discussed in greater detail in Chapter 11.

Another chemotherapeutic agent, mitoxantrone, has been approved for use in adults with secondary progressive multiple sclerosis. Its off-label use in NMO has also been investigated. Mitoxantrone suppresses T-helper lymphocytes and the humoral immune system via both macrophage and B-cell attenuation. Weinstock-Guttman *et al.* described five NMO patients treated with mitoxantrone in a prospective two-year study [88]. Patients received mitoxantrone 12 mg/m^2 monthly for six months followed by three additional treatments every three months. Two patients experienced relapses during the two-year follow-up. EDSS improved from a mean of 4.4 to 2.2 over the same time period. Likewise, annualized relapse rate decreased from 2.4 to 0.4. All of these patients additionally received treatment with methylprednisolone 1000 mg at the time of their mitoxantrone infusion and were started on azathioprine after 18 months of treatment. Mitoxantrone requires special precautions as related to a risk for cardiomyopathy and leukemia. These risks are further discussed in Chapter 11.

A variety of other treatment regimens have been described in case series and cohorts of NMO patients to include children. Such treatments include pulse monthly IVIg 2 g/kg divided over five days followed by monthly booster doses of 500 mg/kg, serial plasmapheresis, and cyclophosphamide [4,5,89,90]. Further clinical trials will be needed to investigate the efficacy and safety of all of these regimens in the pediatric NMO population.

Future directions

Despite the rapid pace of discovery in this novel field of NMO and CNS AQP4 autoimmunity, much remains to be learned about these disorders. Their true prevalence and the seroprevalence of the

NMO-IgG antibody have not been determined in ethnically diverse population-based studies of patients with inflammatory, demyelinating CNS disorders. It also remains to be seen if NMO-IgG antibody values or functional AQP4 antibody assays can predict future attack severity or disease outcome. A recent report has indicated that a laboratory measure of complement-mediated cell injury correlates with NMO attack severity, and may serve as a future marker of disease prognosis [91]. While existing therapies are effective at preventing NMO attacks in most patients, there are other patients who have ongoing relapses despite maximum doses of different antibody-depleting therapies. The discovery of new, effective, and potentially curative therapies for NMO may be expedited by development of validated models of CNS AQP4 autoimmunity in animals and cell culture systems.

References

1. Wingerchuk DM, Hogancamp WF, O'Brien PC, Weinshenker BG. The clinical course of neuromyelitis optica (Devic's syndrome). *Neurology* 1999;**53**:1107–1114.

2. Wingerchuk DM, Lennon VA, Lucchinetti CF, Pittock SJ, Weinshenker BG. The spectrum of neuromyelitis optica. *Lancet Neurol* 2007;**6**:805–815.

3. Banwell B, Tenembaum S, Lennon VA, *et al.* Neuromyelitis optica-IgG in childhood inflammatory demyelinating CNS disorders. *Neurology* 2008;**70**: 344–352.

4. McKeon A, Lennon VA, Lotze T, *et al.* CNS aquaporin-4 autoimmunity in children. *Neurology* 2008;**71**:93–100.

5. Lotze TE, Northrop JL, Hutton GJ, *et al.* Spectrum of pediatric neuromyelitis optica. *Pediatrics* 2008;**122**: e1039–1047.

6. Barbieri F, Buscaino GA. Neuromyelitis optica in the elderly. *Acta Neurol (Napoli)* 1989;**11**:247–251.

7. Lennon VA, Wingerchuk DM, Kryzer TJ, *et al.* A serum autoantibody marker of neuromyelitis optica: Distinction from multiple sclerosis. *Lancet* 2004;**364**:2106–2112.

8. Pittock SJ, Lennon VA, Krecke K, *et al.* Brain abnormalities in neuromyelitis optica. *Arch Neurol* 2006;**63**:390–396.

9. Amiry-Moghaddam M, Ottersen OP. The molecular basis of water transport in the brain. *Nature Rev* 2003;**4**:991–1001.

10. Lennon VA, Kryzer TJ, Pittock SJ, Verkman AS, Hinson SR. IgG marker of optic–spinal multiple sclerosis binds to the aquaporin-4 water channel. *J Exp Med* 2005;**202**:473–477.

11. Hinson SR, Pittock SJ, Lucchinetti CF, *et al.* Pathogenic potential of IgG binding to water channel extracellular domain in neuromyelitis optica. *Neurology* 2007;**69**:2221–2231.

12. Lennon VA, Lindstrom JM, Seybold ME. Experimental autoimmune myasthenia: A model of myasthenia gravis in rats and guinea pigs. *J Exp Med* 1975;**141**:1365–1375.

13. Albutt C. On the ophthalmoscopic signs of spinal disease. *Lancet* 1870;**1**:76–78.

14. Gault F. De la neuromyelité optique aiguë. *Thèse de Lyon serre* 1894;**1**(No. 981).

15. Devic E. Myélite aiguë compliquée de névrite optique. *Bull Med* 1894;**8**:1033–1034.

16. McKee SH, McNaughton FL. Neuromyelitis optica: A report of two cases. *Trans Am Ophthalmol Soc* 1937;**35**:125–135.

17. Galetta SL, Bennett J. Neuromyelitis optica is a variant of multiple sclerosis. *Arch Neurol* 2007;**64**:901–903.

18. Weinshenker BG. Neuromyelitis optica is distinct from multiple sclerosis. *Arch Neurol* 2007;**64**:899–901.

19. Beck G. A case of diffuse myelitis associated with optic neuritis. *Brain* 1927;**50**:687–703.

20. Jeffery AR, Buncic JR. Pediatric Devic's neuromyelitis optica. *J Pediatr Ophthalmol Strabismus* 1996;**33**: 223–229.

21. Krupp LB, Banwell B, Tenembaum S. Consensus definitions proposed for pediatric multiple sclerosis and related disorders. *Neurology* 2007;**68**(Suppl 2): S7–12.

22. Wingerchuk DM, Lennon VA, Pittock SJ, Lucchinetti CF, Weinshenker BG. Revised diagnostic criteria for neuromyelitis optica. *Neurology* 2006;**66**:1485–1489.

23. Ness JM, Chabas D, Sadovnick AD, *et al.* Clinical features of children and adolescents with multiple sclerosis. *Neurology* 2007;**68**(Suppl 2):S37–45.

24. de Seze J, Lebrun C, Stojkovic T, *et al.* Is Devic's neuromyelitis optica a separate disease? A comparative study with multiple sclerosis. *Mult Scler* 2003;**9**: 521–525.

25. Cabre P, Heinzlef O, Merle H, *et al.* MS and neuromyelitis optica in Martinique (French West Indies). *Neurology* 2001;**56**:507–514.

26. Kantarci OH, Weinshenker BG. Natural history of multiple sclerosis. *Neurol Clin* 2005;**23**:17–38.

27. Yuksel D, Senbil N, Yilmaz D, Yavuz Gurer YK. Devic's neuromyelitis optica in an infant case. *J Child Neurol* 2007;**22**:1143–1146.

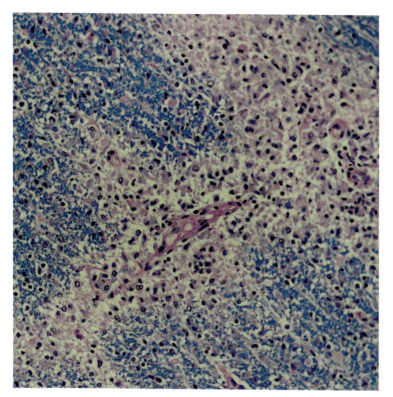

Figure 15.1 Luxol Fast Blue and Cresyl Violet stained autopsy section from the subcortical white matter of a 17-year-old boy with a diagnosis of ADEM (10×). Note the perivascular pattern of myelin loss and inflammatory cell infiltration. Acknowledgments: Department of Pathology, Children's Hospital, Boston.

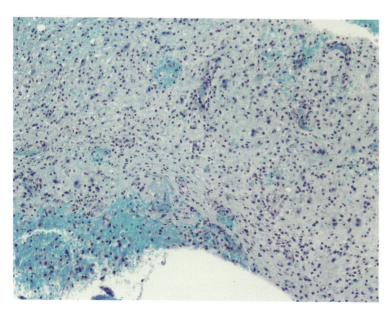

Figure 15.2 Luxol Fast Blue and Cresyl Violet stained biopsy section from the subcortical white matter of a 17-year-old girl with a diagnosis of pediatric multiple sclerosis (10×). Note the diffuse pattern of myelin loss and nodular inflammatory cell infiltration. Acknowledgments: Department of Pathology, Children's Hospital, Boston.

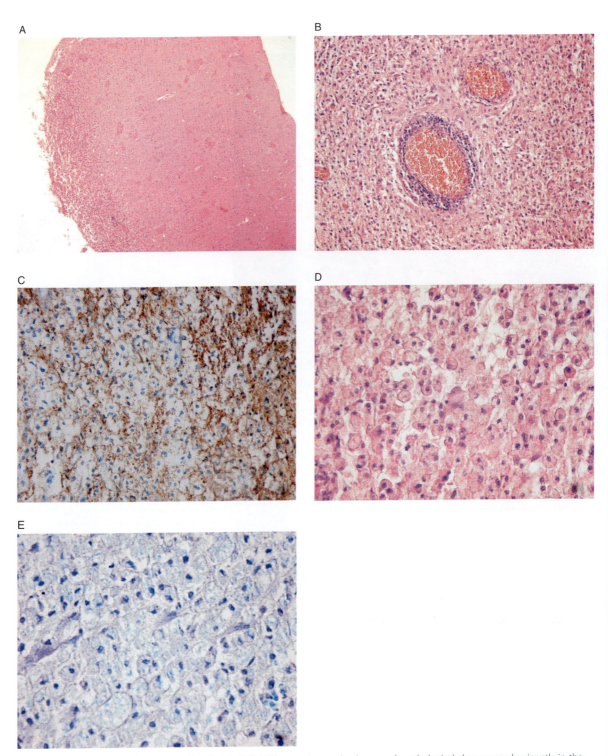

Figure 17.2 Brain biopsy of a 12-year old girl with ADEM. Microscopic examination reveals pathological changes predominantly in the white matter (A, hematoxylin–eosin). The diffuse inflammatory process is characterized by a perivascular infiltration of mononuclear cells, typically around veins and venules (B, hematoxylin–eosin), and reactive astroglial proliferation (C, GFAP). Infiltration of mononuclear cells, comprises mainly macrophages (D, hematoxylin–eosin) containing punctate myelin debris (E, Luxol fast blue–PAS staining). Courtesy of Drs. F. Lubieniecki and A.L. Taratuto, Neuropathology Department, National Pediatric Hospital Dr. J. P. Garrahan, Buenos Aires, Argentina.

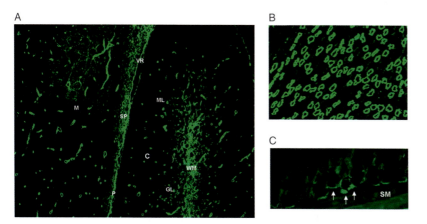

Figure 23.4 Immunofluorescence pattern of NMO-IgG in mouse CNS (A), kidney (B), and stomach (C). (A) Linearly stained pia (P), subpia (SP), and a Virchow–Robin (VR) space divide a section of mouse midbrain (M) on the left and cerebellum (C) on the right. Capillaries in the white and gray matter of the midbrain and cerebellum are stained, and are most prominent in central cerebellar white matter (WM) and in the granular (G) and molecular (ML) layers. The subpial region is stained in a mesh-like pattern. (B) Kidney: a subset of distal urine-collecting tubules in the renal medulla are stained. (C) Mucosa: the basolateral membranes of epithelial cells deep in the gastric mucosa are stained (arrows). SM = smooth muscle (unstained). Images provided courtesy of Dr. Vanda A. Lennon, Neuroimmunology Laboratory, Mayo Clinic, Rochester, MN.

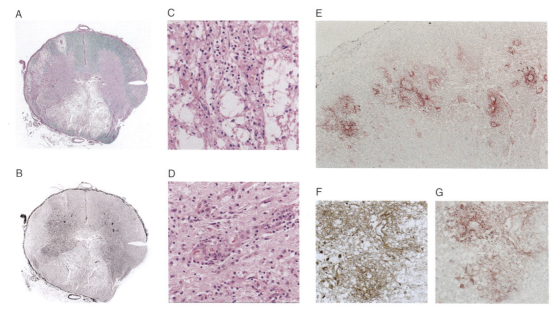

Figure 23.5 Pathological and immunopathological findings in NMO. (A) Extensive demyelination of the gray matter and white matter at the level of the thoracic cord (Luxol fast blue–Periodic acid Schiff stain for myelin; 10×). (B) Extensive axonal injury, necrosis, and associated cavitation (Bielschowsky silver impregnation; 10×). (C, D) The inflammatory infiltrate contains perivascular and parenchymal eosinophils and granulocytes (100×). (E) Prominent vasculocentric complement activation, in a characteristic rosette and rim pattern surrounding thickened blood vessels (immunocytochemistry for C9neo antigen [red]; 200×). (F) Higher magnification (1000×) of rosette pattern of immunoglobulin deposition (immunocytochemistry for IgG). (G) Rosette pattern of C9neo antigen in a similar distribution around the same vessels as in (F). Copyrighted and modified with permission from Elsevier, 2007.

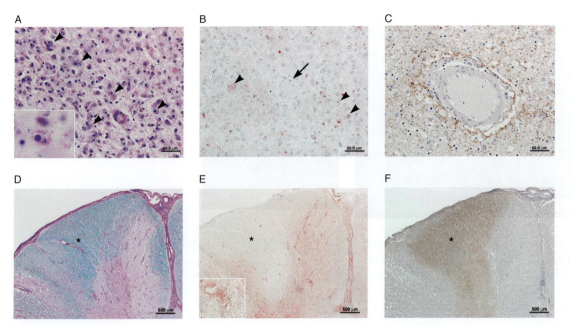

Figure 23.6 AQP4 immunoreactivity in MS (acute pattern II; A–C) and NMO (D–F) lesions. (A) In MS, numerous macrophages containing myelin debris are dispersed throughout the active lesion (arrowheads and inset). (B) C9neo antigen is present within macrophages (arrowheads), but absent around blood vessels (arrow). (C) Higher magnification reveals AQP4 immunoreactivity is prominent in a rosette pattern surrounding a penetrating blood vessel in the lesion. (D) In NMO, there is extensive demyelination involving both gray and white matter, *indicates preserved myelin in the periplaque white matter (PPWM). (E) C9neo is deposited in a vasculocentric rim and rosette pattern (inset) within the active lesions, but not in the PPWM. (F) The lesions lack AQP4, which is retained in the PPWM (*) and gray matter. (A,D), Luxol fast blue–Periodic Acid Schiff stain for myelin; (B,E), C9neo immunohistochemistry; (C,F), AQP4 immunohistochemistry. Copyrighted and modified with permission from Oxford University Press, 2007.

28. O'Riordan JI, Gallagher HL, Thompson AJ, *et al.* Clinical, CSF, and MRI findings in Devic's neuromyelitis optica. *J Neurol Neurosurg Psychiatry* 1996;**60**:382–387.

29. Pittock SJ, Weinshenker BG, Lucchinetti CF, *et al.* Neuromyelitis optica brain lesions localized at sites of high aquaporin 4 expression. *Arch Neurol* 2006;**63**:964–968.

30. Misu T, Fujihara K, Nakashima I, Sato S, Itoyama Y. Intractable hiccup and nausea with periaqueductal lesions in neuromyelitis optica. *Neurology* 2005;**65**:1479–1482.

31. Vernant JC, Cabre P, Smadja D, *et al.* Recurrent optic neuromyelitis with endocrinopathies: A new syndrome. *Neurology* 1997;**48**:58–64.

32. Keefe RJ. Neuromyelitis optica with increased intracranial pressure. *AMA Arch Ophthalmol* 1957;**57**:110–111.

33. Nozaki H, Shimohata T, Kanbayashi T, *et al.* A patient with anti-aquaporin 4 antibody who presented with recurrent hypersomnia, reduced orexin (hypocretin) level, and symmetrical hypothalamic lesions. *Sleep Med* 2009;**10**:253–255.

34. Bergamaschi R, Tonietti S, Franciotta D, *et al.* Oligoclonal bands in Devic's neuromyelitis optica and multiple sclerosis: Differences in repeated cerebrospinal fluid examinations. *Mult Scler* 2004;**10**:2–4.

35. Nakashima I, Fujihara K, Fujimori J, *et al.* Absence of IgG1 response in the cerebrospinal fluid of relapsing neuromyelitis optica. *Neurology* 2004;**62**:144–146.

36. Tenembaum S, Chitnis T, Ness J, Hahn JS. Acute disseminated encephalomyelitis. *Neurology* 2007;**68** (Suppl 2):S23–36.

37. Zuliani L, Blanco Y, Tavolato B, *et al.* Neuromyelitis optica IgG (NMO-IgG) in patients with suspected NMO or limited forms of NMO. *Mult Scler* 2006;**12**:S155.

38. Waters P, Jarius S, Littleton E, *et al.* Aquaporin-4 antibodies in neuromyelitis optica and longitudinally extensive transverse myelitis. *Arch Neurol* 2008;**65**:913–919.

39. Akman-Demir G. Probably NMO-IgG in Turkish patients with Devic's disease and multiple sclerosis. *Mult Scler* 2006;**12**:S157.

40. Marignier R, De Seze J, Durand-Dubief F, *et al.* NMO-IgG: A French experience. *Mult Scler* 2006;**12**:S4.

41. Lucchinetti CF, Mandler RN, McGavern D, *et al.* A role for humoral mechanisms in the pathogenesis of Devic's neuromyelitis optica. *Brain* 2002;**125**:1450–1461.

42. Takahashi T, Fujihara K, Nakashima I, *et al.* Establishment of a new sensitive assay for anti-human aquaporin-4 antibody in neuromyelitis optica. *Tohoku J Exp Med* 2006;**210**:307–313.

43. Waters P, Jarius S, Littleton E, *et al.* Aquaporin-4 antibodies in neuromyelitis optica and longitudinally extensive transverse myelitis. *Arch Neurol* 2008; **4**:202–214.

44. McKeon A, Fryer JP, Apiwattanakul M, *et al.* Diagnosis of neuromyelitis spectrum disorders: Comparative sensitivities and specificities of immunohistochemical and immunoprecipitation assays. *Arch Neurol* 2009;**66**:1134–1138.

45. McKeon A, Chen S, Pittock SJ, *et al.* Comparison of optimized immunohistochemical assay with a novel aquaporin-4-specific ELISA for detection of NMO-IgG. *Ann Neurol* 2009;**66**:S37.

46. Ramagopalan SV, Dyment DA, Valdar W, *et al.* Autoimmune disease in families with multiple sclerosis: A population-based study. *Lancet Neurol* 2007;**6**:604–610.

47. McKeon A, Lennon VA, Jacob A, *et al.* Coexistence of myasthenia gravis and serological markers of neurological autoimmunity in neuromyelitis optica. *Muscle Nerve* 2009;**39**:87–90.

48. Jarius S, Jacob S, Waters P, *et al.* Neuromyelitis optica in patients with gluten sensitivity associated with antibodies to aquaporin-4. *J Neurol Neurosurg Psychiatry* 2008;**79**:1084.

49. Banwell B, Kennedy J, Sadovnick D, *et al.* Incidence of acquired demyelination of the CNS in Canadian children. *Neurology* 2009;**72**:232–239.

50. Weinshenker BG, Wingerchuk DM, Vukusic S, *et al.* Neuromyelitis optica IgG predicts relapse after longitudinally extensive transverse myelitis. *Ann Neurol* 2006;**59**:566–569.

51. Wingerchuk DM, Pittock SJ, Lucchinetti CF, Lennon VA, Weinshenker BG. A secondary progressive clinical course is uncommon in neuromyelitis optica. *Neurology* 2007;**68**:603–605.

52. Matiello M, Lennon VA, Jacob A, *et al.* NMO-IgG predicts the outcome of recurrent optic neuritis. *Neurology* 2008;**70**:2197–2200.

53. Renoux C, Vukusic S, Mikaeloff Y, *et al.* Natural history of multiple sclerosis with childhood onset. *N Engl J Med* 2007;**356**:2603–2613.

54. Wingerchuk DM, Weinshenker BG. Neuromyelitis optica: Clinical predictors of a relapsing course and survival. *Neurology* 2003;**60**:848–853.

55. Papais-Alvarenga RM, Carellos SC, Alvarenga MP, *et al.* Clinical course of optic neuritis in patients with relapsing neuromyelitis optica. *Arch Ophthalmol* 2008;**126**:12–16.

56. Takahashi T, Fujihara K, Nakashima I, *et al.* Anti-aquaporin-4 antibody is involved in the pathogenesis

of NMO: A study on antibody titre. *Brain* 2007;**130**:1235–1243.

57. Jarius S, Aboul-Enein F, Waters P, *et al.* Antibody to aquaporin-4 in the long-term course of neuromyelitis optica. *Brain* 2008;**131**:3072–3080.

58. Yu CS, Lin FC, Li KC, *et al.* Diffusion tensor imaging in the assessment of normal-appearing brain tissue damage in relapsing neuromyelitis optica. *Am J Neuroradiol* 2006;**27**:1009–1015.

59. Rocca MA, Agosta F, Mezzapesa DM, *et al.* Magnetization transfer and diffusion tensor MRI show gray matter damage in neuromyelitis optica. *Neurology* 2004;**62**:476–478.

60. Blanc F, Zephir H, Lebrun C, *et al.* Cognitive functions in neuromyelitis optica. *Arch Neurol* 2008;**65**:84–88.

61. Mandler RN, Davis LE, Jeffery DR, Kornfeld M. Devic's neuromyelitis optica: A clinicopathological study of 8 patients. *Ann Neurol* 1993;**34**:162–168.

62. Lefkowitz D, Angelo JN. Neuromyelitis optica with unusual vascular changes. *Arch Neurol* 1984;**41**:1103–1105.

63. Roemer SF, Parisi JE, Lennon VA, *et al.* Pattern-specific loss of aquaporin-4 immunoreactivity distinguishes neuromyelitis optica from multiple sclerosis. *Brain* 2007;**130**:1194–1205.

64. Lucchinetti C, Bruck W, Parisi J, *et al.* Heterogeneity of multiple sclerosis lesions: Implications for the pathogenesis of demyelination. *Ann Neurol* 2000;**47**:707–717.

65. Roemer S, Parisi JE, Bruck W, *et al.* Neuromyelitis optica brain lesions are pathologically identical to optico-spinal lesions. *Neurology* 2008;**70**:A235.

66. Blanche P, Diaz E, Gombert B, *et al.* Devic's neuromyelitis optica and HIV-1 infection. *J Neurol Neurosurg Psychiatry* 2000;**68**:795–796.

67. Chusid MJ, Williamson SJ, Murphy JV, Ramey LS. Neuromyelitis optica (Devic disease) following varicella infection. *J Pediatr* 1979;**95**:737–738.

68. Ahasan HA, Rafiqueuddin AK, Chowdhury MA, Azhar MA, Kabir F. Neuromyelitis optica (Devic's disease) following chicken pox. *Trop Doct* 1994;**24**:75–76.

69. Heerlein K, Jarius S, Jacobi C, *et al.* Aquaporin-4 antibody positive longitudinally extensive transverse myelitis following varicella zoster infection. *J Neurol Sci* 2009;**276**:184–186.

70. Pittock SJ, Lennon VA. Aquaporin-4 autoantibodies in a paraneoplastic context. *Arch Neurol* 2008;**65**:629–632.

71. Ch'ien LT, Medeiros MO, Belluomini JJ, Lemmi H, Whitaker JN. Neuromyelitis optica (Devic's syndrome) in two sisters. *Clin Electroencephalogr* 1982;**13**:36–39.

72. Yamakawa K, Kuroda H, Fujihara K, *et al.* Familial neuromyelitis optica (Devic's syndrome) with late onset in Japan. *Neurology* 2000;**55**:318–320.

73. Braley T, Mikol DD. Neuromyelitis optica in a mother and daughter. *Arch Neurol* 2007;**64**:1189–1192.

74. McAlpine D. Familial neuromyelitis optica: Its occurrence in identical twins. *Brain* 1938;**61**:430–448.

75. Hinson SR, Roemer SF, Lucchinetti CF, *et al.* Aquaporin-4-binding autoantibodies in patients with neuromyelitis optica impair glutamate transport by down-regulating EAAT2. *J Exp Med* 2008;**205**:2473–2481.

76. Honda K, Yuasa T. A case of anti-aquaporin-4 and anti-glutamate receptor antibodies positive myelitis presented with modest clinical signs. *Magn Reson Med Sci* 2008;**7**:55–58.

77. Vincent T, Saikali P, Cayrol R, *et al.* Functional consequences of neuromyelitis optica-IgG astrocyte interactions on blood–brain barrier permeability and granulocyte recruitment. *J Immunol* 2008;**181**:5730–5737.

78. Ishizu T, Osoegawa M, Mei FJ, *et al.* Intrathecal activation of the IL-17/IL-8 axis in opticospinal multiple sclerosis. *Brain* 2005;**128**:988–1002.

79. Satoh J, Obayashi S, Misawa T, *et al.* Neuromyelitis optica/Devic's disease: gene expression profiling of brain lesions. *Neuropathology* 2008;**28**:561–576.

80. Mandler RN, Dencoff JD, Midani F, *et al.* Matrix metalloproteinases and tissue inhibitors of metalloproteinases in cerebrospinal fluid differ in multiple sclerosis and Devic's neuromyelitis optica. *Brain* 2001;**124**:493–498.

81. Keegan M, Pineda AA, McClelland RL, *et al.* Plasma exchange for severe attacks of CNS demyelination: Predictors of response. *Neurology* 2002;**58**:143–146.

82. Weinshenker BG, O'Brien PC, Petterson TM, *et al.* A randomized trial of plasma exchange in acute central nervous system inflammatory demyelinating disease. *Ann Neurol* 1999;**46**:878–886.

83. Greenberg BM, Thomas KP, Krishnan C, *et al.* Idiopathic transverse myelitis: Corticosteroids, plasma exchange, or cyclophosphamide. *Neurology* 2007;**68**:1614–1617.

84. Watanabe S, Misu T, Miyazawa I, *et al.* Low-dose corticosteroids reduce relapses in neuromyelitis optica: a retrospective analysis. *Mult Scler* 2007;**8**:968–974.

85. Mandler RN, Ahmed W, Dencoff JE. Devic's neuromyelitis optica: A prospective study of seven patients treated with prednisone and azathioprine. *Neurology* 1998;**51**:1219–1220.

86. Cree BA, Lamb S, Morgan K, *et al.* An open label study of the effects of rituximab in neuromyelitis optica. *Neurology* 2005;**64**:1270–1272.

87. Jacob A, Weinshenker BG, Violich I, *et al.* Treatment of neuromyelitis optica with rituximab: Retrospective analysis of 25 patients. *Arch Neurol* 2008;**65**: 1443–1448.

88. Weinstock-Guttman B, Ramanathan M, Lincoff N, *et al.* Study of mitoxantrone for the treatment of recurrent neuromyelitis optica (Devic disease). *Arch Neurol* 2006;**63**:957–963.

89. Jarius S, Aboul-Enein F, Waters P, *et al.* Antibody to aquaporin-4 in the long-term course of neuromyelitis optica. *Brain* 2008;**131**:3072–3080.

90. Mok CC, To CH, Mak A, Poon WL. Immunoablative cyclophosphamide for refractory lupus-related neuromyelitis optica. *J Rheumatol* 2008;**35**:172–174.

91. Hinson SR, McKeon A, Fryer JP, *et al.* Prediction of neuromyelitis optica attack severity by quantitation of complement-mediated injury to aquaporin-4-expressing cells. *Arch Neurol* 2009;**66**:1164–1167.

Index